THE BEST
BABY NAME BOOK

THE BEST
BABY NAME
BOOK

OVER 3,000 NAMES AND
YOUR NEW BABY'S STAR SIGN

LOUISE NICHOLSON

Thorsons

Thorsons
An Imprint of HarperCollins*Publishers*
77–85 Fulham Palace Road,
Hammersmith, London W6 8JB

The Thorsons website address is: www.thorsons.com

and *Thorsons* are trademarks of
HarperCollins*Publishers* Ltd

First published by Thorsons 1985
This revised edition published by Thorsons 2002

3 5 7 9 10 8 6 4 2

© Thorsons 1985, 2002

Louise Nicholson asserts the moral right
to be identified as the author of this work

A catalogue record of this book
is available from the British Library

ISBN 0 00 714548 9

Illustrations by Ingela Paterson

Printed and bound in Great Britain by
Martins the Printers Limited, Berwick Upon Tweed

CONTENTS

INTRODUCTION

M y cousin Filippo grows wine in Tuscany. This Italian branch of the family has produced beautiful girls for generations. So, when he began his family with a daughter, Filippo played the first move of his game. He called her Uliva. Vanozza followed, and then Alessandra arrived. The first letters of his daughters' names spelt *Uva*, the Italian for grape and highly appropriate to Filippo's job.

But grand schemes like that can go wrong. What if Alessandra had arrived as twins? Of if Alessandro had come to spoil the female set? Or if Vanozza was the last born? Certainly, for a chartered accountant to embark upon a similar project to make the word 'mathematics' might be rather ambitious.

There is usually a good reason for parents choosing a particular name – a kindly aunt, a family tradition, a maiden name, a much-loved royal, a local hero, or simply a name that sounds very beautiful. But, perhaps unbeknown to parents, the biggest influence on choice is the prevailing fashion. Kings and queens, soldiers and saints, heroes of fiction and fact, have all brought names into fashion. Anne, Elizabeth, Henry, William, and the names of other British royals have, perhaps, given children a touch of class, and also displayed their parents' loyalty.

Christian missionaries spread stories of the Apostles, disciples and martyrs and soon the enduring popularity of Peter, John and Andrew began. Later, major cults developed around some saints. When pious parents chose the name Francis for their son, they were no doubt remembering the good works of Giovanni Bernardone, known as St Francis of Assisi, and not the derogatory meaning of his nickname, Francesco ('with the airs and graces of a Frenchman'), which he had acquired during a misspent youth. Meanwhile, the romantic medieval legends, revived in the 19th century, put the names of Arthur and his chivalrous knights into the charts of fashion.

Surnames and place names have been honoured as much as first names. After Robert Clive (1725–74) saved the British face in India, proud employees of the East India Company named their sons Clive, not Robert. Surname fashion can also be motivated by status. In the last century, Cecil and the surnames of other ancient aristocratic families appeared as first names in families of more modest backgrounds.

Since the majority of names with fame, prestige, honour or saintly associations were boys' names, the female versions were usually created later. Henrietta then became as royal as Henry, Frances as devout as Francis, and Georgina as patriotic as George, the patron saint of England.

Names also drop out of fashion. After the Norman Conquest in 1066, many Saxon names vanished and names of Continental origin took their place. During the Reformation in the 16th century, parents avoided popish names. In the 17th century, Old Testament biblical names, especially obscure ones, were taken up. And after an abortive attempt by Guy Fawkes and his band to blow up the Houses of Parliament in 1603, no one would call their son Guy.

Revivals also play their part in the fashion game. The English Renaissance of the 15th and 16th centuries revived a whole array of classical names, helped by the popular plays of Ben Jonson and Shakespeare. During the all-pervading medieval revival in the 19th century, parents with their hearts and imaginations back in the romantic Middle Ages turned to names such as Arthur, Elaine, Enid, Gareth and Vivien.

Today, we see a sustained fashion for individuality. Since the 1960s, when Victorian Amys and Emmas began to reappear beside Jade and Moon, the fashion has been simply to be different. Any name can now be revived, from the Old English Ethelbert to the

Greek Eubule, and from the Norman favourite Ella to the saintly Eulalia. Almost any name can be invented – one person has called his son Skylab – so perhaps Perspex and Micro will be going to school soon. Even if parents go for an old favourite, they are quite likely to tease their friends by choosing unfamiliar spellings, such as Jayne for Jane or Jon for John. And if a daughter is to be known as Cass, then it may be Cass, and not the full Cassandra, that goes on to the official birth certificate.

My selection of over 3000 girls' and boys' main names – and the thousands of variant forms and nicknames – includes old favourites as well as many that have been popular in the past but are now almost forgotten. Some unusual names have very beautiful sounds, whatever their meanings may be. Others have fascinating meanings or interesting associations. Many of them will, I hope, appeal to parents searching for a special name, just a little bit different or particularly appropriate in some way.

I am indebted to Professor Chemin Abramsky and Nabil Saidi for their invaluable help with Hebrew and Arabic names. Finally, I would like to dedicate this book to my large and ever-increasing family, for whom I hope it will prove both useful and amusing.

HOW TO USE
THE BEST BABY NAME BOOK

The book lists girls' and boys' names separately: the girls' section comes first, then, after the horoscopes, the boys' section. A main name is in **bold** type; its different forms, spellings and nicknames are listed in alphabetical order at the end of each entry.

It is also indicated if a name within an entry has its own entry elsewhere in the girls' or boys' section. Information is therefore cross-referenced.

Where a name can be given to a girl or a boy, this is indicated in the text. And where the text has '*see under boys ...*' or '*see under girls ...*', the full explanation and meaning will be found in the other section.

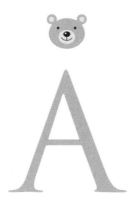

Abigail From the Hebrew, *Avigayil*, 'father of joy', 'source of joy'. In the Bible, one of King David's wives, described as 'of good understanding, and of a beautiful countenance' (1 Samuel 25). Used in Britain from the 16th century. In Beaumont and Fletcher's play, *The Scornful Ladie*(1616), the maid Abigail is the heroine's confidante, initiating the name as a slang term for a trusted lady's maid, hence Abigailship. It was merely coincidence that Queen Anne's lady-in-waiting and confidante was Abigail Masham, an unpopular woman who possibly led to the name's disfavour. **Variants:** Abagael, Abagail, Abaigeal, Abbe, Abbey, Abbie, Abby, Abbye, Abigael, Gael, Gail, Gale, Gayel, Gayl, Gayle.

Abira From the Hebrew, 'strong, heroic'. **Variants:** Adira, Amiza.

Abra Female form of Abraham, thus 'mother of multitudes, mother of the earth', personifying the eternal mother of the cosmos. In the Bible, a favourite of King Solomon. Heroine of the 16th-century romance, *Armadis of Gaul*, and a popular 17th-century name.

Acacia From the Greek, 'thorny', symbolising resurrection and immortality. **Variants:** Cacia, Cacle, Casey, Casia, Kacie.

Acantha From the Greek, 'sharp-pointed, thorny'. The acanthus was a popular motif in Greek architectural decoration.

Accalia Derived from Acca Larentia, a character in Roman mythology who, with her shepherd husband, was a foster-parent to Romulus and Remus, the twin sons of the god Mars who were later to found Rome. A more steamy legend makes Acca Larentia a notorious courtesan who married well and left a large fortune to the Roman people.

Ada A rather complicated derivation: probably a mixture of the Latin, 'of noble birth', the Teutonic, 'joyous, prosperous,

 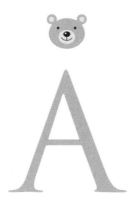

noble', and the old English and old German names, Eda and Etta, 'happy, blessed'. Introduced from Germany into Britain towards the end of the 18th century and very fashionable throughout the 19th. At the height of his popularity, Lord Byron named his daughter (born 1815) Augusta Ada and then wrote of her as 'Ada! sole daughter of my house and heart' in his *Childe Harold's Pilgrimage* (1812–18). The compounds include **Adabelle** and **Adalee. Variants:** Adda, Addie, Addy, Adey, Adi, Aeda, Aida, Eada, Eadda, Eaddu, Eda, Edna, Etta. *See also* Adah, Adela, Adelaide and Adeline.

Adah From the Hebrew, *adah,* 'ornament, beauty', implying a woman's jewel-like preciousness and physical beauty. One of the earliest Hebrew names to be recorded, it is mentioned second only to Eve in the Bible as the name of the wife of Lamech, great-great-great-great-grandson of Adam and Eve (Genesis 4). Familiar in English-speaking countries since the 16th century. The American actress Adah Isaacs Menken (1835–68) lived up to her name, dazzling Dickens, Rossetti, Swinburne, Mark Twain, Alexandre Dumas and more with her countless charms. **Variants:** Ada, Adena, Adene, Adie, Adin, Adina, Adine, Dena, Dina.

Adara From the Arabic, *azra,* 'virgin'.

Adela From the Old German, *athal,* 'noble'. Popular in medieval France, boosted by the veneration of St Adela, Abbess of Pfalzel near Trèves and daughter of Dagobart II. William the Conqueror introduced it to Britain, giving it to his fourth daughter. However, it gained widespread popularity in Britain only under Queen Victoria. **Variants:** Adalia, Addie, Addy, Adel, Adele, Adelia, Adelina, Adella, Adelle, Adila, Akela, Athala, Del, Dela, Dell, Della, Delly, Edila. *See also* Ethel.

Adelaide French form of a compound of two Old German words, *athal,* 'noble', and *haidu,* 'sort', thus Adalhaid, 'noble rank, noble station'. Adapted by the Normans into Adelaide and Alice. St Adelaide (c. 931–1037) was the Empress of Otto the Great, described by a contemporary as 'a marvel of beauty and goodness'. After a period of disuse, the name was revived under the popular Queen Adelaide of William IV (1830–37) after whom the new capital of South Australia was named in 1836. **Variants:** Ada, Adalhaide, Adalheidis, Adalia, Adda, Addi, Addie, Addy, Addison, Adelaida, Adelais, Adelina, Adeline, Adeliz, Adelheid, Dell, Heidi. *See also* Ethel.

Adeline Also derived from the Old German *athal,* 'noble', adapted by the Normans and brought to England. After a period in disfavour, it was revived in the 19th century, rising to popularity after Lord Byron's lines in *Don Juan:* 'Sweet Adeline, amidst the gay world's hum, Was the Queen-Bee, the glass of all that's fair' (1819–1823). The name was linked with 'the flower of my heart' in the lyrics of a popular song at the turn of the century. **Variants:** Adaline, Adelena, Adelin, Adelina, Adelind, Alina, Aline, Alita, Alyna, Athelyna, Della, Dellene, Edelin, Edelina, Edeline, Edolina, Lina. *See also* Ethel.

Adelpha Female form of the Greek, *adelphos, adelphia,* 'brother, brotherhood', thus 'sisterly, sister to mankind'.

Adeola Nigerian name meaning 'crown'.

Adesina Nigerian, meaning 'the arrival of this child has unlocked the path to making a family'. Often given to previously childless parents in the Yaroba tribe.

Adiel From the Hebrew, 'ornament of the Lord'. **Variants:** Addie, Addy, Adie, Adiell, Adiella.

Aditi Indian, ancient Sanskrit for 'abundance, creative power', symbolising rebirth through the life-cycle; also the Hindu mother goddess of all gods on earth.

Adolpha Female form of Adolph. **Variant:** Adolpham.

Adonia Female form of Adonis, thus 'beautiful woman', implying the personification of goodness.

Adora From the Latin and French, 'worthy of divine worship' (not to be confused with Adorna). The compounds include **Adorabelle**. **Variants:** Adorée, Adoria, Dora, Dori, Dorie, Dory.

Adorna From the Middle English, *aourne*, 'embellish, beautify, deck out in splendour', implying a girl adorned by nature with beauty and ability.

Adrian From the Greek, 'rich', and the Latin, 'black, mysterious, dark one'. The Adriatic Sea and one of its ports, Adria, are probably named after their dark-coloured water and sand – hence a later meaning for the name, 'woman from the sea'. Often given to girls with dark eyes and hair. **Variants:** Adrea, Adria, Adriana, Adriane, Adrianna, Adrianne, Adrie, Adrien, Adrienne, Adrina, Hadria.

Affrica From the Anglo-Saxon, *freond*, 'love, beloved, free'. In the 12th century, Affrica became wife and queen to Semerled, Lord of the Isles and King of the Isle of Man.

Afina Rumanian, meaning 'blueberry'.

Afra From the Hebrew, 'young female deer'. A name found in 17th-century Britain. **Variants:** Aphra, Aphrah, Ayfara. *See also* Aphrodite.

Agate From the Old French, *agathe*, and the Greek, *achates*, 'precious stone'; specifically, a precious stone of quartz with bands, stripes or clouds of colour. Small figures were cut into agates in the 16th century, and the word came also to mean a small, diminutive person. The name was believed to give the holder magical properties of eloquence, independence and favour at court. The stone would lead to victory, cure scorpion and snake bites, quell thunder and soothe the mind.

Agatha Female form of the Greek, *agathos*, thus 'good, kind woman'. The beautiful 3rd-century Sicilian Christian martyr, whose veil is supposed to have saved her island from Mount Etna's molton lava, is the patron saint for protection from fire and also of bell-founders. Again, it was the Norman conqueror who gave it to one of his daughters, introducing it to Britain. Revived in the 19th century. **Variants:** Ag, Aga, Agace, Agacia, Agafia, Agas, Agase, Agata, Agathe, Agathie, Agathy, Ageia, Agg, Aggi, Aggie, Aggy, Agueda, Agy, Atka.

Aglaia From the Greek, 'splendid, brilliant'. In Greek mythology, the Three Graces were Aglaia, Euphrosyne and Thalia, children of Zeus and Eurynome. They spread joy in the hearts of men, were the goddesses of gratitude and accompanied Aphrodite. They were also nature-goddesses who presided over the rebirth of life in spring and the ripening of fruits in autumn. **Variant:** Aglae.

Agnes From the Greek, *hagnos*, 'pure, chaste', symbolising purity and chastity, rather than from the Latin, 'lamb'. The 3rd-century Christian saint who was martyred in Rome had as a child refused to marry. Aged about 12, she consecrated her maidenhood to God and offered herself for martyrdom under the persecutions; later elaborate accounts of her life are fictional. A second St Agnes, of Montempulchiano, was equally self-denying, which led to quantities of visions and miracles being associated with her. It was used in England from the 12th to 16th centuries, when it ran close in popularity to Joan and Elizabeth and was pronounced 'annis', leading to confusions with Ann. As it is not a Biblical name, it was hardly used during the Reformation but returned to favour under the Victorians. **Variants:** Ag, Aggi, Aggie, Aggy, Agna, Agnella, Agnesa, Agnese, Agneta, Agnete, Agnetis, Agnetta, Agnette, Agnola, Aigneis, Anese, Anis, Annais, Annes, Anneyce, Anneys, Anneyse, Annice, Annis, Annise, Annot, Annys, Ina, Ines, Inesila, Inez, Nancy, Nessa, Nessi, Nessie, Nest, Nesta, Nevsa, Neysa, Neza, Nezika, Tagget, Taggy, Una, Ynes, Ynez.

Aharona Female form of Aaron. **Variants:** Ahronit, Arni, Arnina, Arninit, Arona.

Ahimsa From the Hindi. Ahimsa is the reverence for all life and the belief in peaceful cures for problems. An appropriate name for pacifists.

Ahulani Hawaiian, meaning 'heavenly shrine'.

Aida From the Latin, *juvare*, and the Old French, *aidier*, 'to help, assist'. In Giuseppe Verdi's tragic opera, *Aida* (1871), the heroine is an Ethiopian princess enslaved in Egypt who, with her hero, dies to save her own people. **Variants:** Aidan, Iraida, Zaida, Zenaida, Zoraida.

Ailene Irish, from the Greek, 'light', thus 'bringing spiritual light into the world'. **Variants:** Aila, Aileen, Aili, Ailina, Ailleen, Aleen, Alene, Aline, Eileen, Eleen, Elene, Ileana, Ileane, Ilene, Iline, Illene, Illine, Illona, Lena, Lina. *See also* Helen and Evelyn.

Ain *See under boys.*

Aislinn From the Gaelic, 'vision, dream'. **Variant:** Isleen, Ashling.

Aithne From the Celtic, *aodnait*, 'little fire'. Popular in Ireland where Aine was queen of the fairies of South Munster–she is now believed to live in County Limerick. Also a female form of Aidan. **Variants:** Aine, Eithne, Ena, Ethne.

Aiyana North American Indian flower name, meaning 'eternal bloom'.

Akako Japanese, meaning 'red'. In Japan, red was believed to have magical powers to cure disease.

Akasma Turkish, meaning 'white climbing rose', that is, the clematis.

Aki Japanese, meaning 'autumn'.

Alana from the Gaelic Irish meaning the 'bright one' or the 'fair one'. The name is the feminine form of Alan and is derived from a term of endearment. **Alternatives include** Alaine, Alanda, Alanis, Alannah, Alayne, Aleina, Alina, Allanah, Allene.

Alamea Hawaiian, meaning 'precious'.

Alarice Female form of Alaric. **Variants:** Alarica, Alarise.

Alaula Hawaiian, meaning 'dawn light' and 'sunset glow'. Also given to boys.

Alberta Female form of Albert. Fashionable in the 19th century in honour of Queen Victoria's husband, the Prince Consort, and of their fourth child, Louise Alberta, after whom Alberta Province, Canada, was named in 1882. **Variants:** Alba, Albertha, Albertina, Albertine, Ali, Allen, Alli, Allie, Ally, Alverta, Auberta, Aubine, Bert, Berta, Berte, Bertie, Elba, Elberta, Elbertina, Elbertine, Elverta.

POPULAR NAMES THROUGH THE YEARS

L ike so many things, names come in and out of fashion over time. Some of the most popular boys' names have remained in the top ten for over a century now – whilst the most popular girls' names tend to change completely every few years. In 1900, the top three boys' names were John, William and James, with the top three girls' names being Mary, Helen and Anna. Skip to 1970 and the popular boys' names are still quite traditional with Michael, David and John topping the list. The most popular girls' names at the start of the 1970s are a whole new set with Jennifer, Lisa and Kimberley topping the list.

More recently, at the start of the new millennium, the top ten for boys and girls was as follows. Starting with the most popular, the boys' names most often picked by new parents were Jacob, Michael, Joshua, Matthew, Andrew, Joseph, Nicholas, Anthony, Tyler and Daniel. The number one girls' name at this same time was Emily, with Hannah, Madison, Samantha, Ashley, Sarah, Elizabeth, Kayla, Alexis and Abigail also being top ten choices.

Albina From the Latin, *albus,* 'white'. Often given to fair or blonde girls. Introduced into Britain from Italy in the 17th century. **Variants:** Albigna, Albinia, Albinka, Alvina, Alvinia, Aubine.

Alcestis In Greek mythology, the King of Thessaly's wife who risked her life to save her husband, thus implying heroism.

Alcina Female form of Alcander. A fairy in Ariosto's *Orlando Furioso* who transformed her admirers into animals and trees, so the name implies strength of will or determination. **Variants:** Alcie, Alcine, Alcinia, Alzina, Elsie.

Alda Female form of Aldous. In the Charlemagne romance, Alda (or Aldabella) was the wife of Orlando. **Variants:** Aldabella, Aldas, Aldina, Aldine, Aldis, Aldona, Aldya, Aldyne, Aldys, Aude, Auld.

Aldith From the Old English, *ealdgyth,* 'experienced in fighting'. Popular in medieval Britain. **Variants:** Adelid, Aethelgith, Ailid, Ailith, Alda, Aldis, Alditha.

Aleph Female form of Aluph. **Variants:** Alufa, Alupha.

Aleria From the Latin, *alerio,* 'eagle', thus implying strength, swiftness and high-flying.

Alethea From the Greek, *aletheia*, 'truth'. Introduced into Britain from Spain in the 17th century when the Prince of Wales, later Charles I, was wooing a Spanish princess. **Variants:** Alatheia, Aleta, Aletea, Aletha, Aletheia, Alethia, Aletta, Alithea, Allathea, Letitia, Letty.

Alexandra Female form of Alexander. Its use for girls dates from at least the 1st century BC when the queen of Judea was Salome-Alexandra. In Britain, the royal connotations began in the 14th century after Edward II married a Danish princess bearing the name. The more recent fashion is in response to another Dane, Edward VII's popular queen (1844–1925), who founded Alexandra Rose Day and Queen Alexandra's Royal Army Nursing Corps. When they married in 1863 the Poet Laureate, Tennyson, wrote of her: 'The sea-king's daughter as happy as fair, Blissful bride of a blissful heir'. Princess Alexandra, Duchess of Kent and cousin of Elizabeth II, continues the tradition today. Many of the variants are also given to boys. **Variants:** Aleixo, Alejandra, Alejandrina, Alejo, Aleksandrina, Alessandra, Alessio, Alex, Alexa, Alexandria, Alexandrina, Alexandrine, Alexe, Alexei, Alexia, Alexina, Alexine, Alexis, Alexscha, Ali, Alisaundre, Alix, Alla, Allesanda, Cesya, Elke, Lesya, Lexi, Lexie, Lexine, Lexy, Lysandra, Sacha, Sande, Sandi, Sandra, Sandy, Sandye, Sondra, Zandra. *See also* Cassandra.

Alfreda Female form of Alfred. **Variants:** Aelfreda, Al, Alberad, Albira, Albirda, Albrad, Albray, Albreda, Alfi, Alfie, Alfy, Alverat, Alvered, Aubrey, Elfreda, Elfrida, Elfrieda, Elva, Freda, Freddie, Freddy, Frieda.

Algoma North American Indian, meaning 'valley of flowers'.

Alice From the same Old German roots as Adelaide, evolving into the High German name, Adelheidis, 'of noble birth', an honorific title for German princesses. Adapted in France to Adaliz, then Aliz, before its import into Britain with the Normans. The *Bele Aaliz* medieval romances quickly established it. Popularity returned with the publication of Lewis Carroll's *Alice in Wonderland* (1865), the birth of Queen Victoria's daughter in 1843 and the fashionable 19th-century romances. Alison, 'son of Alice', is the Gaelic matronymic of Ailis. The compounds include **Allianora**. **Variants:** Aaliz, Adaliz, Adelice, Adelicia, Aeleis, Aelesia, Aili, Ailie, Ailis, Alecia, Aleece, Aleka, Alesia, Ali, Alicea, Alicen, Alicia, Alika, Alikee, Aline, Alis, Alisa, Alisceon, Alise, Alisha, Alison, Alisone, Alissa, Alix, Aliz, Alley, Allie, Allison, Allissa, Allsun, Ally, Alse, Alson, Alyce, Alys, Alyse, Alyson, Alysoun, Alyss, Alyssa, Athelesia, Athelisia, Elissa, Elke, Elsia, Ilysa, Ilyssa, Lexy, Licia, Lissie, Lissy.

Alida Either from the Latin, *alaida*, 'little winged girl' or from the Greek city in Asia-Minor, Alida, where fine clothes were made and also worn by the citizens, thus implying 'dressed in finery'. **Variants:** Aleda, Aleta, Aletta, Alette, Alidia, Alita, Leda, Lita.

Alika Nigerian, implying a girl so beautiful she outshines all other beauties.

Alima From the Arabic, *alimah*, 'skilled in music and dance'. Another meaning is 'sea-maiden'.

Alison *See* Alice.

Aliya From the Hebrew, 'to ascend, rise up'. **Variant:** Aliyah.

Aliza From the Hebrew, 'joy'. **Variants:** Aleeza, Aleezah, Alitza, Alitzah, Alizah.

Allegra From the Latin, *alacer*, and the Italian, *allegro*, 'merry, cheerful, lively, brisk'. Often used to describe music.

Allonia Female form of Alon. **Variant:** Alona.

Alma From the Hebrew, 'maiden, young woman'; from the Celtic, 'all good', or from the Latin, 'kind, bounteous', which led to the Italian and Spanish meaning, 'spirit, soul, warmhearted'. The Romans described Ceres, goddess of agriculture, and Cybele, goddess of nature, as their *Alma Mater*, a term taken up by English universities and schools to mean a foster-mother and now used more generally. During the Crimean War, the victorious battle of Alma (1854) was named after the Spanish river and stimulated a short period of popularity. **Variants:** Aluma, Alumit, Elma.

Almeria Female form of Almeric.

Almita From the Latin, *almities*, 'benign and kindly behaviour'.

Alodie From the Old English, 'wealthy'. **Variant:** Alodi.

Aloha Hawaiian, carrying warm feelings of greeting, kindness and farewell.

Alpha From the Greek, *alpha*, 'first', which in turn comes from the Hebrew, 'leader'. The first letter of the Greek alphabet, thus implying beginning. In the Bible, God is described as the 'Alpha and Omega' of all (Revelations 1). Also given to the chief and brightest star in a constellation.

Alphonsine Female form of Alphonse. **Variant:** Alphonsina.

Alta Spanish, from the Latin, *altus*, 'tall, high', meaning either spiritually or physically tall. **Variants:** Altai, Alto.

Altair From the Arabic, 'bird'. Also given to boys.

Althea From the Greek, *althein*, 'healthy, wholesome'. Also a botanical genus from the Greek, *altheia*, which includes the hollyhock and marsh mallow. In vogue during the 17th century. **Variant:** Altheda.

Alula From the Arabic, *al-ula*, 'the first one', or from the Latin, 'winged one'.

Alura From the Old English, *alhraed*, 'divine or wise counsellor'.

Alva Female form of Alvar. **Variants:** Alevia, Alvan, Alvania.

Alvina From the Old English, *aethel*, 'noble', or *aelf*, 'elf-like, sharp', and *wine*, 'friend', thus a strong and wise woman. **Variants:** Alvinia, Vina, Vinni, Vinnie, Vinny.

Alyssum From the Greek, 'sane, sensible'. Sweet Alyssum is a small plant with white flowers. **Variants:** Alissa, Ilyssa, Lyssa.

Alzena From the Persian, 'woman', implying the personification of love, fidelity and beauty found in woman.

Ama Ghanaian name meaning 'one born on a Saturday'.

Amabel Compound, from the Latin, *amator*, 'lover', and the French, *belle*, 'beautiful'. Alternatively, directly from the Latin, *amabilis*, 'lovable'. Frequently used in medieval Britain, then revived in the 19th century. The Spanish name, Amadis, means 'love of God'. **Variants:** Amabil, Amabilia, Amabilis, Amabilla, Amable, Amadea, Amadis, Amiable, Annabel, Arabel, Bel, Belle, Mabel.

Amalia From the Hebrew, 'the labour of God', implying a child made by God, hence

Amaris, 'promised by God'. **Variants:** Amaliah, Amalthea.

Amalthea From the Greek, 'god-nourishing'. In Greek mythology, the goat that was wet-nurse to the god Zeus. The goat's long horn was the *cornucopia*, 'horn of plenty'. Zeus later rewarded him by placing him with the stars.

Amanda From the Latin, 'worthy of love'. Fashionable during the Restoration and much used by playwrights – it is possible that Vanbrugh invented the name for his fair heroine in *The Relapse* (1697). Its wide use in this century was possibly influenced by another play, Noel Coward's successful comedy, *Private Lives* (1930), which starred himself, with Gertrude Lawrence as Amanda. **Variants:** Manda, Mandi, Mandie, Mandy.

Amandla From the African word meaning 'power'.

Amarinda From the Greek, 'long-lived'. Used by poets to describe the imaginary bloom which, like beauty, never fades. **Variants:** Amara, Amargo, Mara.

Amaryllis From the Greek, *amarullis*, 'refreshing, sparkling'. The poets Theocritus, Virgil and Ovid gave the name to a fictional country girl. In botany, the name of a bright-flowering lily.

Amber From the Arabic, *anbar*, a deep yellow wax-like resin found in tropical seas or as a fossil resin in amber-forests, then polished and made into ornaments and jewellery. Believed to possess powers to cure. **Variants:** Amberlie, Amby.

Ambrosia From the Greek, *ambrosios*, 'immortality, elixir of life'. In mythology, it was the food of the gods and immortals. Later associated with delicious, usually sweet, foods and smells, and used by writers and poets. A name since the 16th century. **Variants:** Ambrosina, Ambrosine.

Amelia From the Latin, *aemulus*, 'toil, work, ambition, earnest striving'. Possibly also from the Latin, *aemilia*, 'persuasive, flattering'. In Shakespeare's *The Comedy of Errors* (1592–94), Aemelia is the mother of the twins. Reintroduced from Germany by the Hanoverian kings and quickly anglicised to the popular Emily. The compounds include **Amelinda**. **Variants:** Amalea, Amalia, Amalie, Amelie, Ameline, Amelita, Amy, Emelie, Emelina, Emelita, Emil, Emilia, Emily, Emelyn, Emmeline, Millie, Milly.

Amelie French name made popular by successful film of this title in 2001.

Amethyst From the Greek, *methustos*, 'intoxicated'. The clear, violet-purple precious stone was believed to prevent intoxication from drink.

Amia Female form of Amory and Ami.

Amina Female form of Amin.

Aminta From the Latin, *amintas*, 'protector'. Coined in the 17th century during the Restoration. **Variants:** Amynta, Arminta.

Amira From the Arabic, 'princess'. **Variants:** Amiret, Amiretta, Emira, Mira.

Amity From the Latin, *amicitia*, 'friendship'.

Amorette From the Latin, 'beloved, sweetheart, little dear'. Probably invented by Spenser for the loving wife character in his *Faerie Queen* (1590). **Variant:** Amorita.

Amy Anglicised form of the French, Aimée, from the Latin, *amor*, 'love'. Widely used in the 17th century, revived in the 19th. The Scottish form, Esme, was taken from the early French form, Esmée, and used for both sexes. **Variants:** Aimee, Amaliya, Amata, Ame, Ami, Amia, Amice, Amie, Amii, Amye, Esme, Esmee, Ismay.

Anastasia From the Greek, *anastasis,* 'resurrection, one who will rise again', thus appropriate for a spring or Easter baby. Used by early Christians to signify the child's entry into new life. A 3rd-century Christian martyr honoured in the Eastern Church. The name was popular in medieval Britain when the cult of the Virgin was at its height and the saint somehow became associated with the Virgin's midwife. **Variants:** Ana, Anastas, Anastase, Anastasie, Anastassia, Anastatia, Anestasia, Annestas, Anstes, Anstey, Anstice, Anstis, Antace, Anty, Asia, Nastassia, Nastassja, Nastasya, Nastenka, Nastia, Nastya, Nastyenka, Nestia, Stacey, Stacy, Stasa, Stasya, Tansy, Tasenka, Tasia, Tasya.

Anatola Female form of Anatole.

Andra From the Old Norse, 'a breath'. *See also* Andrea. **Variants:** Anda, Andria.

Andrea Female form of Andrew. **Variants:** Aindrea, Andee, Andi, Andra, Andreana, Andree, Andrew, Andriana, Andy.

Andromeda In Greek mythology, the beautiful maiden whose mother's pride in her was punished when she was chained to a rock to be devoured by the sea-monster.

Anemone From the Greek, 'wind-flower'. In Greek mythology, the nymph who was transformed into a flower by the wind. Alternatively, the flower that sprang from the blood of the god Adonis when he was killed while hunting. Botanical genus of plants that includes the delicate wind-flower found in Britain.

Angahard From the Welsh, 'much beloved', later anglicised to Ancret. **Variants:** Anchoret, Anchoretta, Ancret, Ancreta, Ancrett, Angharad, Ankerita, Ingaret, Ingaretta.

Angela From the Greek, *angelo,* 'messenger', later meaning an angel bringing good tidings from God to man. The 16th-century saint from Brescia, north Italy, founded the Company of St Ursula, the first teaching order of nuns. Sometimes given to girls born on the festival of St Michael and All Angels, September 29. The name was disapproved of as presumptuous during the Reformation, but recovered towards the end of the 19th century. **Variants:** Aingeal, Angel, Angele, Angeles, Angeleta, Angeletta, Angelica, Angelina, Angeline, Angie, Angiola, Angy, Anjela, Anjelika, Engel, Gelya.

Angelica French, from the Latin, *angelicus,* 'like an angel', thus the perfect woman. Praised by Milton in *Paradise Regained* (1671) as 'the fairest of her sex, Angelica'. *See also* Angela. **Variants:** Angelika, Angeliki, Angelique, Angelita.

Anna Greek form of Hannah. In Virgil's *Aeneid* (1st century BC), Anna is the sister of Dido, Queen of Carthage. A name first popular in Germany and Italy, then very common in Russia. Leo Tolstoy gave it to the heroine of his novel, *Anna Karenina* (1875–8). *See also* Anne. **Variants (many interchangeable with Anne):** Ana, Anca, Anett, Ania, Anica, Anina, Anita, Anitra, Anka, Anne, Annetta, Annette, Anni, Annice, Annie, Annora, Annot, Anusia, Naatja, Nan, Nana, Nance, Nancee, Nancey, Nanci, Nancy, Nanete, Nanette, Nanice, Nanine, Nanita, Nanna, Nannie, Nanny, Nanon, Nansi, Nita, Panna, Panni.

Annabella In England, a compound of Anna and Bella, but well used in Scotland since the 12th century and so possibly derived from Amabel. **Variants:** Anabel, Anabela, Anabill, Anabille, Anabul, Annabel, Annabelle, Annabla, Annable, Annaple.

Anne French form of Hannah. Old English forms include Ann, Annis, Annais and Annys. Although she is not mentioned in the Bible, Anne is the Virgin's mother according to the apocryphal gospels. This led to the name's widespread use in Western Europe after its introduction in the 11th century from Russia and Byzantium where it had long been popular. With the variants Nan and Nanny, Anne was a top favourite name in Britain throughout the 17th century, joined by Anna, with Nancy, in the 18th. The different spellings of Anne and Ann were interchangeable until recently. Anne rose to popularity in Britain again during the reign of Queen Anne (1665–1714), the last of six queens of England to have the name. Later, Lucy Maud Montgomery's novel, *Anne of Green Gables* (1909), encouraged its use, as did the *Diary of Anne Frank*. A further boost came when Elizabeth II chose Anne Elizabeth Alice Louise as the names for her daughter born in 1950. *See also* Anna. The many compounds using Anne and Anna include **Annalise, Ann-Maria, Annemarie** and **Annarose**. **Variants (many interchangeable with Anna):** An, Ana, Anais, Ani, Anica, Anicka, Ann, Annais, Annette, Anni, Annice, Annie, Annis, Anny, Annya, Annys, Anuska, Anya, Hanon, Nan, Nancy, Netti, Nina, Ninette, Ninon. *See also* Amabel.

Annunciata From the Latin, *annunciatio*, 'bearer of news'. In the Bible, the Annunciation was the occasion when an angel told the Virgin she would give birth to Christ. Appropriate for a March baby, the month the Virgin conceived, or for a Christmas baby. **Variant:** Nunciata.

Anthea From the Greek, *antheios*, 'flowery', thus maiden of the flowers. As with many soft-sounding Greek names, favoured by the 17th-century pastoral poets. **Variant:** Anthia.

Antigone Compound from the Greek, *anti*, 'contrary', and *gonos*, 'born'. In Greek legend, the heroic but tragic daughter of Oedipus.

Antoinette French female form of Anthony. Made lastingly famous by Louis XVI's queen, Marie Antoinette (1755–93), who was famed for her beauty, wit, extravagance, intelligence and knowledge of the arts. But she is also credited with remarking, 'Let them eat cake,' when told that her people could no longer afford bread. Several saints named Antonia gave popularity to the Italian form. **Variants:** Antonetta, Antonette, Antonia, Antonias, Antonica, Antonie, Antonietta, Antoninas, Antonma, Netta, Nettie, Netty, Tanya, Toinette, Toni, Tonia, Tonneli, Tony, Tonya, Tuanette.

Anzu Japanese, meaning 'apricot', the emblem of woman. In the West, the apricot symbolises timid love.

Aphrodite From the Greek, 'born of foam'. The Greek goddess of love, fertility and beauty rose up out of the sea as daughter to Zeus, the supreme god. She was the essence of feminine beauty, seduction and grace, and was officially judged the most beautiful goddess of all by Paris. She later fell deeply in love with, amongst others, the beautiful Adonis.

Appoline From the Greek, *appolonia*, 'concerning or belonging to Apollo'. Adapted from Apollonia, the 3rd-century saint from Alexandria whose teeth were pulled out before he was martyred by fire – hence he is invoked against toothache. **Variants:** Abbelina, Apollonia, Appolina, Appollonia.

April From the Latin, *apricus*, 'open to the sun', the second month of the year in the Roman calendar, signifying springtime and the earth softening and opening for growth and life. **Variants:** Aprilette, Averil, Averyl, Avril. *See also* Averil.

Arabella Compound from the German, *ara*, 'eagle', or the Latin, *ara*, 'altar', and *bella*, 'beautiful'. Its use began in 13th-century Scotland where it was possibly related to the Latin, *orabilis*, 'moved by prayer'. Compounds include **Araminta. Variants:** Ara, Arabel, Arabela, Arabelle, Arable, Arbel, Arbela, Arbell, Bella, Belle, Orabell, Orabilis, Orable, Oriabel.

Arachne From the Greek, *arakne*, 'spider, spider's web'. The name implies the floating, delicate fineness of gossamer. In Greek mythology, Athena's revenge on Arachne was to transform her into a spider destined to weave for ever the thread produced from her own body.

Arazie Armenian, referring to a river which is supposed to inspire poets.

Ardelia Female form of Arden. **Variants:** Ardelle, Ardis, Ardith.

Arethusa In Greek mythology, a wood nymph loved and pursued by Alpheius whose passion carried him across the seas to join her after she was transformed into a spring. **Variants:** Aretha, Aritha.

Argenta From the Latin, *argentum*, 'silver'. The Welsh form is Arianwen. *See also* Silver.

Aria From the Latin, 'melody, air, tune'. Ario was a Greek poet and musician who lived in the 7th century BC. In opera, an aria is usually sung by a single voice.

Ariadne From the Greek, 'extremely divine'. In Greek mythology, the daughter of King Minos who helped Theseus escape from the Labyrinth after he had slain the Minotaur. She later married the god Dionysius who, on her death, cast the crown he had given her into the heavens where it became a constellation. **Variants:** Ariana, Ariane, Arianna.

Ariel *See under boys*. **Variants:** Ariela, Ariella, Arielle.

Arista Female form of Aristo. May also be from the Latin, 'grain', implying harvest time.

Arline From the German, 'girl'; from Adeline; or the female form of Arlen, from Arles. **Variants:** Arilita, Arla, Arlana, Arleen, Arlen, Arlene, Arleta, Arlette, Arleyne, Arlie, Arliene, Arlise, Arlyne, Arlynn, Arlyss, Lene, Lena.

Armilla From the Latin, 'bracelet'.

Armina Female form of Herman. **Variants:** Armine, Arminel.

Armona Female form of Armon. **Variants:** Armonit.

Arnoldine French female form of Arnold. **Variants:** Arnalda, Arnolde.

Arta Female form of Arthur.

Artemis In Greek mythology, goddess of the moon, the hunt and animals. Fond of roaming the countryside as well as making music, she is twin sister of Apollo and daughter of Zeus. Also given to boys. **Variants:** Arta, Arte, Artema, Artemas, Artemisa, Artemisia. *See also* Selena.

Aruna Indian, meaning 'dawn light'.

Arva From the Latin, *arva*, 'countryside, fields, pastureland'. Also given to boys. **Variants:** Arvelle, Arvilla.

Asa *See under boys.*

Asenath From the Egyptian, 'possession of, belonging to'. In the Bible, the wife given as thanks to Joseph after he interpreted Pharaoh's dreams (Genesis 41).

Ashira From the Hebrew, 'wealthy'.

Asoka Indian, meaning the 'non-sorrow tree' which is supposed to blossom scarlet flowers when touched by a good maiden. Ashok was the great emperor of the Mauryan empire (3rd century BC). **Variants:** Ashok, Ashoka.

Aspasia From the Greek, 'welcome'. The name of the witty and clever mistress of the Greek statesman, Pericles (495–429 BC). Brought into modern use by Beaumont and Fletcher's play, *The Maid's Tragedy* (1619), in which the disguised heroine is killed by her lover after he rejects her. **Variant:** *Spase*.

Asphodel The Greek name for the family of lilies including the Daffodil and Narcissus. In Greek mythology, asphodels grew in the Elysian fields (*see* Elysia).

Astera From the Greek, *aster*, 'star'. In early Greek mythology, Asterius, 'starry', was a name for the chief deity, the Universal Mother. Also a delicate, star-shaped flower. **Variants:** Asta, Asteria, Asterius, Astor, Astra, Astraea, Astrea, Astred, Astrid, Esther, Hester, Hadassah. *See also* Nancy.

Astrid Norse, from the Old German name, Ansitruda, a compound of *ansi*, 'god, divine', and *drudi*, 'strength'. Its royal connotations come from both the mother and the wife of Olaf, King of Norway (c. 995–1030), a zeal-

ous Christian who was finally slain by King Knute. *See also* Astera.

Atalanta Female form of Atlas. In Greek mythology, the skilled and beautiful huntress. Her admirers competed in the fields to beat her at hunting and so win her hand. **Variant:** Atlanta. *See also* Melanie.

Athena From Athene, the Greek virgin goddess of wisdom, industry, the household arts and civilisation in general. She was also the well-armed protectress of heroes. **Variant:** Athene.

Atida From the Hebrew, 'the future'.

Audrey From the Old English name Ethel. In the early 16th century St Etheldreda was known in Britain as St Audrey. The word tawdry comes from the cheap necklaces that were sold on her festival. A name given to poor and country people until its fashion grew in the 17th century. **Variants:** Addie, Addy, Audey, Audra, Audre, Audrie, Audry, Audrye, Awdrey, Awdrie.

Augusta Female form of Augustus. Introduced as an exclusively royal name from Germany by the Hanoverian kings: the name of both the mother and the daughter of George III (1738–1820). **Variants:** Agostina, Aste, Auguste, Augusteen, Augustin, Augustina, Austine, Gus, Gussie, Gusta, Guste, Gustel.

Aura From the Greek, 'gentle breeze, zephyr'. **Variant:** Aural.

Aurelia Female form of Aurelius. **Variants:** Arelia, Aura, Aurea, Aurel, Aurelea, Aurelie, Aureola, Auria, Aurie, Auriol, Ora, Oralia, Oralie, Orel, Orelee, Orelia, Orelie.

Aurora From the Latin, 'dawn', thus the threshold of life. In Roman mythology, the beautiful maiden goddess of the dawn encouraged into unhappy love affairs by the jealous Venus. Morning dew originated in the daily tears she shed after her son's death. **Variants:** Alola, Aurore, Ora, Rora, Rori, Rorie, Rory.

Avalon From the Latin, 'island'. In Celtic mythology, King Arthur and his heroes went after death to this island in Paradise. A name revived last century amid the Victorian vogue for medievalism; *see* Arthur. **Variant:** Avallon.

Averil Compound of the Old English, *eofor*, 'boar', and *hyld*, 'favour, protection', carrying a religious meaning because wild boars were hunted for their heads and offered to pagan gods. The name has also taken on some of the associations of April. **Variants:** Eberhilda, Everild.

Avis From the Old German name, Haduwig, 'refuge in war', brought to England as Havoise by the Normans. An alternative origin is from the Latin, *ava*, 'bird', implying swiftness and song. **Variants:** Amice, Aveis, Aves, Avice, Avicia, Avison, Havoise.

Avital *See under boys*. In the Bible, one of David's wives. **Variant:** Abital.

Aviva From the Hebrew, 'springtime, spring-like', implying youth. **Variants:** Abibi, Abibiti, Avivah, Avivi, Avivit.

Ayeesha Asian name meaning 'life'. **Alternatives include** Aisha, Esha, Lisha.

Azelea From the Greek, *azaleos*, 'dry'. Large shrubs that thrive in dry soil and produce clouds of fragrant-scented blossoms. **Variants:** Azalee, Azalia.

Aziza From the Arabic, *azizi*, 'beloved, dear'; also an African name, from the Swahili, meaning 'precious'. **Variant:** Asisa.

Azura From the Persian, *lazward*, 'lapis lazuli', the semi-precious stone that was much prized for grinding to use as a rich blue dye, hence an adjective for a cloudless sky. **Variants:** Azora, Azure, Azurine.

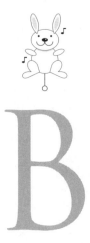

B

Bairn From the Scottish, 'child'.

Bakula Indian; in Hindu mythology, a plant that blossoms if sprinkled with wine by a beautiful maiden.

Bambalina Italian, meaning 'little child'. **Variant:** Bambi. *See also* Fawn.

Baptista Female form of Baptist. **Variants:** Baptiste, Batista, Battista, Bautista.

Barbara From the Greek and Latin, 'foreign, strange, unknown quantity'. St Barbara is possibly a fictional saint, but the legend and cult surrounding her was very strong from the 9th century onwards. Her father imprisoned her for her beauty, tried to kill her for becoming a Christian, had her publicly tortured, then killed her himself and was immediately struck by lightning and turned to ashes. She is patron saint of gunners, miners, architects and engineers and protects against lightning. With the Reformation, the name fell out of use, to be revived this century. The compounds include **Barbarette** and **Barbarella**. **Variants:** Bab, Babb, Babbie, Babes, Babette, Babie, Babola, Babs, Babson, Bara, Barb, Barbary, Barbata, Barbe, Barbi, Barbica, Barbie, Barbo, Barbot, Barbota, Barbraa, Barby, Barica, Barra, Baubie, Bob, Bobbe, Bobbie, Bobby, Bobs, Bonnie, Bonny, Boris, Vara, Varina, Varinka, Varvara.

Basilia Female form of Basil; St Veronica is also called Basilia in some texts. **Variants:** Basil, Basilie, Bassilly.

Bathild The 7th-century saint, Queen Bathild, was born in England, captured by pirates and sold as a slave to King Clovis II of the Western Franks. She rose to become his wife and, after his death, regent for Chlotar III, when she fought against the slave-trade. She encouraged monasticism, and symbolises fighting for honour and truth. **Variants:** Bathilda, Batilda.

Bathsheba From the Hebrew, 'daughter of an oath' or 'of too much pleasure, of fulfilment' or 'seventh daughter'. In the Bible, wife first of Uriah and then of King David, by whom she bore Solomon (2 Samuel 11–12). Fashionable in medieval Europe. **Variants:** Barsabe, Bathshua, Bathsua, Batsheva, Batsua, Sheba, Sheva.

Batya From the Hebrew, 'daughter of God'. **Variants:** Basya, Bethia, Bithia, Bitya.

Beata From the Latin, *beatus*, 'blessed, happy'. Associated with Beata Virgo, the Blessed Virgin Mary. Found occasionally from the 12th to 18th centuries.

Beatrice From the Latin, *beatrix*, 'bearer of happiness and blessings'. Popular in the Middle Ages as the unattainable heroine who personified spiritual love in Dante's epic poem, *La Divina Commedia* (c. 1300). Later, the witty character in Shakespeare's *Much Ado About Nothing* (1598–9). The name then fell out of use, to be revived by the Pre-Raphaelite Movement of the 19th century when it also acquired royal overtones as that of Queen Victoria's ninth and last child (born 1854). Beatrix Potter (1866–1943) wrote and illustrated children's books and created the characters Peter Rabbit, Jeremy Fisher and Squirrel Nutkin. **Variants:** Bea, Beah, Beat, Beate, Beaten, Beathy, Beatie, Beatrica, Beatrice, Beatriks, Beatrisa, Beatrix, Beatriz, Beatty, Beautrice, Bebe, Bee, Beitris, Bertrice, Beton, Bettris, Bettrys, Betune, Bice, Trix, Trixie, Trixy.

Behira From the Arabic, *bahira*, 'dazzling'.

Belinda Compound from the Latin, *bel*, 'beautiful', and the Old Norse, *lindi*, 'snake' – snakes were respected as sacred and symbolised both wisdom and immortality. A character in the romantic Charlemagne legends. Introduced into Britain in the 18th century when Alexander Pope gave it to the heroine of his satirical poem, *The Rape of the Lock* (1712–14). **Variants:** Bellalinda, Blenda, Linda, Lindi, Lindy, Line, Lynda, Lynde, Velinda.

Belle From the French, 'beautiful'. This and the Italian form, Bella, are now full names in their own right, although formerly they were suffixes or prefixes for compound names or otherwise considered as pet names. **Variants:** Bel, Bela, Bell, Bella, Belvia, Bill, Billi, Billie, Billy.

Belva Female form of Belveder.

Bena From the Hebrew, 'wise'. **Variants:** Bina, Buna, Bunie.

Benedicta Female form of Benedict. Used in Britain from the 13th century. **Variants:** Bendetta, Bendite, Benedetta, Benedictine, Benedikta, Benet, Benetta, Benita, Bennet, Bennie, Bennitt, Benoite, Betta, Bettina, Binnie, Binny, Dixie.

Benjamina Female form of Benjamin. **Variants:** Benay, Jamima, Jemima.

Berenice From the Greek, *phere*, 'bearer', and *Nike*, goddess of victory, thus 'bearer of victory or good news'. Widespread in the Greek and Roman empires. When Racine and Corneille entered a play-writing competition in Paris in 1670, they both chose the Judaean princess, Berenice, as heroine; Racine won. Found in Britain from the 19th century. **Variants:** Barrie, Bernelle, Bernice, Berniece, Bernine, Bernita, Bunni, Bunnie, Bunny, Neigy, Nicia, Nixie, Pherenice, Vernice. *See also* Veronica.

Bernadette Female form of Bernard. Rose to popularity after Bernadette Soubirous (1844–79), aged 14 and sickly, had a vision in which the Virgin revealed the healing

 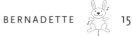

powers of the local waters at Lourdes. **Variants:** Berna, Bernadina, Bernadine, Bernadot, Bernadotte, Bernarda, Bernardina, Bernela, Berneta, Bernetta, Bernette, Bernine, Bernita.

Bertha From the Old High German, *beraht*, 'bright, illustrious'. Charlemagne's beautiful mother made the name fashionable in medieval Europe. As Berta, a favourite with the Normans in Britain, then again in the 19th century. **Variants:** Berta, Berte, Berthe, Bertie, Bertina, Bertine, Berty, Bird, Birdie.

Bertilde From the Old English, *beorht* and *hilde*, 'gleaming battle maid'.

Beryl A word found in several old languages. In Sanskrit, it means 'precious stone'; in Arabic, 'crystal, very clear'; and in Greek, 'sea-green jewel'. Whatever its origins, it implies gleaming with purity. The stone was believed to bring good fortune. Also given to boys. **Variants:** Berura, Beruria, Berylla.

Beta The second letter of the Greek alphabet and the second most important star in a constellation.

Beth Although usually a variant of Elizabeth, it can be an independent name, from the Hebrew, 'house', or *bethia*, 'worshipper of God'. As used in Scotland, it comes from the Celtic, *beathaq* 'breath of life', as in Macbeth. **Variants:** Bethany, Bethesda, Bethseda.

Bethel From the Hebrew, 'house of God'.

Bettula From the Persian, *bettule*, 'maiden, young girl'.

Betty *See* Elizabeth.

Beulah From the Hebrew, 'she who is to be married, ruled over'. Also used to refer to Israel in the Bible, and to the land of heavenly joy near the end of man's journey through life in Bunyan's allegory, *The Pilgrim's Progress* (1678).

Beverley From the Old English, 'meadow of the beaver' – the industrious animal is skilled at cutting down trees, building huts and constructing dams. Also given to boys. **Variants:** Bev, Beverie, Beverlee, Beverly, Buffy.

Bevin From the Irish Gaelic, 'sweet-singing maiden'.

Bibi From the French, *beubelot*, 'toy, bauble'.

Bijou From the French, 'jewel', which in turn comes from the Old English, *bizou*, 'ring'.

Bilhah From the Hebrew, 'old, weak'. In the Bible, Jacob's wife and Rachel's servant. **Variant:** Baila.

Billie Female form of William. Also a full name, from the Old English, *willa*, 'resolution, determination'.

Binnie From the Celtic, 'crib, wicker basket'.

Bira From the Hebrew, 'fort, capital'.

Bird From the Anglo-Saxon, *bridd*, 'bird'. **Variants:** Birdella, Birdena, Birdie, Byrd, Byrdie. *See also* Bertha.

Blair From the Celtic, 'place, field, battle'. Also given to boys.

Blanche From the French, 'white'. Widely used in France and then carried to Britain by Blanche of Artois when she married Edmund, Earl of Lancaster (died 1296). Revived in the 19th century as part of the romantic medieval fashion. **Variants:** Balaniki, Blanca, Blanch, Blandina, Blinnie, Bluinse. From the Italian, Bianca, the variant is Biancha. From the Spanish, Blanca, the variants are Bellanca, Blanka, Blinni, Blinnie, Blinny, Branca.

 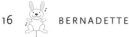

NORMA OR MARILYN?

When actress Lucille Le Sueur's Hollywood studio sponsored a contest to find her a better name, the winning entry was 'Joan Crawford'. Lucille was accordingly renamed, even though she thought it sounded like 'crawfish'. Grace Stansfield's theatrical agent was adamant that the future star's name was too long to fit on the front of a theatre in big neon lettering – so she opted for Gracie Fields. Marilyn Monroe's alliteration certainly sounds more powerful than her real name, which was Norma Jean Baker – just as Doris Day is more memorable than Doris Kappelhoff, Sophia Loren than Sophia Scicoloni and Stan Laurel than Stanley Jefferson. Would Rudolph Valentino have won quite so many hearts as Rudolpho Guglielmi, or Cary Grant as Archibald Leach? By choosing George Eliot, Mary Anne Evans avoided all sorts of potential prejudices against women writers. The French writer, philosopher and pamphleteer, François Marie Arouet, used more than 50 pseudonyms to preserve his anonymity before finally settling on Voltaire. And the British writer Daniel Foe switched to Defoe, and then published his most successful novel, *Robinson Crusoe*, as 'written by himself, Robinson Crusoe'.

Blandina From the Latin, 'seductive, flattering, affable'.

Blaze From the Old English, 'torch, shining', and the Middle English, 'to blow, proclaim'. Occasionally given to boys. **Variants:** Blaise, Blasia.

Bliss From the Old English, 'happiness and joy'.

Blodwen From the Welsh, *blod-yu*, 'flower', and *gwen*, 'white', hence white flower.

Blossom From the Old English, 'a plant or tree in flower'. The German form is **Bluma**.

Blythe From the Old English, *blithe*, 'mild, gentle, kind'. Also given to boys. **Variants:** Bliss, Blisse.

Bo Chinese, meaning 'precious'.

Bona From the Arabic, *bana*, 'builder'.

Bonita From the Spanish, 'pretty'.

Bonnie From the Latin, *bonus*, 'good'. Used in Scotland to imply beautiful, as in 'bonnie lass'. **Bonita** is the Spanish form. **Variants:** *Bonnee, Bonni, Bonny*.

 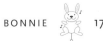

Brandy From the Dutch, *brandewijn*, 'brandy-wine', a fiery spirit distilled from wine. **Variants:** Brandi, Brandie.

Brenda Female form of Brendan. Especially popular in Scotland, it was then spread further afield by the sweet-natured character in Sir Walter Scott's novel, *The Pirate* (1821). **Variants:** Bren, Brenna.

Brian *See under boys.* **Variants:** Breanne, Briana, Brianne, Brina, Brine, Briney, Briny, Brione, Briony, Bryan, Bryanna, Bryn, Bryna, Brynie, Brynja, Brynn, Bryony.

Bridget From the Celtic, *briganti*, 'strong, high'. Brighid was the Celtic goddess of fire, light and poetry, daughter of the sun-god. The cult of the Irish St Brigid (c. 450–c. 523) spread throughout Britain and built a strong, gay and compassionate character around her, based more on old legends about Brighid than on the few known facts about the saint, although she did found a community of women at Kildare. As St Brigid ranked with St Patrick and St Columba in Ireland, her name was possibly too sacred to use. It is rarely found before the 15th century and not wide-spread until the 17th. Then it rose and, with Mary, became the most popular name in Ireland, still true today. **Variants:** Bedelia, Beret, Berget, Biddie, Biddu, Biddy, Bidu, Birgit, Birgitta, Birte, Brid, Bride, Bridgit, Bridie, Brietta, Briget, Brighde, Brighid, Brigid, Brigida, Brigit, Brigitta, Brigitte, Brit, Brita, Britte, Bryde.

Brilliant From the French, *brilliant*, 'sparkling'. **Variant:** Brilliana.

Britannia The Latin name for Britain; introduced as a name in the 18th century. **Variant:** Britain.

Britney Originally meaning 'from Britain', this name has become popular since the late 1990's after Britney Spears, one of the world's most successful female pop stars.

Bronwen From the Welsh, 'fair-bosomed'. In Welsh legend, the daughter of Llyr, god of the sea. Also from the Middle English, *braun*, 'fleshy, muscular', and *wyn*, 'friend', thus a well-built friend. **Variant:** Bronwyn.

Brook From the Old English, *brucan*, 'to enjoy, be rewarded by'; alternatively, from the Old English, *broc*, 'marsh, small stream'. **Variant:** Brooke.

Brunella From the Old French, 'brown-haired'. The Italian form is **Brunetta**.

Brunhild From the Old High German, *brunna*, 'armour', and *hilti*, 'fight', implying someone well-prepared for life's struggle. In German legend, one of the Valkyries, restored to fame with *The Ring of the Nibelung*, the epic four-part opera by Richard Wagner (1813–83) which introduced the name to Britain. **Variants:** Brunhilda, Brunhilde, Brunnhilde, Brynhild, Brynhilda, Brynhilde, Hilda, Hilde.

Bryna From the Irish Gaelic, 'strength, honour'.

Bubbles From the Old French, *beubelot*, 'toy, bauble'. **Variant:** Bibi.

Bunty Probably from bunny, 'little rabbit'. Made famous on the London stage by the successful popular comedy, *Bunty Pulls the Strings* (1911).

Butterfly The name of this colourful, large-winged insect has been used for girls since the Middle Ages.

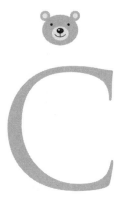

Cadence From the Latin, *cadere*, 'to fall', as in the pleasant rise and fall of the rhythms of music and speech. **Variants:** Cadina, Cadenza.

Calandra From the Greek, *kalandros*, 'lark'. **Variants:** Cal, Calander, Calandre, Calandria, Calli, Callie, Cally, Kallie.

Calantha From the Greek, 'beautiful blossom'. **Variants:** Cal, Calanthe, Callie, Cally.

Calida Spanish, meaning 'warm, ardent'. **Variant:** Callida.

Calista From the Greek, 'most beautiful'. **Variants:** Calesta, Calisto, Calla, Calli, Callie, Callista, Cally, Calysta, Kallista.

Callan From the Old High German, *kallon*, 'to chatter', or the Old Norse, *kalla*, 'to cry out, summon loudly'.

Calliope From the Greek, 'beautiful-voiced'. In Greek mythology, the muse of eloquence and heroic poetry. Also the name of a musical instrument made up of steam whistles, like an organ, and formerly played on Mississippi steamboats on arrival at a town.

Callula From the Latin, 'beautiful little girl'.

Calpurnia From the Greek, *kallos*, 'beauty', and *porne*, 'prostitute'. Known in Britain through Caesar's wife in Shakespeare's tragedy, *Julius Caesar* (1599).

Calypso From the Greek, *kaluptein*, 'to cover, conceal'. In Homer's epic poem, *The Odyssey* (8th century BC), a sea nymph who kept Odysseus on her island, Ogygia, for seven years.

Camellia Botanical genus of shrubs, mostly from Japan and China, and the name of a flower (also known as japonica), both called after botanist Joseph Kamel (1661–1706). The tantalising, beautiful courtesan in Alexandre Dumas Jnr's novel, *La Dame Aux Camellias* (1852), was called Marguerite.

Cameo Italian, from the Latin, *cammaeus*, usually a precious stone of different coloured layers finely carved so that the figures are one colour, the background another. Hence the further meaning of a tiny but important part in a play, and the name's implication of the part a person plays in the world.

Camilla From the Latin, *camillus*, 'messenger, attendant at a religious rite'. In Roman ritual, the boy and girl attendants were called *Camilli* and *Camillae* respectively. In Roman mythology, the swift-footed huntress and attendant to Diana; thus the name came to imply a noble and pure virgin. Used in Europe in the Middle Ages, then re-introduced in the 18th century, stimulated by Madame D'Arblay's hugely popular novel, *Camilla* (1796). **Variants:** Cam, Camala, Camel, Camila, Camille, Cammie, Cammy, Milli, Millie, Milly.

Canace From the Greek, 'daughter of the wind'.

Candide From the Latin, *candere*, 'to be white, glow with heat'. Popularised with the success of Voltaire's play, *Candide* (1759), in which the hero remains unaffected by the disasters he encounters. Then revived again in G. B. Shaw's play, *Candida* (1898), in which the heroine is one of his most sympathetic characters. Candace is the official title and name of the queens of Ethiopia. **Variants:** Candace, Candance, Candase, Candee, Candice, Candida, Candie, Candis, Candra, Candy, Candyce, Kandace, Kandy.

Caprice From the Latin, *caput*, 'head', and *ericius*, 'hedgehog'. From the evolved the Italian word, *capriccio*, 'head with hair standing on end', meaning an erratic, impulsive personality.

Cara From the Celtic, 'friend', the Italian, 'dear', or the Vietnamese, 'diamond, precious jewel'. The compounds include **Carabelle**. **Variants:** Carina, Carine, Carrie, Kara.

Cari From the Latin, 'keel'. One of the five stars in the constellation Orion, each of which names a part of a boat. **Variants:** Carin, Carine, Caryn.

Carita From the Latin, *caritas*, 'charity, kindness'. **Variant:** Carity. *See also* Charity.

Carla Female form of Charles. **Variants:** Arla, Carley, Carlia, Carlita, Carly.

Carma From the Arabic, *karm*, 'a field of fruit, vineyard'; hence Carmia, 'vineyard of the Lord'. **Variants:** Carmania, Carmel, Carmela, Carmelina, Carmelit, Carmen, Carmia, Carmie, Carmine, Carmit, Carmita, Carmiya, Carmy, Kaarmia, Karma, Karmel, Karmela, Karmelit, Karmit, Lita, Melina.

Carmen From the Latin, 'to sing, praise, be lyrical'. The beautiful and sensuous heroine of Bizet's opera, *Carmen* (1873–4), is taken from Prosper Mérimée's novel. **Variants:** Carmencita, Carmia, Carmine, Carmita, Charmain, Charmaine, Charmian, Charmion.

Carmine From the Latin, *carminium*, 'deep vivid red', a pigment obtained from cochineal. *See also* Carmen.

Carna From the Latin, 'flesh'; or the Hebrew, 'horn', hence Carniela, 'horn of the Lord'. **Variants:** Carniella, Carnit, Karniela, Karniella, Karnit.

Carnation From the Latin, *careu*, 'flesh', thus flesh-coloured. In botany, the genus of herbs and flowers that includes sweet william.

Carnelian From the Latin, *carne*, 'flesh'. A red, translucent, semi-precious stone.

Carol From the Old French, 'round dance, dance-song, to celebrate in song'. *See also* Caroline. **Variants:** Carel, Carey, Carola, Carole,

Carolee, Carolin, Carrie, Carroll, Carry, Caryl, Charla, Karel, Sharyl, Sherrie, Sherry, Sherye, Sheryl.

Caroline Italian female from of Charles. Introduced to England and made immediately fashionable by Caroline of Brandenburg-Anspach, wife of George II (1683–1769). *See also* Charlotte. **Variants:** Arla, Cara, Carey, Carla, Carlana, Carleen, Carlen, Carlene, Carley, Carlia, Carlin, Carline, Carlite, Carley, Carly, Carlyn, Carlynne, Caro, Carol, Carola, Carole, Caroleen, Carolina, Carolly, Caroly, Carolyn, Caron, Carona, Carri, Carrie, Carry, Cassie, Charla, Charlayne, Charleen, Charlen, Charlena, Charlene, Charlet, Charlot, Charo, Cherlene, Karla, Karlene, Karole, Karolina, Karoline, Karolyn, Lina, Lolo, Sharleen, Sharlene, Sharline.

Carpathia From the Greek, *karpos,* 'fruit'.

Casey From the Irish Gaelic, 'brave'. **Variants:** Casie, Kacie.

Cassandra From the Greek, 'entangler of men'. In Greek mythology, Priam's beautiful daughter (sometimes called Alexandra), to whom Apollo gave the powers of prophecy in order to win her love. When she cheated on him, he changed the gift to a curse, making her prophecies always disbelieved. Popular in medieval romances. **Variants:** Caasi, Casandra, Case, Cash, Caso, Cass, Cassander, Cassandre, Cassandry, Cassie, Casson, Sandi, Sandie, Sandra, Sandy.

Cassia From the Greek, *cassia,* 'herb', and the Hebrew, *kesiah,* 'cinnamon bark', a family of trees and shrubs highly prized for their fragrant perfume and medicinal properties. Also a female form of Cassius. **Variant:** Caswell.

Casta From the Latin, 'pious, modest'.

Catherine From the Greek, *katharus,* 'pure'. The 4th-century St Katherine of Alexandria escaped martyrdom on a spiked wheel but was then beheaded, when milk flowed from her veins and angels carried her body to Mount Sinai. She stimulated a great cult and many later saints, churches, hospitals, pealing bells and queens were named after, keeping the name popular. Another saint, Catherine of Siena (1347–80), was an adviser to church leaders in Rome and is now patroness of Italy and of the Order of Dominicans. The powerful Catherine de Medici was wife of Henry II of France (1519–59) and mother of three more monarchs. It is the wild Katherina, or Kate, whom Petruchio conquers in Shakespeare's comedy, *The Taming of the Shrew* (1594). When introduced into Anglo-Saxon Britain by Crusaders returning from the Holy Land, it was given a 'C', since the alphabet then lacked 'K'. The nickname Katy received a boost with the publication of Susan Coolidge's novel, *What Katy Did* (1872). **The many variants include:** Caitlin, Caitrin, Caren, Carin, Carina, Carita, Carolly, Caroly, Caronia, Caryn, Casey, Cassie, Casy, Catalina, Catarina, Cate, Caterina, Cath, Catharine, Cathee, Cathie, Cathleen, Cathlene, Cathlin, Cathrine, Cathryn, Cathy, Cati, Catie, Caton, Catlin, Catling, Catriona, Cattie, Caty, Caye, Ekaterina, Gaton, Kaki, Kara, Karen, Karin, Karina, Kasia, Kassia, Kat, Katalin, Katarina, Kate, Katelin, Katerina, Katerine, Kateryn, Kath, Katha, Katharine, Katharina, Kathchen, Kathe, Katherine, Kathi, Kathleen, Kathlene, Kathline, Kathrene, Kathrina, Kathryn, Kathy, Kati, Katie, Katina, Katinka, Katja, Katrina, Katrine, Katrinka, Katty, Katy, Katya, Kay, Kaye, Kerry, Ketty, Kinny, Kit, Kitty, Kytte, Thrine, Treinel, Trinette, Trini.

REGISTERING A BABY'S BIRTH

T he law requires that a baby is registered once it is born. Every major town has a register office and a baby must be registered where it is born.

At the registration the child's date and place of birth are recorded, as are its given names, surname and sex. There are however various concessions to modern customs. If the first names are undecided the father's occupation and the mother's maiden name are all required to be recorded; there is also provision to record the mother's occupation. However, if the child is born outside of wedlock the father's details are only recorded if he either goes with the mother to register the birth or provides written recognition of his child.

In the UK, you can obtain further information from: the Family Records Office, 1 Myddelton Street, London EC1R 1UW (020 8399 5300)

Cecilia Female form of Cecil. The Italian saint was supposed to have consecrated her virginity to God on her wedding day, impressing her pagan husband so much that he was converted; later they were both martyred. Widely honoured from the 6th century and patroness of music since the 16th because she sang to God while musicians played at her wedding. The name was introduced to England by a daughter of William the Conqueror. **Variants:** Cacilia, Cacilie, Cecelia, Cecely, Cecil, Cecile, Cecilie, Cecille, Cecillia, Cecily, Cecilya, Ceil, Cele, Celia, Celie, Ces, Cicely, Cicily, Ciel, Cilka, Cis, Cissie, Cissy, Cycalye, Cycly, Kikelia, Sela, Sely, Sile, Sileas, Sis, Sisile, Sisley, Sissela, Sissi, Sissie, Sissy. *See also* Celeste and Sheila.

Celandine From the Greek, *cheladon*, 'swallow'; also a yellow-flowered plant.

Celena In Greek mythology, one of the seven daughters of Atlas who were called the Pleiades. They were turned into stars by Zeus and can be seen in the sky in May.

Celeste From the Latin, *caelum*, 'heaven, abode of gods and angels, divine'. Very popular with Tudor poets. In his poem, *To Celia*, Ben Jonson (1573–1637) wrote: 'Drink to me only with thine eyes, And I will pledge with mine.' **Variants:** Caelia, Cele, Celesta, Celestia, Celestine, Celestyn, Celestyna, Celia, Celie, Celina, Celinda, Celine, Celinka, Celka, Selen, Selina, Sheila, Sile.

Celosia From the Greek, *keleos*, 'flame', or from the Latin, *cella*, 'store-room, main body of a temple'.

Ceres From the Latin, 'of the spring'. In Roman mythology, goddess of the cultivation of corn and the growth of fruits. Astrological name for girls born under the spring zodiac signs of Aries, Taurus and Gemini. **Variants:** Cerelia, Cerella.

Ceridwen From the Welsh, *cerdd*, 'poetry', and *gwyn*, 'fair, white', thus beautiful poetry. The Welsh goddess of poetic inspiration.

Chandelle From the French, 'candle'.

Chandra From the Sanskrit, 'eminent, illustrious', hence 'moon, moonlike' because the moon outshines the stars.

Chantal Female form of Chanticleer.

Charity From the Greek, *karis*, 'favour, grace, talent', via the Latin, *caritas*, 'dear, affection, brotherly love'. The Charities were three Roman goddesses of grace, charm and beauty – both intellectual and spiritual. In the Bible, Faith, Hope and Charity are considered the great Christian virtues, 'but the greatest of these is charity' (1 Corinthians 13). The 3rd-century St Sophia named her triplets thus, and all three remained popular, especially during the Reformation. **Variants:** Carita, Charis, Charissa, Charita, Charito, Charry, Chattie, Cherry. *See also* Louise.

Charlotte French female form of Charles. Introduced into England by the wife of the 12th-century Earl of Derby. Made popular by the heroine of Goethe's *Sorrows of Werther* (1774) and by George III's wife, who gave him fifteen children. *See also* Caroline. **Variants:** Cara, Carla, Carlota, Carlotta, Char, Charil, Charla, Charlayne, Charleen, Charlen, Charlena, Charlene, Charlet, Charlie, Charline, Charlot, Charlotta, Charlotty, Charyl, Cheryl, Karlene, Karlotta, Karlotte, Lola, Loleta, Lolita,

Lotta, Lotte, Lottie, Lotty, Sharlene, Sharline, Sharyl, Sheree, Sherrill, Sherry, Sherrye, Sheryl, Totly, Totti, Totty.

Charmian From the Greek, 'drop of joy'. The name of Cleopatra's sweet-natured attendant, made known in England through Shakespeare's play, *Antony and Cleopatra* (1607). *See also* Carmen.

Chastity From the Latin, *castus*, 'pure, virtuous, decent', in both the moral and physical senses.

Chaya Female form of Chaim.

Cheera From the Greek, *kara*, 'face', implying a happy and warm expression.

Chelsea Recently popularised in the USA after the daughter of former president Bill Clinton, Chelsea Clinton.

Chenetta From the Greek, *chen*, 'goose', or the French, *chene*, 'oak tree', implying strength and longevity.

Chenoa North American Indian, meaning 'white dove'. *See also* Dove.

Chere From the French, *chere*, 'dear, beloved', thus Cherami, 'dear friend'. **Variants:** Cher, Cherami, Cheri, Cherie, Cherrie, Cherry, Chery, Cherye, Cheryl, Cheryle, Cherylie, Sharol, Sher, Sheral, Shere, Sheree, Sherelle, Sheri, Sherrelle, Sherri, Sherry, Sherye, Sheryl, Sheryle.

Cherry From the Old French, *cherise*, the sweet, red fruit.

Chesna Slavic, meaning 'peaceful'. **Variant:** Chessy.

Chilali North American Indian, meaning 'snowbird'.

Chimene French, derived from the Greek, 'hospitable'. *See also* Ximenia.

Chita From the Middle English, *kitte*, 'kitten'.

Chizu Japanese, meaning 'a thousand storks'. The bird is a symbol of longevity.

Chloe From the Greek, *kloe*, 'green, verdant'. In Greek mythology, goddess of young crops. In use since the 17th century, especially in pastoral poetry to name country girls; *see also* Daphne. In Harriet Beecher Stowe's novel, *Uncle Tom's Cabin* (1851), the wife of Uncle Tom. **Variants:** Clea, Clo, Cloe.

Chloris From the Greek, *kloros*, 'blooming, fresh'. In Greek mythology, goddess of flowers. Again, favoured by poets in the 17th and 18th centuries. **Variants:** Chlorine, Cloris, Lorice.

Cho Japanese, meaning both 'born at dawn' and 'butterfly'.

Choomia English gypsy name, meaning 'kiss'.

Christabel Compound of Christian and Bella. Used in medieval romances. **Variants:** Christa, Christabell, Christabella, Christable, Christey, Christie, Christobelle, Christobella, Christy, Cristehildis, Cristemberga, Cristemia, Cristie, Cristy.

Christine Female form of Christian. Christine comes from the Old English, *christen*. Christiana comes from the Latin, *christianus*. Both mean Christian and have been in use with many variants since at least the 11th century. **Variants:** Cairistine, Cairistiona, Cauline, Chris, Chrissie, Chrissy, Christal, Christeena, Christen, Christian, Christiana, Christiane, Christiania, Christel, Christie, Christina, Christy, Chrystal, Chryste, Ciorsdan, Crete, Crissie, Cristi, Cristin, Cristina, Cristine, Karstin, Kersti, Kina, Kirsteen, Kirsten, Kirstin, Kirsto, Kirsty, Kris, Kriss, Krissie, Krista, Kristel, Kristi, Kristian, Kristin, Kristina, Kristine, Kristyan, Krystyan, Krystyna, Teenie, Tina, Tine, Tiny, Xena, Xina.

Christmas Compound from the Latin, *Cristes* and *masse*, thus 'mass of Christ' the festival of the birth of Christ, December 25. Since medieval times, a name given to both boys and girls born on that day but superseded by Noel in the last century. *See also* Natalie and Noel.

Chrysanthemum From the Greek, *Krusos*, 'gold', and *anthenon*, 'flower'. In botany, the genus of large, autumn-blooming flowers, originally from China. In Greek mythology, Chryseis was a priestess of Apollo who was given as a slave to Agamemnon. **Variant:** Chryseis.

Chrysogon From the Greek, *krusogonos*, 'born of gold'. The 3rd-century saint was adviser to St Anastasia. **Variants:** Chrisogone, Grisegond, Grisigion, Grisigon, Grisogonia, Grissecon.

Cinderella From the French, *cendre*, 'ashes'. In the fairy-tale, the down-trodden but beautiful younger step-sister who finally marries Prince Charming. **Variants:** Cindy, Ella.

Clare From the Latin, *clarus*, 'clear, bright, shining, distinct, evident, famous'. St Clare of Assisi (1194–1253) was a follower of St Francis and founded the order of Poor Ladies, later called Poor Clares. She was considered the best expression of the evangelical perfection that St Francis describes. Because of an account that she once 'witnessed' a mass being celebrated far away, she is patron saint of television. The name has been popular in England ever since her death, with the latinised form, Clara, gaining equal attention

GOOD QUEEN BESS

Nicknames are usually a sign of affection during childhood, but sometimes they are given later. Queen Elizabeth II grew out of her childhood nickname of Lilibet. But Queen Elizabeth I attracted a string of names while she was on the throne. They ranged from the simple Good Queen Bess to the elaborate poetical compliments in Edmund Spenser's epic poem, *The Faerie Queene*. He openly admitted that his heroine fairy was in fact 'the most excellent and glorious person of our sovereine the Queene'. One name was not enough to describe her attributes. He called her Astraea (star), Belphoebe (beautiful moon), Gloriana (glory, praised) and Mercilla (kindness, mercy).

---

in the last century. The many compounds include **Claramae, Claribele, Clarabella, Clarimond, Clarinda. Variants, some also given to boys:** Chiara, Chiarra, Claira, Claire, Clairene, Clare, Clares, Clareta, Claretha, Clarette, Clarey, Clari, Clarice, Claricia, Clarie, Clarinda, Claris, Clariscia, Clarissa, Clarisse, Clarita, Clarrisse, Clarus, Clary, Clatie, Clerissa, Clorinda, Klara, Klarika, Klarrisa, Larisa, Sorcha.

Clarette From the French, *claret*, 'clear red', referring to the red wine of Bordeaux.

Claudia French female form of Claudius. Carried to England by the Romans in the 1st century. **Variants:** Claude, Claudella, Claudette, Claudie, Claudina, Claudine, Clodia, Gladys, Gwladys.

Cleantha From the Greek, *kleio*, 'praise, glory', and *anthenon*, 'flower'. **Variants:** Cleanthe, Cliantha.

Clemence Female form of Clement. In Roman mythology, the goddess of pity. **Variants:** Clem, Clemency, Clemense, Clementia, Clementina, Clementine, Clemmie, Clemmy, Klementine, Tina.

Cleopatra From the Greek, 'glory of her father'. The attractive, intelligent and ambitious Cleopatra VII (69–30 BC) was twice Queen of Egypt and took Julius Caesar and Mark Antony as lovers. **Variant:** Cleta.

Clio From the Greek, *kleios*, 'to praise, acclaim'. As one of the nine muses presiding over music and poetry in Greek mythology, Cleo watched over history. Also given to boys. **Variants:** Cleo, Cleon, Cleona, Cleone, Cleora.

Cloelia In Roman mythology, the courageous heroine who escaped captivity with the Etruscans by swimming the Tiber. **Variant:** Clolia.

Clorinda From the Latin, 'renowned, verdant, beautiful'. A fictional name invented by the 16th-century Italian poet, Tasso.

Clotilda From the Old German, *chlotichilda*, 'renowned in battle'. **Variants:** Clothild, Clothilde, Clotilde, Klothilde.

Clove From the Latin, *clavus*, 'nail'. Cloves are the dried flower buds of an East Indian tree, highly prized for their aromatic and medicinal properties.

Clover From the Old English, *cloefre*, 'to cling'. A lush pasture plant with three-lobed leaves; four-lobed leaves are believed to bring good luck.

Clymene From the Greek, *klymene*, 'famous'. A name given to many Greek heroines.

Clytie From the Greek, *klytai*, 'splendid'. In Greek mythology, a maiden who died of despair from her unrequited love for Helios, god of the sun. Her body took root and became the heliotrope plant whose flowers always turn towards the sun.

Colette French female variant of Nicholas. Sidonie Gabrielle Colette (1873–1954) was the French novelist famed for her sensuous and idyllic evocations of childhood and nature, such as *Gigi* (1944); she was always known simply by her surname. **Variants:** Colecta, Colet, Coleta, Collect, Collett, Collette, Cosette, Cosetta, Kalotte.

Colleen From the Irish, *cailun*, 'girl'. **Variants:** Coleen, Colena, Colene, Collice.

Columbine From the Latin, *columba*, 'female dove', symbol of peace. In botany, the flowers resemble a cluster of doves. In pantomime, the sweetheart of Harlequin. *See also* Columba. **Variants:** Columba, Columbia, Columbina.

Comfort From the Latin, *confortare*, 'to strengthen, give solace, ease pain'. Given to both boys and girls by the Puritans.

Conception From the Latin, *conceptio*, 'conceive, reproduce, begin'. Usually used referring to the Virgin Mary of the Immaculate Conception. **Variants:** Concepcion, Concha, Conchita. *See also* Dolores.

Concha From the Greek, 'shell'. **Variant:** Conchata.

Concordia From the Latin, 'harmony, agreement, state of peace'. In Roman mythology, the goddess of peace after war.

Constance Female form of Constantine. Introduced into Britain by one of William the Conqueror's daughters and quickly adopted. Widely used until the 17th century; revived by the Victorians. **Variants:** Conetta, Connie, Conny, Constancia, Constancy, Constanta, Constantia, Constantina, Constanza, Conte, Custance, Custancia, Custans, Custins, Konstanze.

Consuela From the Latin, *consolari*, 'to free from sadness, comfort'. Another Puritan favourite. **Variants:** Consolata, Consuelo.

Content From the Latin, *contentus*, 'completely satisfied, fulfilled'. Again, common with the Puritans.

Cora From the Greek, *kore*, 'maiden'. In Greek mythology, a name for the beautiful goddess Persephone who was abducted by Pluto, god of the dark underworld, but later permitted to spend half of each year on earth. Corinna, the Greek poetess (5th century BC) was one of the most beautiful and talented women of her age and won the major poetry prize five times. Popular in 19th-century American. The compounds include **Corabelle**.

Variants: Coralie, Corella, Corene, Coretta, Corette, Cori, Corie, Corinna, Corinne, Corita, Correne, Corrina, Corrine, Corry, Cory, Kora.

Coral From the Greek, *korallion*, 'pebble'. The red, orange, pink or white substance secreted by tiny animals living on the seabed which, when hardened, is collected for jewellery and ornaments. **Variants:** Coralie, Coraline.

Cordelia From the Celtic, 'daughter of the sea'. In Shakespeare's *King Lear* (1606), the youngest and only faithful one of the king's three daughters. **Variants:** Cordeilia, Cordelie, Cordell, Cordelle, Cordie, Cordula, Cordy, Delia, Della, Kordel, Kordula.

Cornelia Female form of Cornelius. The Roman women of the Cornelius family were regarded as the epitome of female virtue and motherhood. **Variants:** Cornela, Cornelie, Cornelle, Cornie, Corny, Neely, Neila, Nelia, Nell, Nellie, Nelly.

Corona From the Spanish, 'crown'.

Cosima From the Greek, *kosmos*, 'universe, order, harmony'.

Courtney *See under boys.*

Creola From the French Provencal, *crioulo*, 'home-bred, home raised', originally from the Latin, *creare*, 'to create'. In the West Indies, it means someone born there who is of European descent, while in the USA it usually describes a person born there who is of either European or African negro race, or a mixture of both.

Crescent From the Latin, *crescere*, 'to grow, increase'. The shape of the moon at the beginning and end of its cycle.

Cressida In Greek mythology, a Greek woman called Briseis forsakes her Trojan lover, Troilus, for the Greek, Diomedes. Popularised in medieval legend, with Cressida taking on Briseis' role, and then by Shakespeare in *Troilus and Cressida* (1602).

Crystal From the Greek, *krustallos*, 'ice', hence the transparent and brilliantly clear quartz rock. Used since the Renaissance and very fashionable at the end of the 19th century.

Cuthberga Female form of Cuthbert. The 8th-century English saint was a princess-turned-abbess, the wife of King Aldred of Northumbria. She founded the nunnery at Wimborne.

Cybele In early Greek mythology, the mother-goddess of Anatolia, who watched over fertility, health and nature and whose strong cult drove worshippers into states of ecstasy and prophetic rapture. Not to be confused with Sibyl. **Variants:** Cybebe, Cybela, Cybill.

Cymbeline The English name for Cunobelinus (died AD 42), chief of the Catuvellauni tribe and ruler of modern Hertfordshire, and the hero of Shakespeare's play, *Cymbeline* (1610). **Variant:** Cymbaline.

Cymry The Cymry are the branch of the Celts that include the Welsh, Cornish and the Bretons of north-west France. Today, it usually means just Welsh. **Variants:** Cymri, Kymry.

Cynara From the Greek, 'thistle, artichoke', implying well-protected.

Cynthia In classical mythology, another name for Artemis (or Diana) who was born on Mount Cynthus on the island of Delos in the Aegean Sea. A term given to Elizabeth I by poets. **Variants:** Cinda, Cindee, Cindi, Cindie, Cindy, Cyndie, Cyndy, Cynth, Cynthiana, Cynthie, Kynthia, Sindee, Sindy. *See also* Hyacinth.

Cypris From the Greek, 'from Cyprus'. In Greek mythology, a name for Aphrodite who was born on that island. Her cult made it renowned for gaiety and licentiousness. **Variants:** Ciprian, Cipriana, Cyprian.

Cyr Female form of Cyril. **Variants:** Ciri, Cirilla, Cyra, Cyrilla.

Cytherea In classical mythology, another name for Aphrodite (or Venus), who came from the island of Cytherea, or Cyprus; *see* Cypris.

D

Daffodil From the Greek, *asphodelos*. The bright yellow spring flower is also known as the Lent Lily.

Dagania From the Hebrew, *daga*, 'corn, ceremonial grain'. In Phoenician mythology, Dagon was the chief deity, represented as half man and half fish. **Variants:** Daganya, Degania, Deganya.

Dagmar From the Danish, *dag* and *mar*, 'joy of the Dane'.

Dahlia In botany, the family of Mexican and Central American plants with big, bright-coloured flowers, named after the 18th-century Swedish botanist, Anders Dahl.

Daisy From the Old English, *doegeseage*, 'day's eye'. European plant, some species of which open their flowers to reveal yellow discs in the morning and close up again at night. Also a form of Margaret, because the daisy was the symbol of St Margherita of Italy. Heroine of Henry James's novel *Daisy Miller* (1878). In common with most other flower names, popular only since the last century, when Harry Dacre wrote the song, 'Daisy, Daisy, give me your answer, do! I'm half crazy, all for the love of you!' **Variant:** Daisie.

Dale From the Old English, *dael*, 'valley'. Also given to boys. **Variants:** Dael, Daile, Dallas, Dayle.

Dama From the Latin, *domina*, 'gentle and noble lady', the female counterpart of Lord. **Variants:** Damara, Damaris, Dame, Damita.

Damalis From the Greek, 'tamer, conqueror'.

Damaris From the Greek, 'heifer', implying its gentleness. **Variant:** Damara.

Dana Female variant form of Daniel. **Variants:** Danae, Danella, Danelle, Danette, Dania, Danice, Daniela, Daniele, Daniella, Danielle, Danit, Danita, Danni, Danny, Dannye, Danya.

Danica From the Old Slavic, 'morning star'.

Danielle Female form of Daniel.

Dantel Female form of Dante. **Variant:** Dantia.

Daphne From the Greek, 'laurel, bay tree'. In Greek mythology, the goddess of music and poetry who refused to requite Apollo's love. As she fled from his embrace she was saved by the earth goddesses who transformed her into a tree. A Laurel crown is a symbol of victory. The name has been common only in this century. **Variants:** Daff, Daffy, Dafna, Dafne, Dafnit, Daph, Daphna, Daphnit.

Dara From the Middle English, 'compassion' and 'to have courage, daring'. Also from the Hebrew, 'source of wisdom'. **Variants:** Daralice, Daralis, Dare, Darelle, Dareth, Daria, Darice, Darryl, Darya, Daryl.

Darcey From the old French meaning 'dark'. This name has recently become popular in the UK after the ballet dancer Darcey Bussell.

Daria Female form of Darius; *see also* Dara. **Variants:** Darice, Darya.

Darleen From the Old English, *deorling*, 'beloved, highly valued, worthy, favourite'. **Variants:** Darelle, Darla, Darlene, Darline, Darlyn, Darragh, Daryl.

Daron Female form of Dareen.

Davene Female form of David. Devina is a Scottish form; Davita is Spanish. **Variants:** Davi, Davida, Davina, Davita, Devina, Vida, Veda, Veta, Vita, Vitia.

Dawn From the Old High German, *tagen*, via the Old English, *dagian*, 'daybreak'. A name first used in the 19th century and now superseding the long-popular Latin form, Aurora, while taking over its nicknames. **Variants:** Orrie, Rora.

Daya From the Hebrew, 'bird'. **Variant:** Dayah.

Deborah From the Hebrew, 'a bee', which later also meant 'to speak with eloquence'. In the Bible, Rebecca's faithful, much-loved nurse (Genesis 35); also, a substantial character, both prophetess and judge, who predicted that the Israelites would win freedom from the Canaanites and then helped them to achieve it (Judges 4). A name very popular with the 17th-century Puritans. **Variants:** Deb, Debbe, Debbee, Debbi, Debbie, Debby, Debera, Debi, Debir, Debo, Debor, Debora, Debra, Debs, Deva, Devera, Devora, Devorah, Devorit, Devra, Dobra, Dovra, Dvera, Dvorit.

Decima Female form of Decimus. Often given to the tenth daughter or child–more common when families were larger. Deka is the Greek form. **Variants:** Declan, Deka.

Dee From the Welsh, *du*, 'black, dark'. Thus suitable for a daughter with dark complexion or hair. **Variants:** Dede, Dee Dee, Didi.

Degula From the Hebrew, 'outstanding, excellent'.

Deirdre From the Celtic, *derdriu*, 'raging one', or the Gaelic, *deoirid*, 'broken-hearted one', or even Middle English, *der*, 'young girl'. In Irish mythology, the beautiful daughter of an Ulster harper who eloped to Scotland with her lover, Naoise. When Naoise was murdered by King Conchobar, to whom she was officially betrothed, she took her own life. Hence, a popular romantic name for Irish poets and writers. **Variants:** Dede, Dee, Deerdre, Diedra, Dierdra, Dierdre, Dorcas.

Delia Female form of Delius, from Delos. Another name for Artemis, who was born on the island of Delos. In his *Sonnets to Delia*, Samuel Daniel (1562–1619) wondered 'whether Delia's eyes Are eyes, or else two

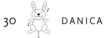

radiant stars that shine'. **Variants:** Dede, Dee, Dehlia, Delinda, Della, Didi. *See also* Cynthia.

Delicia Italian, from the Latin, *delectare*, 'to allure, charm, give pleasure'. **Variants:** Delight, Delizia.

Delilah From the Arabic, 'guide, leader', or the Hebrew, 'poor' or 'hair'. In the Bible, the seductive Philistine mistress of Samson who was persuaded by her people to betray him. She discovered that his strength came from his long hair, and cut it off as he slept (Judges 16). Hence the term Delilah for a seductive, treacherous woman. **Variants:** Dalila, Delila, Lila, Lilah.

Delma From the Spanish, *delmar*, 'of the sea'. **Variant:** Delmar.

Delpha From the Greek, *delphis*, 'dolphin'. In Greek mythology, symbol of a calm sea. In botany, delphinium is the genus for several tall garden plants, such as larkspur, whose blue flowers have dolphin-shaped nectaries. In astronomy, a constellation in the northern hemisphere. **Variants:** Delfine, Delphina, Delphine, Delphinie, Delphinium.

Demelda From the Greek, *melden*, 'to proclaim, speak out loud'.

Demetria Female form of Demetrius. In Greek mythology, an earth mother goddess of fertility and cultivated land, especially of corn and the harvest. **Variants:** Demeter, Demetra, Demetris, Dimitra, Dimity.

Demi A diminutive form of the Latin Demetria, this name has become popular with the fame of actress Demi Moore.

Denise Female form of Denis. Popular in the Middle Ages, then out of fashion until this century. **Variants:** Deney, Denice, Deniece, Deniese, Denis, Dennet, Dennie, Denny, Denyse, Deonysia, Dinnie, Dinny, Dion, Dione, Dionetta, Dionis, Dionise, Dionycia, Dionysia, Diot.

Denna From the Anglo-Saxon, 'glen, valley'. **Variants:** Deana, Deanna, Dene, Dena, Dina.

Derora From the Hebrew, 'flowing stream', implying total freedom. **Variant:** Derorit.

Desdemona From the Greek, *dusdaimonia*, 'woman of bad fortune'. In Shakespeare's tragedy, *Othello* (1604), the honest wife whose husband is tricked into falsely believing that she has been unfaithful; in a jealous rage he murders her. **Variant:** Desmona.

Desire From the Latin, *desiderare*, 'to long for, crave, wish'. **Variant:** Desirée.

Desma From the Greek, *desmos*, 'bond, pledge'.

Deva From the Sanskrit, 'god, divine'; Hindu name for the goddess of the moon. **Variant:** Devaki.

Dextra From the Latin, *dexter*, 'right-hand side', implying someone skilful with her hands.

Deziree From the Native American meaning 'the desired one'. **Alternatives include** Dezira, Deziray, Dezyrae.

Diamanta From the Greek, *adamas*, 'unconquerable', because a diamond is so hard that it can be cut or polished only by another diamond.

Diana From the Latin, *dius*, 'god-like, divine, the bright one'. In Roman mythology, the woodland goddess of chastity, hunting and the moon. She protected wild animals and was distinctly uninterested in men: when

Acteon espied her bathing, she turned him into a stag. Nevertheless, she was especially honoured by women, who associated her with fertility and childbirth. A name introduced into Britain in the 16th century but common only since the mid-18th. Recently boosted when Prince Charles, Prince of Wales, married Lady Diana Spencer. **Variants:** Deana, Deane, Deanna, Deanne, Deannis, Dede, Dee, Dena, Di, Diahann, Dian, Diandra, Diane, Dianna, Dianne, Didi, Diona, Dione, Dionne, Dionetta, Dyan, Dyana, Dyane, Dyann, Dyanna, Dyanne.

Diantha From the Greek, *dios* and *anthos*, 'heavenly flower'. In Greek mythology, the flower of the supreme god, Zeus. **Variants:** Diandra, Dianthe.

Diara From the African word meaning 'a gift'. **Alternatives include** Diera, Dierra, Dyara.

Dickla From the Hebrew, 'palm or date tree'. Also given to boys. **Variants:** Dicey, Dicia.

Dido In Roman mythology, the foundress of Carthage. In Virgil's epic poem, *The Aeneid* (70–19 BC), she falls deeply in love with Aeneas and when he leaves her she commits suicide by burning.

Dillian From the Latin, *idolom*, 'image for worship, apparition', thus the object of deep love or devotion. **Variants:** Dilli, Dilliana, Dillo.

Dilys From the Welsh, 'genuine, perfect, true'.

Dimitra Female form of Demetrius. **Variant:** Dimity.

Dinah From the Hebrew, 'vindication, judgement'. In the Bible, the beautiful daughter of Jacob and Leah. Another Puritan favourite. **Variants:** Deanna, Deanne, Deena, Dena, Dina.

Dione From the Greek, 'divine queen'. In Greek mythology, mother of Aphrodite. A favourite poetic name for a beautiful and loved woman. **Variants:** Dion, Dionée, Dionis.

Ditza From the Hebrew, 'joy', **Variants:** Ditzah, Diza.

Dixie From the Old Norse, *diss*, 'active sprite'. The name of a Nordic fairy guardian. Dixieland is a term for the southern United States of America, probably inspired by a ten-dollar bill issued in French-influenced New Orleans which had *dix*, 'ten', printed boldly on each side – hence 'a girl from Dixie'. **Variants:** Disa, Dix.

Doda From the Hebrew, 'friend, aunt'. **Variants:** Dodi, Dodie, Dody. *See also* Dorothea.

Dolcila From the Latin, *dolcilis*, 'gentle, amenable'. **Variants:** Docila, Docilla.

Dolores From the Latin, 'lady of sorrows'. The sorrows are the seven sad episodes of the Virgin's life. In the Latin countries of southern Europe, one name for the Virgin was Santa Maria de los Dolores. As Mary was considered too sacred to use, girls were often christened this or Carmen, Consuelo, Mercedes (from Mercy) and other names associated with the life of the Virgin. **Variants:** Dalores, Delora, Delores, Deloris, Delorita, Dolorita, Doloritas, Dolours, Lo, Lola, Lolita.

Dominica Female form of Dominic. **Variants:** Domenica, Domeniga, Domina, Dominick, Dominique, Dominga.

Donalda Female form of Donald.

Donata From the Latin, *donum*, 'gift, deserving of gifts'. **Variants:** Donia, Donica. *See also* Donatus *under boys*.

NAMES AND THE LAW

Every birth must be registered. The Registration Act of 1836 took effect on July 1, 1837, since when every child born in Britain must be registered within 42 days of its birth (penalties for failing to register a child were introduced in 1874). However, the name options do not close then. Further names can be added to the bottom of the certificate for another 12 months. So, if Nicholas seems on reflection to be a little warlike, Henry could be added to encourage hopes of future wealth and power. Of course, a person can later re-name himself or herself absolutely anything, from Broom-Broom for a car fanatic to Floppy Disc for a computer-programmer. The original birth record cannot be changed, but if documents are to be registered in the adopted names, the Inland Revenue must be told.

Changing a surname is different: it is done by Deed Poll. For a small fee, a Commissioner for Oaths (usually a solicitor) draws up the deed which is then sworn and stamped. The two areas to be careful about when changing names are infringing copyright or the obscenity laws. Incidentally, when a couple marry, the woman is not legally required to change her surname to that of her husband.

Donna Italian, from the Latin, *domina*, 'lady, woman worthy of respect, mistress of a house-hold'. **Variants:** Domella, Donalie, Donella, Donelle, Donita, Donni, Donnis, Donny.

Dorcas From the Greek, *dorkas*, 'gazelle', implying a delicate, light-footed girl. **Variant:** Dorcia.

Doris From the Greek, 'bountiful, from the ocean'; also the word for 'sacrificial knife'. In Greek mythology, daughter of Oceanus, god of the sea, and wife of the just and kind Nereus, 'Old Father of the Sea'. On their marriage, she bore him fifty golden-haired, beautiful daughters who became the sea nymphs of the Mediterranean, and they all lived happily together deep in the Aegean Sea. A popular name towards the end of the last century and the early years of this. Amy Dorrit was the heroine of Charles Dickens' *Little Dorrit* (1857). The compounds include **Dorinda. Variants:** Dorea, Dori, Doria, Dorice, Dorie, Dorisa, Dorit, Dorita, Dorith, Doritt, Dorrie, Dorris, Dorrit, Dory, Rinda. *See also* Nerine.

Dorit From the Hebrew, *dor*, 'generation'. **Variant:** Dorrit.

Dorma From the Latin, *dormire*, 'to sleep'.

Doronit From the Aramaic, 'gift'.

Dorothea From the Greek, *doron*, 'gift', and *theos*, 'God', thus 'gift of God, divine gift'. After the martyrdom of St Dorothy in the 4th century, a child miraculously appeared with a basket of apples and roses to present to the lawyer who had mockingly asked her to send him fruits from the heavenly garden. Of the many variants, Dorothy was in vogue from the 15th century and gave the word to a child's doll. Dora gained in popularity in the last century and the Irish Doreen was introduced to England at the beginning of this century. The many compounds include **Doralyn, Dorann, Dorinda and Dorothy-Anne**. **Variants:** Dahtee, Dasha, Dasya, Dede, Derede, Dode, Dodi, Dodie, Dodo, Dody, Doe, Doirean, Doll, Dolley, Dollie, Dolly, Dora, Doralane, Doraleen, Doralene, Doralia, Doralice, Doralyn, Dorat, Dore, Doreen, Dorelia, Dorene, Doretta, Dorette, Dori, Dorinda, Dorisia, Dorita, Dorka, Dorlisa, Doro, Dorolice, Dorota, Dorotea, Doroteya, Dorothee, Dorothy, Dorri, Dorrie, Dorthea, Dorthy, Dory, Dosi, Dot, Dotti, Dottie, Dotty, Tiga, Tigo, Tio, Totie. *See also* Doris and Theodora.

Dova Female form of Dove.

Dreama From the Old English, *dream*, 'to sing, to make a happy and joyful noise'.

Druella From the Old German, *drugiself*, 'elfin vision' – elves were believed to be very clever, spry, and quick-thinking.

Drusilla From the Greek, 'soft-eyed'. **Variants:** Dru, Druci, Drucie, Drucilla, Drusa, Drusie, Drusus, Drusy.

Duana From the Irish Gaelic, *duan*, 'song'. **Variants:** Duan, Swana.

Dudee English gypsy name, meaning 'star, bright light'.

Dulcie From the Latin, *dulcis*, 'sweet'. **Variants:** Delcina, Delcine, Dulce, Dulcea, Dulcee, Dulcia, Dulciana, Dulcine, Dulcinea, Dulcy.

Dusha Russian, meaning 'soul'.

Dymphna From the Irish, *damhnait,* 'one fit to be', often referring to the Virgin. **Variant:** Dympna.

Dysis From the Greek, 'sunset'. Thus suitable for a child born at dusk or born to older parents.

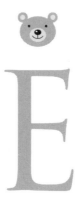

Eartha From the Old High German, *erde*, 'ground, this country, or the world (as distinct from heaven)'. **Variants:** Erda, Erde, Ertha, Herta, Hertha.

Easter From the Middle English, *ester*, 'where the sun rises', from the Old High German, *ostarun*, 'eastern'. The Anglo-Saxon monk and scholar, Bede (673–735) took the name of a goddess whose feast was celebrated at the vernal equinox and gave it to the Christian festival of the resurrection of Christ. *See also* Esther.

Ebony From the Greek, *ebenos*, 'ebony tree'. A hard, dark, durable and highly-valued heartwood. **Variants:** Ebonee, Eboney, Eboni, Ebonie.

Edda From the Old Norse, 'poetry'.

Edga Female form of Edgar.

Edith From the Old English, *ead*, 'wealthy, fortunate', and *gyo*, 'war'. St Eadgyth (962–84) made it a favourite Anglo-Saxon name. Also the wife of Henry 1 (1068–1105), who was known as Metilda or Mold, but whose name was probably altered to Edith by the Normans who found Anglo-Saxon names difficult to pronounce. The name underwent a 19th-century revival. The variant, Edda, is also an Old Norse word, meaning 'poetry'. **Variants:** Ardith, Eade, Eadita, Eady, Eda, Edda, Edde, Ede, Edie, Edine, Edita, Editha, Edithe, Edon, Edy, Edythe, Eidita. *See also* Mathilda.

Edna From the Old English, *edana*, 'happiness, rich gift'; a female form of Edwin; a female form of Edan; or from the Hebrew, 'delight, rejuvenation'. The 19th-century best-seller novelist, Edna Lyall, brought the name into fashion. **Variants:** Adena, Adina, Edana, Ednah.

Edwina Female form of Edwin. **Variants:** Edina.

Efrata From the Hebrew, 'distinguished, respected'.

Efrona From the Hebrew, 'sweet-singing bird'.

Eileen Either from the Irish name, Eibhlin, developed from Evelyn, or the Irish form of Helen. Introduced to Britain early this century. Elain and Elaine are the French forms. Elaine was Sir Galahad's mother in Arthurian legend, raised to popularity once more by Alfred Tennyson's epic poem, *The Idylls of the King* (1859); *see also* Arthur. **Variants:** Aileen, Eila, Eilidh, Eily, Elain, Elaine, Elane, Elayne, Elie, Ilene.

Eiluned From the Welsh, *eilun*, 'idol'. The French variant, Linet, was a heroine in the medieval Arthurian legend, as retold by Tennyson; *see* Eileen. **Variants:** Elined, Eluned, Linet, Linnet, Lyn, Lynette, Lynn, Lynne.

Eirene From the Old Norse, 'peace'.

Elana From the Latin, *elan*, 'spirited'; or from the Hebrew, 'tree'. **Variant:** Ilana.

Eldora From the Spanish, *el dorado*, 'gilded', from the fabled land or city overflowing with gold and riches that was believed to lie on the Amazon in South America.

Eleanor The Provençal form of Helen, Alienor, was carried to England via France when Eleanor of Aquitaine married Henry II (1133–89). Popularised when Edward I erected memorial crosses to his wife, 'Good Queen Eleanor' (died 1290). 'Little Nell', in Charles Dickens' novel *The Old Curiosity Shop* (1841), brought that form into vogue. Leonora was the original title of Beethoven's opera, *Fidelio* (1805). **Variants:** Alianora, Alienor, Alienora, El, Ele, Eleanora, Eleanore, Elen, Elenor, Eleonora, Eleonore, Eli, Elianor, Elianora, Elie, Elien, Elin, Ellnor, Elinore, Elinorr, Ella, Ellen, Ellenor, Ellette, Ellie, Ellin, Ellyn, Elnore, Elnora, Elyenora, Elyn, Elynn, Heleanor, Leanor, Lennie, Lenora, Lenore, Leonora, Leonore, Leora, Nelda, Nell, Nella, Nellie, Nelly, Nora, Norah, Noreen, Norene, Norina, Norine, Nureen.

Electra From the Greek, *elekron*, 'amber, one that shines brilliantly'. Electricity is so named because the property for developing it was first observed in Amber. In Greek mythology, Electra and her brother avenged the murder of their father, Agamemnon, by killing their mother and her lover. **Variant:** Elektra.

Elizabeth From the Hebrew name, *Elisheva*, 'oath of God', which becomes Elisabet in Greek and Elizabetha in Latin. The English spelling usually prefers 'z'. In the Bible, Elisheva is first found as the wife of Aaron (Exodus 6). In the New Testament, she appears as the elderly mother of John the Baptist (Luke 1). Introduced into Britain at the end of the 15th century, the name was sometimes confused with Isabel. It gained royal aplomb and huge popularity from the strong personality of Elizabeth I (1533–1603), known as 'Good Queen Bess', named after her grandmother, Elizabeth of York. In the 18th century, Betty became so common that it lost its prestige value and was kept for chambermaids, and Bess was revived to replace it. In this century, the Queen Mother (born 1900), popular consort of George VI, gave her name to their child, Elizabeth II (born 1926) who was crowned in 1953 and celebrated her silver jubilee in 1977–her childhood nickname was Lilibet. **One of the most consistently popular names in Britain with countless variants, including:** Bab, Babette, Bela, Belita, Bess, Bessie, Bessy, Bet, Beth, Betsey, Betsie, Betssy, Bett, Betta, Bette, Bettina, Bettine, Betty, Ealasaid, Eilis, Elese, Elisa,

Elisabet, Elisabeta, Elisabeth, Elisabetta, Elise, Elisheba, Elisheva, Elissa, Eliza, Elizabet, Elizabez, Elize, Elsa, Elsabet, Else, Elsebin, Elsie, Elspet, Elspeth, Elspie, Elsye, Elysa, Elyse, Elyssa, Erzebet, Helsa, Ila, Ilisa, Ilise, Ilsa, Ilse, Ilyse, Isabel, Letha, Lety, Libbie, Libby, Lili, Lilian, Lilibet, Lilla, Lillah, Lisa, Lisbet, Lisbeth, Lise, Liselotte, Lisenka, Lisette, Lisl, Lista, Liz, Liza, Lizabeth, Lizbeth, Lize, Lizette, Lizzie, Lizzy, Orse, Tetsy, Tetty, Tibby, Ysabel.

Ella From the Old English, *aelf*, 'fairy maiden' or the Old German, *alja*, 'all'. Popular with the Normans, and later with the Victorians. **Variants:** Ala, Ela, Ella, Ellen, Hela, Hele.

Ellen *See* Helen.

Elma Turkish, meaning 'apple'.

Elsa From the Anglo-Saxon, 'swan'. Alternatively, from the Old German, 'noble maiden'. The heroine of *Lohengrin*, the opera by Richard Wagner (1813–83), brought the medieval name back into vogue. **Variants:** Ailsa, Elsie. *See also* Alice and Elizabeth.

Elva From the Old English, *aelf*, 'spry, quick-witted, clever, mischievous'. In folklore, elves are the small, supernatural beings with magical powers. **Variant:** Elvia.

Elvira Spanish, probably from the German name, Alverat, 'wise counsel', which became Alvery and Aubrey in English. **Variants:** Elva, Elvia.

Elysia From the Greek, *elision*, 'blissful, ideal happiness'. In Greek mythology, the Elysian fields were in the paradise abode of the dead.

Elza From the Hebrew, 'God is my joy'. **Variant:** Aliza.

Emerald Originally from the Greek, *smaragdos*, via the Middle English, *emeraude*. A bril- liant green, transparent precious stone which gave its name to the vivid green colour – hence the term Emerald Isle for Ireland. Esmeralda was the heroine of Victor Hugo's novel, *The Hunchback of Notre Dame* (1831). **Variants:** Emeralda, Emeraldine, Emerlin, Emerline, Esmeralda, Esmeraldah, Meraud.

Emily *See* Amelia. Rose to popularity in the last century, when it was sometimes confus- ingly shortened to Emma. **Variants:** Amelia, Em, Emaline, Eme, Emele, Emelin, Emeline, Emelina, Emilia, Emilie, Emm, Emma, Emmaline, Emmeleia, Emmie, Emmy, Imma, Millie, Milly, Ymma.

Emma From the Old German, *ermin*, 'univer- sal, whole'. Carried to Britain by the Normans and consistently popular – Queen Emma, 'Fair Maid of Normandy', married the English King Ethelred the Unready in 1002 and then his successor, Knute, in 1017. It was shortened to Em or Emm until the 18th century. The young women of two immensely successful novels, Jane Austen's *Emma* (1816) and Flaubert's *Madame Bovary* (1856), pushed the name further into the limelight. **Variants:** Em, Ema, Emengarde, Emm, Emme, Emmete, Emmie, Emmot, Emmota, Emmote, Emmy, Ermegardel, Imma, Irma, Ymma.

Emuna From the Arabic, *eman*, 'faith'. **Variants:** Emunah, Iman.

Ena From the Old Irish, *aodh*, 'fire', via the Irish name, Eithne, then anglicised to Ena or Hannah. Widespread since the end of the last century. **Variants:** Aine, Aithne, Eithne, Ina.

Enid From the Celtic, 'soul, purity, flawless'. In Arthurian legend, the patient and loyal wife of Geraint. Like Eileen, it was popularised by Tennyson's poem. Occasionally given to boys.

Eolande From the Greek, *eos*, 'dawn', thus 'land to the east'. In Greek mythology, Eos is goddess of dawn, counterpart to the Roman Aurora, ushering in each new day. **Variants:** Iolanthe, Yolanda, Yolande.

Erica Female form of Eric. **Variant:** Erika.

Erin From the Old Irish, *Erinn*, 'Ireland, peace'. A poetic term. **Variant:** Errin.

Ermintrude From the Old German name, Ermentrudis, from *ermin*, 'whole, universe', and *drudi*, 'strength'. Adopted by 18th-century British Romantic writers. **Variants:** Armigil, Ermegarde, Ermengarde. *See also* Emma.

Esme From the Anglo-Saxon meaning 'protector', this name is the feminine form of Edmund. **Alternatives include** Esmé and Edmee.

Esperanza From the Spanish for 'hope'.

Estelle From the French, *etoile*, 'star'. Heroine of Charles Dickens' novel *Great Expectations* (1861). **Variants:** Essie, Estella, Estrella, Estrellita, Stella, Stelle.

Esther From the Hebrew, *hadassah*, 'myrtle'; or, less likely, from the Persian, *esthar*, 'star'. In Assyro-Babylonian mythology, the somewhat violent goddess of morning, evening, love and desire. In Phoenician mythology, goddess of the moon. In the Bible, the story of Esther, Queen of Persia, bravely saving her people from massacre is recounted in the book of her name. Not to be confused with Easter. **Variants:** Eister, Essa, Essie, Esta, Estee, Estella, Ester, Estralita, Estrella, Ettie, Etty, Heddy, Hedy, Heidi, Heiki, Hester, Hesther, Hettie, Hetty, Trella.

Ethel From the Old German, *athal*, 'noble'. A 19th-century shortening of several Anglo-Saxon names, such as Etheldreda, Ethelburg, Ethelinda. Two successful novels spread the name: Thackeray's *The Newcomers* (1853–55) and Charlotte M. Yonge's *The Daisy Chain* (1856). **Variants:** Adal, Adale, Alice, Edel, Ethelda, Etheldreda, Ethelinda, Etheline, Ethelyn, Ethyl. *See also* Adela, Adelaide, Adeline and Audrey.

Euclea From the Greek, *eukleia*, 'glory'.

Eudora From the Greek, *eu*, 'good, pleasant', and *doron*, 'gifted'.

Eugenia From the Greek, 'excellent, well-born, fortunate'. Used in the Middle Ages, then brought back into vogue by Eugénie (1826–1920), the influential consort of Napoleon III of France, who acted as regent during his absence from France. After his capture at Sedan in 1870, she fled to England where she lived at Farnborough until her death 30 years later. **Variants:** Ena, Eugenie, Gene, Genie, Ina.

Eulalia From the Greek, 'sweetly spoken', a term given to Apollo. The 4th-century saint was for some time the most celebrated virgin martyr in Spain. **Variants:** Eula, Eulalie.

Eunice From the Greek, *eu* and *vike*, 'good victory'. A favourite of the 17th-century Puritans. **Variants:** Niki, Nikki, Unice, Younice.

Euphemia From the Greek, 'well-spoken, speech that brings honour and good fortune'. In use since the 12th century but now found mostly in Scotland. **Variants:** Eadaoine, Effie, Effim, Effum, Epham, Eppie, Eufemia, Eupham, Eupheme, Phamie, Phemie.

Eustacia Female form of Eustace. **Variants:** Stacey, Stacia, Stacie, Stacy.

Evangeline From the Greek, *euangelos*, 'to bring good tidings' and thus 'to preach the Christian faith'. A name made up by Longfellow for his poem, *Evangeline* (1847). **Variants:** Angela, Eva, Evangelia, Evangelina, Eve, Lia, Litsa. *See also* Angela.

Eve From the Hebrew, *hawwah*, 'breath of life'. In the Bible, Eve is the first woman, so named by Adam 'because she is the mother of all living' (Genesis 3). Found in Britain since the 12th century, when it was believed that the name would bring longevity to the bearer. It was probably boosted in the last century by the character of the angelic but delicate white child in Stowe's *Uncle Tom's Cabin* (1852). The Irish form, Eveleen, may also come from the Gaelic, *eiblin*, 'pleasant'. **Variants:** Aoiffe, Eeve, Eubha, Ev, Eva, Evadne, Evalina, Evaline, Evie, Eviene, Evita, Evleen, Evonne, Evota, Evy, Ewa, Yeva, Zoe.

Evelyn From the Old German and French, 'hazel-nut', a Celtic fruit of wisdom. Introduced by the Normans. Also given to boys. **Variants:** Avelina, Aveline, Avelyn, Avi, Avila, Evalina, Eve, Evelina, Eveline, Eveling, Evette, Evie, Eviene, Evonne, Evy.

 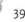

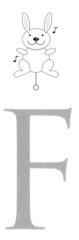

F

Fabia Female form of Fabius.

Faith From the Latin, *fides*, 'trust, loyalty, devotion'. One of the three foremost virtues of a good Christian; *see* Charity. In Latin mythology, Fides, 'good faith', was one of the three goddesses who watched over public transactions – the other two personified hospitality and oaths. **Variants:** Fae, Fay, Faye, Fayth, Faythe, Fidelity, Fidella.

Faline From the Latin, *feles*, 'cat'. **Variant:** Feline.

Fancy From the Greek, *phantazein*, 'to make visible', thus to visualise or imagine fantasies, to have whims, to wish for dreams to come true. **Variant:** Fancie.

Fanny *See* Frances and Myfanwy.

Farrah From the Middle English, 'beautiful, pleasant'; or from the Arabic, 'happiness'. **Variant:** Farah.

Fawn From the Latin, *fetus*, 'offspring', via the French, *feon*, 'offspring of an animal', hence the English meaning of a young deer less than a year old. In Walt Disney's famous cartoon, the young deer was called 'Bambi' (1942).

Fay From the Old French, *fei*, 'fairy', or the French, 'fidelity'. Also given to boys. **Variants:** Fae, Faye, Fayette, Fayina. *See also* Faith.

Fayme From the Latin, *fama*, 'reputation, public esteem, acclaim'. **Variant:** Faym.

Felicia From the Latin, *felicitas*, 'great happiness'. In Roman mythology, goddess of good fortune, luck and happy events. Another popular Puritan name, not to be confused with Phyllis. **Variants:** Falice, Falicia, Felcia, Felecia, Felice, Felicia, Feliciana, Felicidad, Felicie, Felicite, Felicity, Felis, Felise, Felisia, Felisse, Felita, Feliza, Filisia, Fillys.

Fern From the Old English, *fearn*, a flowerless plant with large, feathery, green fronds. Like

WHAT IS A CHRISTIAN NAME?

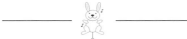

In the Church of England, the names given at baptism, the ceremony of welcoming a person into the Christian faith, are the Christian names. Canon law, the law of the church, does not lay down which names are suitable; that is left for the parents and minister to agree between them. The baptism ceremony is usually during a family service, so the whole congregation welcomes the child. The godparents (usually three) assume responsibility for the child's upbringing in the Christian faith. In the eyes of the church, a Christian's baptismal names remain the lifelong legal names, to be altered or added to only by a bishop at confirmation (and this is not a common practice). The Roman Catholic Church follows much the same path, preferring baptism to be performed during the morning mass. But there are differences between the churches' customary practices. At least one of a Catholic's given names must usually be a saint's name: there are normally just two godparents; and most people take an additional name at confirmation. *See also* Baptist *under boys.*

---

other plant names, popular at the end of the last century. Also a female form of Ferdinand. **Variant:** Ferne.

Filomena *See* Philomela.

Filomena From the Greek, *philos*, 'beloved' and *armonia*, 'harmony', thus, 'loving harmony' or 'devoted to music'. **Variant:** Philomena.

Fiona From the Celtic, *finn* and *fionn*, 'white, fair'. Probably made up by the Irish romantic writer, William Sharp (1855–1905). In Irish legend, Fionnuala was transformed into a swan and condemned to wander the lakes and rivers until Christianity came to Ireland. In Scotland, Fiona may also come from the Gaelic, *finghin*, 'beautiful child'. **Variants:** Fee,

Fenella, Finella, Finnuala, Finola, Fionna, Fione, Fionnuala, Fionnula, Nuala. *See also* Penelope.

Flavia From the Latin, *flavus*, 'golden yellow, blonde'. Thus suitable for a fair daughter or, as Flavius, for a son. **Variant:** Flavus.

Fleta From the Anglo-Saxon, 'clean, beautiful' or 'inlet of water'.

Flora From the Latin, *floris*, 'flower', implying a person who will flourish herself and also bring out the best in others. In Roman mythology, goddess of blossoming plants and of fruits and vines. The annual Floralia celebrations at her temple on April 28 included highly indecent plays. The French form, Fleur, was made popular by

Galsworthy in his novel, *The Forsyte Saga* (1922). **Variants:** Eloryn, Fflur, Fiora, Fiore, Fleur, Fleurette, Flo, Flor, Flore, Florella, Floria, Florida, Florie, Floris, Florrie, Florry, Flossie, Flower.

Florence From the Latin, *florentia*, 'blossoming, flourishing'. Given to boys and girls during the Middle Ages. Later, a visit to the Renaissance city in Italy became essential for persons of culture and education. Florence Nightingale (1820–1910), 'The Lady with the Lamp', was born there; as nurse and champion of medical reform, she made the name fashionable throughout the world. Compounds include **Florarose** and **Florinda**. **Variants:** Fiorella, Fiorenza, Flo, Flonda, Flor, Flora, Florance, Flore, Floreen, Floren, Florencia, Florentia, Florenz, Florina, Florinda, Florrie, Flory, Floryn, Floss, Flossi, Flossie, Flossy.

Fonda From the French, *fondre*, 'to melt'; or from the Spanish, 'profound'. Also given to boys. **Variants:** Fon, Fondea.

Fortunata From the Latin, *fortuna*, 'luck, chance'. In Roman mythology, Fortuna (also called Fors) was goddess of good luck and also the bringer of fertility–hence her attraction for both gardeners and would-be mothers. **Variants:** Faustine, Fortuna.

Frances From the Old Middle Latin, *franciscus*, 'a free man'. The Franks were the German tribes who fought for freedom against the yoke of the Romans and then settled in Gaul, which became known as France. St Frances Cabrini (1850–1917) founded the Missionary Sisters of the Sacred Heart, helped Italian immigrants in America, and in 1950 was the first American citizen to be canonised as a saint. She is patron saint of all emigrants. A favourite name among the Tudor aristocracy, then more widely used since the 18th century. **Variants:** Fan, Fanchette, Fanchon, Fancy, Fanechka, Fania, Fanni, Fannie, Fanny, Fannye, Fanya, Fran, France, Francesca, Francie, Francina, Francine, Francisca, Franciska, Francoise, Franconia, Francyne, Frania, Franika, Frank, Frankie, Franja, Franny, Franziske, Fronia, Ranny. *See also* Francis.

Frayda From the Yiddish, 'joy'. **Variants:** Frayde, Fraydyne, Freida, Freide.

Frederica Female form of Frederic. Used in England as a girls' name since the last century. **Variants:** Farica, Federica, Feriga, Fred, Fredda, Freddi, Freddie, Freddy, Fredericka, Frederika, Frederique, Frerika, Friederike, Fritze, Frydryka, Rica, Ricki, Ricky, Rike, Rikki.

Freya From the Old Norse, *freyja*, 'noble lady'. In Norse mythology, goddess of love and beauty. Her male counterpart, Frey, was god of peace, prosperity, fertility and good weather. **Variant:** Freyja.

Frieda From the Old High German, *fridu*, 'peace'. **Variants:** Freda, Fredda, Fredie, Fredyne, Freida, Freide, Friede, Fritzi. *See also* Winifred.

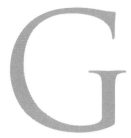

Gabriela From the Hebrew, 'strong man of God'. Female form of Gabriel who, in the Bible, was first seen by Daniel in a vision and was later the Archangel from God who told the Virgin Mary she would give birth to Christ (Luke 1). Most common during the Middle Ages. **Variants:** Gabay, Gabby, Gabel, Gabell, Gabey, Gabi, Gabie, Gabriele, Gabriella, Gabrielle, Gabryell, Gaby, Gavi, Gavra, Gavrila, Gavrilla.

Gaia The Greek word for 'earth' is often used to refer to the notion of the spirit of mother earth, and has become a popular girls' name since the beginnings of the environmental movement. **Alternatives include** Kaia.

Gail *See* Abigail.

Gal From the Hebrew, 'spring, fountain, hill', or from the Irish, 'courageous'. **Variants:** Gali, Galit.

Gana From the Hebrew, 'garden'. **Variants:** Ganit, Ganya.

Gardenia In botany, a genus of evergreen plants with glossy leaves and large, fragrant, usually pale-coloured blooms, such as Cape jasmine. It was named after the American botanist, Alexander Garden (1730–91).

Garland *See under boys.*

Garnet From the Latin, *granum*, 'grain', via the Old French, *pome grenate*, 'pomegranate'. The deep red juice of the fruit gave the name to a rich, dark red colour and also to the gemstones, which may be red, black, green, yellow or white. **Variant:** Grania.

Garniata From the French, *garnir*, 'to provide for, embellish, garnish'.

Gay From the Old French, *gai*, 'lively, full of joy, exuberantly cheerful'. **Variants:** Gae, Gaye.

Gayora From the Hebrew, 'valley of light'.

Gazelle From the Arabic, *ghazal*, 'small antelope', implying delicacy, nimbleness and swiftness. **Variant:** Gazella.

Gedual From the Hebrew, 'greatness, big'. **Variant:** Gedulah.

Gemma From the Latin, *gema*, 'fullness, swelling' as in a plant bud, or 'a precious stone'. Thus a precious child who will blossom into life. The child saint, Germaine of Pibra, near Toulouse (c. 1579–1601), was accused by her step-mother of giving bread to a beggar. When she opened her apron, it was full of spring flowers. She died soon afterwards and her grave became a place of pilgrimage and miracles. **Variant:** Germaine.

Genevia From the Latin, *juniperus*, 'junipertree'. **Variants:** Geneva, Genna.

Genevieve French, from the German, *geno*, 'race' and *wefa*, 'woman', thus 'womankind'. The 5th-century saint is protectress and patroness of Paris. **Variants:** Gena, Gene, Genevra, Genie, Gennie, Genny, Genovefa, Genovera, Gina, Guenevere, Guinevere, Janeva, Jennie, Jenny.

Georgia Female form of George. This and other variants became popular under the Hanoverian kings, who began with George I in 1714. **Variants:** Georgea, Georgeanna, Georgeanne, Georgeen, Georgeene, Georgena, Georgess, Georgett, Georgette, Georgiana, Georgianna, Georgianne, Georgie, Georgina, Georgine, Georgie.

Geraldine Literally, 'one of the Fitzgeralds'. A name made up by the Earl of Surrey, a romantic poet who was in love with Lady Elizabeth Fitzgerald and wrote about her beauty in about 1540. When another romantic poet, Coleridge, gave the name to a mysterious stranger in *Christabel* (1816), the name spread quickly. **Variants:** Deena, Dina, Geralda, Geraldene, Geraldina, Gerardene, Gerardine, Gererdine, Gerhardine, Geri, Gerldine, Gerrie, Gerry, Giralda, Jeralee, Jere, Jeri, Jerrie, Jerry.

Germain *See* Gemma.

Gertrude From the Old High German, *ger*, 'spear', and *drudi*, 'strength, wizard'. In Norse mythology, one of the Valkyries, goddesses who escorted slain heroes to Valhalla, the place of bliss. Introduced to Britain from the Low Countries, where the 13th-century mystic saint was a cult, but really popular only late in the last century. **Variants:** Gatt, Gatty, Gerda, Gert, Gerte, Gertie, Gertruda, Gertrudis, Gerty, Jara, Jera, Jerica, Truda, Trude, Trudel, Trudi, Trudy, Trula, Truta.

Gigi Female variant of Gilbert.

Gila From the Hebrew, 'joy'. **Variant:** Ghila.

Gilana From the Hebrew, 'joy'. **Variants:** Geela, Geelan, Ghila, Gila, Gilah, Gili, Gilia, Giliah.

Gilda From the Old English, *gyldan*, 'to gloss over, make superficially attractive', usually the art of applying a thin layer of gold leaf to an inferior metal.

Gillian *See* Julia.

Gina From the Hebrew, 'garden'. **Variant:** Ginat.

Giselle From the Anglo-Saxon, 'sword', implying a shining protector. **Variants:** Giselda, Giselle, Ghislaine.

Gladys From the Welsh, Gwladys, which is derived from *gwledig*, 'ruler, princess'; or the Welsh form of Claudia. Familiar in England since the 1870s. **Variants:** Glad, Gladi, Gleda, Gwladys.

Glenda Probably a female form of Glen, a popular American name. Found in the USA at the end of the 19th century, then in Australia, but only quite recently in Britain. See also Gwendolen and Gwyneth.

TEDDY BEARS' PICNIC

The soft, squashy and cuddly toy bear is named after Theodore Roosevelt, President of the United States of America from 1901 to 1909, whose nickname was Teddy. A keen huntsman, he nevertheless once spared the life of a bear cub while on the chase. After a cartoon of the event appeared, the lifesaver's name was given to bear cubs and their toy versions soon appeared. Other famous teddy bears going down to the woods to the picnic might include honey-loving Winnie-the-Pooh, Fuzzy Wuzzy (the bear with no hair), and the Three Bears – but probably without Goldilocks.

Gloria From the Latin, 'fame, renown, praise, honour'. A widespread name only since the end of the nineteeth century. **Variants:** Glora, Glori, Gloriana, Gloriane, Glorianna, Glorianne, Glory.

Glynis From the Irish Gaelic, *gleann*, 'narrow mountain-valley'. **Variant:** Glennis, Glyn, Glynnis.

Golda From the Old English, *gold*, the most precious metal, of a brilliant yellow-white colour. It is soft, conducts heat well, is unlikely to rust and is the symbol of a person's or a country's wealth. Golda Meir (1898–1978), Prime Minister of Israel from 1969 to 1974, was born in Kiev in Russia. **Variants:** Goldarina, Goldia, Goldie, Goldina.

Gozala From the Hebrew, 'young bird'.

Grace From the Latin, *gratus*, 'pleasing, attractive, effortlessly charming'. In Greek mythology, the Three Graces were nature-goddesses who nourished the fruits and spread joy throughout the world. Fashionable with the Puritans, then the Victorians. The Irish forms, Grainne and Grania, may also come from the name Graidhne. **Variants:** Engracia, Gracia, Gracie, Grainne, Grania, Grata, Gratia, Gratiana, Grayce, Grazia, Graziella, Grazina. *See also* Garnet and Kelly.

Gracilia From the Latin, *gracilis*, 'slender'.

Greta A diminutive form of the name Margaret, the name comes from the German/Swedish for 'pearl'. Greta has become particularly popular following the success of film actress Greta Garbo.

Griselda Possibly from the Old German, *gris-ja*, 'grey', and *hild*, 'battle'. Introduced into Britain through the patient heroine of the Clerk's Tale in Chaucer's *The Canterbury Tales* (begun 1386). **Variants:** Chriselda, Criselda, Griseldis, Grishilda, Grishilde, Grissel, Grittie, Grizel, Grizelda, Grizzel, Selda, Zelda.

Guinevere From the Welsh name, Gwenhwyvar, from *gwyn*, 'fair, white', and *hwyvar*, 'phantom'. In Arthurian legend, the beautiful wife of King Arthur and mistress of Lancelot. **Variant:** Guenevere. *See also* Jennifer.

Gwawr Welsh, meaning 'dawn'.

Gwendolen From the Gaelic, *gwen*, 'fair'. The name probably means 'white circle' and refers to a moon-goddess. In Arthurian legend, King Arthur fell in love with the fairy, Gwendolen. **Variants:** Guendolen, Gwen, Gwenda, Gwendaline, Gwendoline, Gwendolyn, Wendi, Wendy, Wyn, Wynelle, Wynette, Wynne. *See also* Winifred.

Gwyneth From the Celtic, *gwynedd*, 'blessed'; Gwynedd is Welsh for North Wales. The actress, Nell Gwyn (1650–87), was mistress to Charles II and bore him two sons. **Variants:** Gwen, Gwenda, Gwenith, Gwenn, Gwenne, Gwenny, Gwenth, Gwyn, Gwynne, Venetia, Wendi, Wendie, Wendy, Winnie, Winny, Wynne.

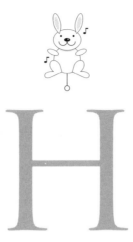

H

Habiba From the Arabic, *habib*, 'lover'; the male form is Habib.

Hadara From the Hebrew, 'deck out with beauty'.

Hadassah From the Hebrew, 'myrtle tree'; a symbol of victory. **Variants:** Dasi, Dassi Hadassa. *See also* Esther and Laurel.

Haley From the Norse, *haela*, 'hero'. **Variants:** Haile, Halie, Hallie, Hally, Hayley, Hailie.

Halina Hawaiian, meaning 'likeness, resemblance'.

Hana Japanese, meaning 'flower, blossom'.

Hannah From the Hebrew, *Hanani*, 'God favoured me', thus implying mercy and good fortune. **Variants:** Chana, Chanah, Chani, Hana, Hanita, Hanna, Hanni, Hannie, Hanny, Nan, Nana. *See also* Anna, Anne, Jane and John.

Harmony From the Greek, *armonia*, 'agreement in feelings, concord'. In Greek mythology,

the beautiful virgin, Harmonia, daughter of Aphrodite, married Cadmus, founder of Thebes. **Variants:** Harmonia, Harmonie.

Harriet Female form of Harry, from Henry. Developed during the Middle Ages, when Harry was highly popular. Henriette Marie, named after her father, Henry IV of France, carried her version to Britain when she married Charles I in 1625. **Variants:** Enrica, Enrichetta, Enriqueta, Etta, Etti, Ettie, Etty, Haliaka, Jarri, Harri, Harrie, Harrietta, Harriette, Harriot, Harriott, Hatti, Hattie, Hatty, Hendrike, Henka, Henrie, Henrieta, Henriete, Henrietta, Henriette, Henrinka, Henriqueta, Hetta, Hetti, Hetty, Minette, Yetta, Yettie, Yetty.

Hasia From the Hebrew, 'protected by the Lord'. **Variant:** Hasya.

Hawa From the Hebrew and Arabic, 'breath of life'. *See* Eve.

Hayat From the Arabic, *hayat*, 'life'.

Hazel From the Old English, *haesel*, 'hazelnut'. A wand of hazel symbolises protection and authority. The nut gives its name to a reddish-brown colour, used to describe pretty brown eyes or hair. With Heather and all the other flower names, it was in vogue at the end of last century. **Variants:** Hasse, Hazelle. *See also* Evelyn.

Heather From the Middle English, *haddre*. The small heathland shrub thrives especially in Scotland.

Hebe From the Greek, 'youth'. In Greek mythology, daughter of Zeus and goddess of youth.

Helen From the Greek, *elene*, 'the bright one, light'. Its widespread popularity in medieval times is due to St Helen (255–330), a fervent champion of the faith and also the British royal mother to Constantine the Great. In Greek mythology, the daughter of Zeus and Leda, who was judged the most beautiful of all women. She married the King of Sparta but eloped with a Trojan, Paris, which initiated the 10-year Trojan War. During the English Renaissance, this classical association put the name back in favour again, to be further promoted in two of Shakespeare's comedies. *A Midsummer Night's Dream* (1596) and *All's Well That Ends Well* (1595). In Christopher Marlowe's play, *Faustus* (1589), the appearance of Helen prompts Faust to exclaim, 'Was this the face that launched a thousand ships?' She is described as 'fairer than the evening air, Clad in the beauty of a thousand stars'. More recently, the remarkable Helen Keller (1880–1968) overcame deafness and blindness, learning to read, write and speak; she then worked with blind people. **Variants:** Eileen, Elaine, Eleanor, Elena, Elene, Elin, Elinor, Ellen, Ellin, Ellyn, Elyn, Helaine, Helayne, Helena, Helene, Helina, Hella, Jelena, Jelika, Leonora, Lina, Lino, Liolya, Nel, Nella, Nellene, Nelly, Yelena. *See also* Ailene, Alaina, Eileen and Eleanor.

Helga From the Old Norse, 'pious, religious'.

Hephziba From the Hebrew, 'my desire is in her'. **Variants:** Hephzibah, Hepzi, Hepziba, Hepzibah, Hesba.

Herma From the Latin, *herma*, 'square stone pillar', often used for milestones, thus the name implies strength and leadership.

Hermione Female form of Hermes who, in Greek legend, protected travellers and was a speedy, efficient and eloquent messenger for the gods. **Variants:** Erma, Hermia, Hermina, Hermine, Herminia. *See also* Cadmus.

Hero In Greek mythology, the beautiful priestess of Venus; *See* Leander.

Hesper From the Greek, *hesperos*, 'evening, evening star'. The Greek name for Italy. **Variant:** Hespera.

Hester *See* Esther.

Hestia In Greek mythology, goddess of the hearth. In early times the hearth would burn continuously, symbolising life. The one belonging to the chief or ruler had magical and religious significance.

Hilary From the Greek, *hilaros*, 'jovial, lively, cheerful, boisterous'. Quite a common name from the 13th to 16th centuries, then revived last century, when it was given to both boys and girls. **Variants:** Hilaire, Hilaria, Hilarie, Hillary.

Hilda From the Old German, *hild*, 'battle'. In Norse mythology, the chief of the Valkyries; see Gertrude. St Hilda (614–680), grand-niece of King Edwin of Northumbria, founded

Whitby Abbey, and the name is still popular in that area. **Variants:** Hild, Hilda, Hilde, Hildie, Hildy, Hylda.

Hisa Japanese, meaning 'long-lasting, longevity'. **Variants:** Hisae, Hisako, Hisayo.

Holly From the Old English, *holen*, 'holly-tree'. Twigs of the evergreen tree, with bright red berries, symbolising life, are hung on doors at Christmas to bring good luck. **Variants:** Holli, Hollye.

Honey From the Old English, *hunig*, 'honey'. The sweet liquid produced by bees from nectar has overtones of love and harmony.

Honor From the Latin, 'recognition, acknowledgment'. **Variants:** Honey, Honora, Honoria, Honorine, Nora, Norah, Noreen, Norine, Norrie, Nureen.

Hope From the Old English, *hopian*, 'to wish with optimism'. One of the three great Christian virtues; see Charity. Much favoured by the Puritans. Also given to boys.

Hortense From the Latin, *hortus*, 'garden', implying a place that will mature and blossom under careful attention. **Variants:** Hortensia, Ortense, Ortensia.

Hoshi Japanese, meaning 'star'.

Hula From the Hebrew, 'to make music'.

Hyacinth From the Greek, *huakinthos*, 'precious blue stone', probably a sapphire. In Greek mythology, a purple flower sprung from the blood of the slain youth, Hyacinthus – hence the name of the strongly-scented bulbous plant. **Variants:** Cinthie, Cynthie, Giancinta, Hyacintha, Hyacinthe, Hyacinthia, Jacenta, Jacinda, Jacinta, Jacintha, Jacinthe, Jackie, Jacky.

I

Ianthe In Greek mythology, a sea-nymph goddess with a pedigree genealogy. She is the daughter of Oceanus, supreme god of the seas and of cosmic power. She is therefore grand-daughter of Uranus and Ge, rulers of the sky and earth.

Ida From the Old English, *ead*, 'protection', and *id*, 'possession'; alternatively, from the Old Norse, *idh*, 'to labour', or from *itis*, 'woman'. In Norse mythology, Idhuna was a goddess of spring and guardian of the magical youth-giving apples of the gods. Idane was a successful Norman import, revived in the last century first with Tennyson's poem *The Princess* (1847) and then with its adaptation for opera by Gilbert and Sullivan, *Princess Ida* (1880). The compounds include **Idalee, Idalou** and **Idana**. **Variants, some of which are also given to boys:** Edonia, Edony, Idalia, Idalina, Idaline, Idande, Idane, Iddes, Idel, Idelle, Idena, Ideny, Idette, Idhuna, Idina, Idona, Idonea, Idonia, Idony, Ita, Ydonea.

Idra From the Aramaic, 'fig-tree, flag'. The fig-tree was the Hebrew symbol of a scholar.

Idris Welsh, meaning fiery lord. In Irish legend, Idris the Giant was an astronomer and magician; the mountain, Cader Idris, was believed to have been his observatory.

Ignatia Female form of Ignatius. **Variant:** Ignacia.

Ilka Scottish, from the Middle English, *ilke*, 'of that same standing'.

Ilona Hungarian, meaning 'beautiful'. **Variant:** Ilonka.

Imogen From the Latin, *imago*, 'image, likeness, imitation'. A more fanciful theory is that when the manuscript of Shakespeare's play *Cymbeline* (1610) was copied, the romantic character Innogen was mis-read. **Variants:** Emogene, Imagina, Immy, Imogene, Imogine, Imojean.

India A popular girls' name that reflects British ideas about the romance of this continent.

Inge From the Old Norse, *eng*, 'meadow'; also from the Old English, *ling*, 'to extend, belong to, be descended from'. In Norse mythology, Ing was god of fertility and peace; Ingrid means 'Inge's ride' and refers to the golden-bristled boar he rode. **Variants:** Inga, Ingaberg, Inger, Ingerith, Ingrede, Ingrid, Ingunna, Inky. *See also* Ingram.

Iola From the Greek, *ion*, 'dawn cloud, violet colour'. **Variants:** Iole, Ione.

Iona A small island of the Inner Hebrides, rich in Celtic remains. It was the burial place for countless rulers of Scotland, Ireland, Norway and Denmark, and was where St Columba founded his monastery in 563. **Variants:** Ione, Ionia.

Iora From the Latin, *aurum*, 'gold'.

Iphigenia In Greek mythology, the daughter of Agamemnon who was sacrificed to Artemis before the Greek fleet sailed to wage war on Troy.

Irene From the Greek, *eirene*, 'peace'. In Greek mythology, goddess of peace. Although well-used in literature, it became popular only at the end of the last century. **Variants:** Eirene, Erena, Ira, Irena, Irenee, Irenka, Irina, Rena, Rene, Renette, Renie, Renny, Rina.

Iris From the Greek, *iris*, 'rainbow' and 'iris of the eye'. In Greek mythology, goddess of the rainbow and a messenger of the gods, crossing between them and mortals on a multi-coloured bridge. In botany, the genus with sword-shaped leaves and many-coloured blooms. **Variants:** Irisa, Irita, Iryl, Irys.

Irma From the Old High German, Irmin, another name for Tiu, god of war. **Variants:** Erma, Irmina, Irmintrude.

Isabel *See* Elizabeth. This was the popular variant in Spain, France and Scotland of the Middle Ages. It reached Britain in the 12th century, when royal bearers of it included the wives of the three kings, John, Edward II and Richard II. **Variants:** Bel, Belia, Belicia, Belita, Bell, Bela, Bella, Ezabel, Ib, Ibbot, Ibby, Isa, Isabeau, Isabele, Isabella, Isabelle, Isbel, Isobel, Isopel, Issabell, Issie, Issy, Izabel, Nib, Tibbi, Tibbie, Tibbs, Tibby.

Isadora From the Greek, *Isis* and *doron*, 'gift of Isis'. In Egyptian mythology, Isis was goddess of the moon and of fertility, later identified with Aphrodite by the Greeks. **Variants:** Isadore, Isidora, Isidore, Izzy.

Ismenia Possibly an Irish form of Ismay (see Amy) or Jesmond (see Jasmin). Used from the Middle Ages until the 18th century, then rare. **Variants:** Emmanaia, Ismania, Ismena.

Isolde From the Old High German, 'to rule', or from the Celtic, 'fair maiden'. In Celtic and German legend, Princess Iseult (or Isolde) married Mark, King of Cornwall, but loved his nephew, Tristam. In some versions Tristam returns her love and they eventually marry; in others, they never unite. As with other names from German legends, it was Wagner who revived it in the last century, in his opera *Tristan und Isolde* (1865). **Variants:** Isaut, Iseult, Iseut, Isola, Isolda, Isolt, Yseult.

Ivy From the Middle English, *ivye*, the clinging vines with evergreen leaves and black, berry-like fruits, symbolising faithfulness. With other flower names, in vogue at the turn of the century.

J

Jacqueline French female form of Jacques, from Jacob. Brought to England by the sister-in-law of Henry V (1387–1422), Jacqueline of Hainault (in Belgium), who was known as Jack. **Variants:** Jacket, Jackelyn, Jackey, Jacki, Jackie, Jacklyn, Jaclyn, Jacoba, Jacobina, Jacquelyn, Jacquelynne, Jacquenetta, Jacquenette, Jacquetta, Jacquette, Jacqui, Jacquie, Jakolina, Jaqualine, Jaquetta, Jaquith.

Jade From the French, the name both for nephrite, a hard translucent gemstone of light green or blue colour, and the similar stone, jadite. Also from the Middle English, 'inferior or worn-out horse' – hence the term 'jaded' for worn-out. Jade has been increasingly popular since musician Mick Jagger gave this name to one of his daughters.

Jael From the Hebrew, 'mountain goat' and 'to go up, ascend'. Popular with the Puritans.

Jaffa From the Hebrew, *yafeh*, 'beautiful, attractive'. Also the name of a city founded by the Phoenicians, taken by the Israelites in the 6th century BC and now part of Tel Aviv. The juicy oranges were originally grown near there. **Variants:** Jafit, Yaffa, Yafit.

Jaime Female form of James. **Variants:** Jaimee, James, Jamesena, Jamesina, Jamie, Jymie.

Jamila From the Arabic, *jamilah*, 'beautiful, lovely'. Jamil is the male form.

Jane Female form of John. Jane and its variants probably derive from the Old French name, Jehane. The widespread use of Joan in the Middle Ages was supplanted in the Tudor period by Jane which has remained in vogue ever since, its popularity generating quantities of compounds and variants. Jane Frances de Chantal founded The Order of the Visitation for single women and widows in 1610 at Annecy. *See also* Hannah, Janet, Jean and Joan. The many compounds include Mary Jane and Sarah Jane. **Variants:** Giovanna, Hanne, Janee, Janel, Janella, Janelle, Janerette,

Janet, Janette, Janey, Jani, Jania, Janice, Janie, Janina, Janine, Janis, Janita, Janith, Janka, Jantina, Jasisa, Jatney, Jayne, Jaynie, Jean, Jehane, Jene, Jenine, Jennie, Jenny, Jessie, Joan, Joanna, Johanna, Jovanna, Juana, Juanita, Sheena, Shena, Sine, Vania, Zaneta.

Janet Scottish form of Jane, derived from the French variant, Jeannette. **Variants:** Jan, Janella, Janelle, Janeta, Janete, Janetta, Janette, Janot, Jenetta, Jennit, Jessie, Netta, Nettie. *See also* Jessie.

Japonica From the New Latin, *japonia*, 'Japan'. A climbing plant from Japan that bears quince fruits and bright red flowers; part of the Camellia family.

Jarita Sanskrit name meaning 'bird'.

Jardena From the Hebrew, *yarod*, 'to flow downward, descend'. The male form, Jordan, is the name of the river bank that flows from Syria down to the Dead Sea.

Jasmin From the Persian and Arabic, *yasmin*, 'an olive flower'. In botany, the genus of shrubs from Asia bearing tiny fragrant flowers, white, yellow or red. Their scents are used for perfumes and teas. **Variants:** Jasmina, Jasmine, Jesmond, Jess, Jessamine, Jessamy, Jessie, Yasmin, Yasmina, Yasmine.

Jean This and Janet are the Scottish form of Jane, derived from the French variant, Jehane. The most renowned Jeanne was Madame de Pompadour (1721–64), the influential and beautiful mistress of Louis XV and patron of the arts. Her full name was Jeanne Antoinette Poisson ('fish'), Marquise de Pompadour. The compounds include Jenalyn. **Variants:** Gene, Genie, Genna, Gianina, Giovanna, Jeane, Jeanette, Jeani, Jeanice, Jeanie, Jeanine, Jeanne, Jeannette, Jeannine, Jen, Jenat, Jenda, Jenica, Jenni, Jennie, Jenny, Jinny, Netta, Nettie, Netty.

Jemima From the Arabic, *jonina*, 'dove'. Its peak of popularity was in the last century. Also associated with Jemina, the female form of Benjamin. **Variants:** Jem, Jemimah, Jemma, Jona, Jonati, Jonina, Jonit, Mima, Yonina, Yemima.

Jennifer English form of the Welsh name, Guinevere, which later became Winifred. Its use spread out from Cornwall only in this century. Compounds include **Jennelle** and **Jennilee**. **Variants:** Ganor, Gaynor, Ginevra, Guenevere, Guinevere, Gwinny, Gwyneth, Jen, Jenefer, Jenifer, Jennie, Jennifer, Jenny, Jinny, Vanora.

Jerusha From the Hebrew, 'inheritance'. Much favoured by 17th-century Puritans.

Jessie From the Hebrew, *yishai*, 'riches, a gift'. In the Bible, Jesse was the father of David (1 Samuel) and the Tree of Jesse is the genealogy of Christ traced back to this ancestor. However, the use of the female form in Scotland is as a variant of Janet. **Variants:** Jesse, Jessica. *See also* Jasmine.

Jesusa Spanish, contracted from 'Maria de Jesus'. *See also* Dolores.

Jethra Female form of Jethro.

Jetta From the Greek, *gagates*, 'stone of Gagai' (a town in Lycia), via the Old French, *jaiet*. A hard, deep black gemstone that can be highly polished. **Variant:** *Jet*.

Jewel Possibly originally from the French, *jeu*, 'game, jest', but now implying something or someone of great preciousness. **Variant:** Jewell.

Jezebel From the Hebrew, 'impure, not respected'. In the Bible, wife of King Ahab.

Jill A variant form of Gillian; *see* Julia. **Variant:** Jilly.

ANDY PANDY AND LOUBY LOU

W̶ith the common desire to find a nickname for every name, new ones have had to be found for the most popular names. Rhyming nicknames were natural solutions, offering countless new possibilities. Richard went beyond Rich and Rick to Dick and Hick. Robert moved on from Rob to Bob and Margaret from Molly to Polly. There is an especially intimate and friendly ring about two rhyming names, both ending in 'y'. When J. M. Barrie's young friend Margaret called him her 'fwend', or perhaps 'fwendy Wendy', he invented the name Wendy for her as the heroine of his Peter Pan stories. And her name lives on today in children's playhouses – Wendy houses.

Joan Both this and Joanna are from the French variants of Jane, Johan and Jhone, which are both contractions of Johanna. Jhone, daughter of Henry II (1133–89), brought one of the carliest forms of Jane to Britain – hence the English translation of Jeanne d'Arc as Joan. Joan of Arc (1412–31), 'Maid of Orleans', was a patriotic peasant from Champagne who as a teenager fought in the army to save France from the English. She was captured, tried for witchcraft and heresy, and burned in Rouen market-place. Joan was supplanted by Jane in Tudor times, and by Joanna during the Reformation; both these forms are used regularly now. Siobhan is the favourite Irish form. *See also* Hannah and Jane. The compounds include Jo-Anne. **Variants:** Giovanna, Giovannina, Hanne, Ione, Ivanna, Jane, Janis, Janna, Jean, Jehane, Jenise, Joann, Joanna, Joanne, Joeann, Johan, Johanna, Johanne, Johna, Johnna, Johnnie, Jonet, Joni, Jonie, Jonnie, Jovana, Jovanna, Juan, Juana, Juanita, Nita, Siobhan, Zaneta.

Jobina Female form of Job. **Variants:** Jobey, Jobie, Joby.

Jocelin From the Old German, *gauzelen*, 'descendant of the Goths'; from the Celtic, *josse*, 'champion'; or the German female form of Jacob. Introduced as a male name by the Normans, as Jocelin and Josse, and used for girls only since the end of the last century. **Variants:** Jacoba, Jacobina, Joceline, Jocelyn, Jocelynd, Jocelyne, Joscelin, Joscelind, Josceline, Joscelyn, Josette, Josie, Joslyn. *See also* Joyce.

Jody Hebrew name meaning 'a woman from Judea'. **Alternatives include** Jodene, Jodette, Jodi, Jodia.

Joel From the Hebrew, 'God is willing'. In the Bible, one of the twelve minor prophets. Also given to boys. **Variants:** Joela, Joella, Joelle.

Jolene *See* Jolie. The name Jolene has been popularised by Dolly Parton's successful song of this title.

Jolie French, from the Middle English, *joli*, 'high spirited'. **Variants:** Jolene, Joletta, Joliet, Jolly.

Jora From the Hebrew, 'autumn rain'; also the astrological name for a child born under the zodiac sign of Scorpio. **Variant:** Jorah.

Josephine French female form of Joseph. Popular for Catholic girls ever since the pope created the festival of St Joseph on March 19 in 1621. Further boosted by Napoleon's first wife, the able Empress Josephine (1763–1814), whose full name was Marie Josephe Rose. She continued to advise Napoleon on state matters after he had repudiated their marriage because she was barren. **Variants:** Fife, Fifine, Jo, Jodi, Jodie, Joe, Josepha, Josephina, Josette, Josie, Pepita, Peppy, Pheeny, Yoseb, Yosepha, Yosifa.

Jovita From the Latin, *jovis*, 'jovial' or 'born under the influence of Jupiter'. In Roman mythology, Jove was a name for Jupiter, the supreme god, the counterpart for the Greek god, Zeus. The planet named after him is the largest in the solar system and was believed to be the source of all happiness.

Joy From the Latin, *jocosa*, 'merry'. Found in medieval Britain, then revived first by the Puritans and then the Victorians. **Variants:** Joia, Joya, Joye.

Joyce From Joisse, the French popular form of the Latin name, Jocosa, 'merry'. Made famous throughout the Low Countries and northern France by a 7th-century saint who was a Breton prince turned hermit. The Breton popular form was Josse (see Jocelin). In vogue until the 15th century, revived at the end of the 19th. Also given to boys. **Variants:** Jocea, Jocey, Jocosa, Joice, Jolia, Jooss, Jossy.

Jubilee *See* Yovela.

Judith From the Hebrew, 'praise'. In the Bible, Esau's wife. The male form, Judah, was the name of one of Jacob and Leah's sons. The courage of Judith of Bethulia, who saved her countrymen by slaying the enemy general, Holofernes, was recounted in the Apocrypha and already a popular story in medieval times. Shakespeare named his daughters Judith and Susanna. **Variants:** Eudice, Jodette, Jodi, Jodie, Jody, Judi, Judie, Judy, Yehudit, Yudit, Yuta. See also Garland under boys.

Julia Female form of Julius. The forms Julian and Gillian, with countless nicknames, were very widespread in Britain from the 12th to the 15th centuries – hence the nursery rhyme, 'Jack and Jill'. Juliet is from the Italian form, Giulietta, given its English form and made lastingly famous by Shakespeare in his play, *Romeo and Juliet* (1595), the tragic romance of a young couple from Verona (see Romeo). Gillian became so popular in the 17th century that it was debased to mean 'wench, flirt' and a Gill-flirt was a 'giddy young girl'. The compounds include **Julieanne** and **Julinda**. **Variants:** Gill, Gillian, Gillot, Giula, Giulia, Giulietta, Jill, Juet, Juetta, Jule, Jules, Julian, Juliana, Julie, Julienne, Juliet, Juliette, Julitta, Julka, Julyan, Sheila, Utili.

June From the Latin, Junius, which derives from *juvenior*, 'young'. In Roman mythology, the goddess who united with a fabulous flower to produce her son, Mars. The sixth month of the year was named after the Roman family, Junius. **Variant:** Unella.

Justina Female form of Justine. **Variants:** Jussy, Justine.

 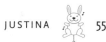

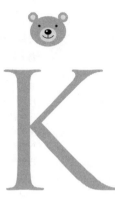

K

Kagami Japanese, meaning 'mirror', signifying the reflection of the parents' love.

Kaimana Hawaiian, meaning 'diamond'.

Kalila From the Arabic, 'beloved, sweetheart'.

Kalyca From the Greek, 'rosebud'. **Variants:** Kalica, Kalika, Kaly.

Kameko Japanese, meaning 'tortoise'. One of several Japanese symbols of longevity. *See also* Kiku and Koko.

Kanani Hawaiian, meaning 'a beauty'.

Kara In Norse mythology, the Valkyrie who took the form of a sweet-singing swan to follow her beloved warrior hero, Helgi, to war.

Karla Female form of Karl, from Charles. **Variants:** Karleen, Karlene. *See also* Caroline.

Karima Female form of Karim.

Karmiti Banti Eskimo, meaning 'trees'.

Karniela From the Hebrew, 'horn of the Lord'. **Variants:** Carniela, Carniella, Karna, Karnit, Karniella. *See also* Carna.

Kasimira Slavonic, meaning 'commands peace', implying someone whose presence encourages a peaceful atmosphere.

Kasota North American Indian, meaning 'clear sky'.

Katherine *See* Catherine.

Kay From the Greek, 'rejoice'.

Kaya Native American meaning 'older sister'.

Kedma From the Hebrew, *kedem*, 'towards the East'.

Keely From the Irish Gaelic, 'beautiful girl'.

Kefira From the Hebrew, 'young lioness'.

Kelda From the Old Norse, *kelda*, 'well, fountain, spring' and 'a still, deep area of river', meaning a source of life.

Kelila From the Hebrew, 'crown of laurel'; see Laurel. **Variants:** Kaile, Kayle, Kelula, Kyla, Kyle, Kylene, Lylia.

Kelly From the Greek, *keltoi*, referring to the ancient Celtic warriors of Western Europe, including the Bretons, Welsh and Irish. The American actress, Grace Kelly (1929–82), became a fairy-tale princes when she married Prince Rainier II of Monaco in 1956. **Variants:** Kaley, Keely, Kellee, Kelli, Kelton.

Kemba From the Old English, *cymaere*, 'Saxon lord'. **Variants:** Kem, Kemp, Kemps.

Kenna From the Old English, *cennan*, 'to make known, tell' and also 'to know how, to have ability'. **Variants:** Ken, Kendis, Kendra.

Keren From the Hebrew, 'animal horn'. **Variants:** Kaaren, Kareen, Karen, Karin, Karon, Karyn, Kyran.

Kerry From the Irish Gaelic, *ciarda*, 'dark one', and thus appropriate for a girl with a dark complexion. The name given to the southwest country of Ireland, renowned for its beautiful countryside of mountains and lakes. **Variants:** Ceri, Kerrie.

Keshet From the Hebrew, 'rainbow, bow'.

Keshisha From the Aramaic, 'an elder', implying wise and worthy of respect.

Ketifa From the Arabic, *gatafa*, 'to pluck a flower'.

Ketzia From the Hebrew, 'ground up, sweet-scented bark', such as cinnamon. **Variants:** Kerzia, Keziah, Kezzie, Kezzy.

Kichi Japanese, meaning 'fortunate'.

Kiku Japanese, meaning 'chrysanthemum'. A Japanese symbol of longevity. **Variants:** Kikuko, Kikuyo.

Kimi Japanese, meaning 'sovereign, the best'. **Variants:** Kimie, Kimiko, Kimiyo.

Kin From the Old English, *cyn*, 'related, of the family'. **Variants:** Kinchen, Kinsey, Kyn, Kyna.

Kineta From the Greek, *kinetikos*, 'active person'.

Kirsten From the Old English, *cirice*, 'church', which is derived from the Greek, *kuriakos*, 'of the Lord'. **Variants:** Kirby, Kireen, Kirstie, Kirsty.

Kismet From the Arabic, *quismah*, 'destiny, fate'.

Kitra Possibly from the Hebrew, *keter*, 'crown'.

Koko Japanese, meaning 'stork'. Like Kiku, a symbol of longevity.

Koren From the Greek, *kore*, 'maiden'. **Variants:** Cora, Corey, Corie, Kora, Kori, Korrie, Kory.

Korenet From the Hebrew, 'to shine out'.

Kylie Feminine version of Kyle, made internationally popular by Australian pop singer Kylie Minogue.

Kyna From the Irish Gaelic, 'wisdom, intelligence'.

Kyra Female form of Cyrus. **Variants:** Cyra, Kira.

Kyrene From the Greek, *kyrios*, 'lord'.

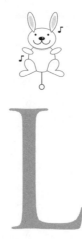

L

Laila From the Persian and Arabic, *laylah*, 'night' or 'dark-haired'. Byron popularised the Persian romance about Leila and Majnun through his poem, *The Giaour* (1813). **Variants:** Laili, Lailie, Laleh, Layla, Laylie, Leila, Lela, Lelah, Lelia, Leyla.

Lala Slavonic, meaning 'tulip flower'.

Lalita From the Sanskrit, 'honest, charming, straightforward'.

Lamorna From the Middle English, *morn*, 'morning', thus suitable for a girl born early in the day.

Lana From the Latin, *lanatus*, 'woolly, downy'. **Variants:** Lanette, Lanne, Lanny.

Lani Meaning 'heavenly'.

Lara In Roman mythology, the nymph daughter of the god of the river, Almo, whose tongue was cut out by Jupiter because she talked too much.

Larisa From the Latin, *lascivia*, 'playfulness, jollity', a word that also carried overtones of licentiousness and petulance. **Variants:** Lacey, Laris, Larissa, Lissa. *See also* Clare.

Lark From the Middle English, *larke*. Several species of the *Alaudidae* family of birds are larks, characterised by their sustained and melodious song.

Lass Scottish form of the Middle English, *lasce*, 'young girl, sweetheart'. **Variant:** Lassie.

Laulani Hawaiian, meaning 'heavenly branch', implying a precious, divine offspring.

Laurel From the Latin, *laurus*, 'laurel, bay tree'. Under the Greeks and Romans, a wreath of laurel symbolised victory, honour and achievement and was conferred upon the best soldiers, poets and athletes. Known in Britain by the 13th century. The beautiful Laura, who inspired the fine love-poems by the Italian Petrarch (1304–74), sustained its popularity through the Renaissance. **Variants:** Lara, Laraine, Lari, Larinda, Laura, Lauraine, Lauran, Laurane, Laure, Laureen, Laurel, Lauren, Laurena, Laurencia, Laurene, Laurentia, Laurestine, Lauretta, Laurette, Lauri, Laurice, Laurie, Laurinda, Lawrie, Lolly, Lora, Lorain, Loraine, Loral, Lorann, Lorayne, Loree, Loreen, Lorell, Loren, Lorena, Lorene, Lorenza, Loretah, Loretta, Lorette, Lori, Lorinda, Lorine, Lorita, Lorna, Lorraine, Lorri, Lorrie, Lorry, Loura, Lourana. *See also* Daphne.

Lauve From the Old English, *hlaf*, 'loaf', and *weard*, 'bread', thus 'keeper of the bread, lord of the manor'.

Lavender From the medieval Latin, *lavendulia*. In botany, the genus of aromatic plants whose clusters of tiny pale mauve flowers are dried or pressed for their fragrance.

Lavinia In Roman mythology, the wife of Aeneas. He was the ancestor of the Romans and son of Aphrodite and Anchises, and thus the link between mortals and gods. Through this, Lavinia came to mean 'woman of Rome'. In vogue during the Renaissance, revived to become a favourite in the 18th century. **Variants:** Lavena, Lavina, Lavinie, Vin, Vina, Vinia, Vinnie, Vinny.

Layla Meaning 'born at night'. This name has become increasingly well-known following Eric Clapton's successful song of this title.

Leah From the Hebrew, 'to be weary'. In the Bible, the first of Jacob's wives. Another favourite of the 17th-century Puritans. The compounds include **Leandra**. **Variants:** Lea, Lee, Leigh, Lia.

Leala From the Old French, *loiol* and *leial*, 'faithful to obligations, loyal'. **Variant:** Lela.

Leda In Greek mythology, the beautiful queen of Sparta. The god Zeus came to her disguised as a swan and fathered Helen and Pollux. The same night, Leda's husband fathered Castor and Clytemnestra. **Variants:** Lida, Lidia.

Lee From the Old English, *leah*, 'meadowland', or *hleo*, 'shelter, cover'. **Variants:** Leann, Leanna, Leigh.

Leeba From the Yiddish, 'beloved'. **Variants:** Liba, Luba.

Leilani Hawaiian, meaning 'heavenly flower'. **Variants:** Lei, Lelani.

Lena From the Hebrew, 'to dwell, sleep'. *See also* Eleanor, Helen and Magdalene. **Variants:** Leena, Lenea, Lenette, Lina.

Leoma From the Old English, 'light, brightness'.

Leona Female form of Leo. A name found in Britain since the 13th century. **Variants:** Leola, Leoma, Leonarda, Leone, Leonel, Leonia, Leonie, Leonina, Leonine, Leonora, Leontine, Leontyne, Leota. *See also* Fidel.

Leora From the Hebrew, 'light'. **Variant:** Liora. *See also* Eleanor.

Lera Female form of Leroy.

Lesley From the Scottish Gaelic, 'low-lying meadow'. The ancient Scottish family, Leslie, came from Leslie in Aberdeenshire and were ennobled in 1457. Its use as a first name began only in the last century. **Variants:** Lea, Lesli, Leslie, Lesly, Lezlie.

Letifa From the Arabic, *latif*, 'gentle'. As Allatif, one of the 99 names given to God in the Qur'an. Also given to boys. **Variants:** Letipha.

 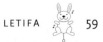

Letitia From the Latin, *laetitia*, 'unrestrained joy'. As Lettice, it was in England by the 12th century, and a favourite until the 18th, when it was replaced by Letitia. **Variants:** Laetitia, Lece, Lecelina, Lecia, Leta, Lethia, Letice, Leticia, Letisha, Letizia, Lettice, Lettie, Letty, Loutitia, Tish, Tisha, Titia.

Levanna From the Latin, *levana*, 'lifting up, rising sun'. In Roman mythology, the goddess Levana lifted up new-born babies from the ground. **Variants:** Levona, Livana, Livona.

Levia From the Hebrew, 'to join, be attendant upon'. In the Bible, the descendants of Jacob's third son, Levi, were priests and Levites serving in the temple in Jerusalem. **Variants:** Livia, Liviya.

Levina From the Middle English, *levene*, 'lightning'.

Lewanna From the Hebrew, *lebhanah*, 'the beaming white one, the moon'. In early Greek mythology, Lebanon was one of four giants who ruled the mountain ranges. As the mountains were known for their fragrant woods, the gods were thought to have invented incense.

Liana From the French, *lier*, 'to bind'. Used to describe high-climbing, light-seeking, tropical vines. **Variants:** Leana, Leanne, Lianna, Lianne.

Liberty From the Latin, *libertas*, 'freedom', meaning freedom of body, will and spirit.

Lilac From the Persian, *nil*, 'indigo, blue', via the Arabic, *lilak*. In botany, shrubs and trees cultivated for their delicate clusters of bluish-purple or white blooms. **Variants:** Lila, Lilah.

Lilian From the Latin, *lilium*, 'lily'. In botany, the genus of some 80 species whose flowers are often large, boldly-coloured and trumpet-shaped. The flower is a symbol of purity in Christian art. The compounds include Lilybeth; *see also* Elizabeth. **Variants:** Lil, Lili, Lilia, Liliane, Lilias, Lilibet, Lilion, Lilli, Lillian, Lillie, Lillis, Lilly, Lily, Lilyan.

Lilith From the East Semitic, 'belonging to the night'. In Assyro-Babylonian mythology, a female demon who haunts the wilderness on stormy nights and is especially dangerous to children. **Variants:** Lilis, Lilita, Lillith, Lillus.

Lilo Hawaiian, meaning 'generous'.

Linda *See* Belinda and Rosalind. As an independent name, Linda emerged at the end of the nineteenth century and reached its height of popularity during the 1950s.

Linden From the Old English, *lind*, 'lithe, pliable, flexible'. The wood of the linden, or lime, tree was very suitable for shields, so the name implies a shield of protection. **Variants:** Linde, Lindi, Lindy.

Lindsey From the Old English, 'waterside linden trees', implying a place suitable for pitching camp. Like Lesley, Lindsey is an old Scottish family name, that of the Earls of Crawford. Also given to boys. **Variant:** Lindsay. *See also* Linden.

Linnea The small blue national flower of Sweden, named after the Swedish botanist, Carolus Linnaeus (1707–78), who created the system of classification of plants and animals. **Variant:** Lynnea.

Linnett From the Latin, *linum*, 'flax'. The name of a small, pink-breasted songbird whose favourite food is linseed. Alternatively, a medieval French form of the Welsh name, Eiluned. In Arthurian legend, Gareth was in love with Lynette, a romance popularised by

Tennyson's poem, *The Idylls of the King* (1859); see also Lynn and Arthur. **Variants:** Eiluned, Lanette, Linet, Linnet, Linnette, Luned, Lynette, Lynnet, Lynnette.

Lioba The English saint led 30 nuns to help St Boniface with his missionary work in Germany. They became well-loved and known for their domesticity, hard work and intelligence. In addition, Abbess Lioba was beautiful, generous and always calm. See also Leo. **Variant:** Leona.

Lirit From the Greek, *lurikos*, 'like a lyre', meaning the smooth clear rhythms of music and poetry. *See also* Lyris.

Liron From the Hebrew, 'song is mine', implying great happiness. Also given to boys. **Variant:** Lirone.

Lodemai From the Old English, *ladman*, 'pilot, guide'. **Variant:** Lodema.

Lois From the Greek, 'good, desirable'. Probably first used in Britain by the Puritans who sought out unusual Biblical names.

Lolita See Caroline, Charlotte and Dolores. **Variants:** Lita, Lola, Loleta, Lurchel, Lurleen, Lurline.

Lora From the Latin, 'a thin wine made from the husks of grapes'. **Variants:** Laraine, Loraine, Lorraine.

Lorelei From the German, 'song, melody'. In German legend, Lorelei was the cliff on the River Rhine from which a siren mysteriously sounded to lure sailors on to the rocks. **Variants:** Lorelie, Lorilee, Lura, Lurette, Lurleen, Lurlene, Lurline.

Lorice From the Latin, *lorum*, 'thong, slender vine branch'. In Roman mythology, Venus' girdle. **Variant:** Loris. *See also* Chloris.

Loris From the Dutch, *loeres*, 'clown'.

Lorna A name made up by R. D. Blackmore for the romantic heroine of his novel, *Lorna Doone* (1869), a bestseller when it was published. The name has been popular ever since. **Variant:** Lona.

Lotus From the Greek, *lotos*, the fruit eaten by an imaginary North African tribe described in Homer's *Odyssey* (8th century BC). The fruit made them perpetually drugged and indolent, hence the term 'lotus-eater' for someone who avoids work in favour of self-indulgent pleasure. The name was given to a real aquatic plant native to Africa and Asia, with large circular leaves and delicate, fragrant blooms. It often carried sacred symbolism for the local religion: in China, the name Lien (lotus) symbolises the past, present and future. *See also* Padma and Sadira.

Louise French female form of Louis. The intelligent and sympathetic St Louise de Marillac (1591–1660) co-founded with St Vincent de Paul the Daughters of Charity who look after the sick poor. A favourite name in Europe in the 17th and 18th centuries. It won the royal stamp of approval in Britain when Charles II (1630–85) created his favourite, Louise de Kérouaille, Duchess of Portsmouth. The American novelist, Louisa May Alcott (1832–88), based *Little Women* (1868) on her own family and childhood. Today, Louise is one of the most popular names. The compounds include **Loudella, Loudonna, Louella** and **Ludella. Variants:** Alison, Allison, Aloise, Aloisia, Alouise, Aloys, Aloyse, Aloysia, Eloisa, Eloise, Heloise, Lewes, Lisette, Lois, Loise, Lola, Lolita, Lou, Louie, Louisa, Louisette, Lova, Loyce, Lu, Luisa, Luise, Luiza, Lula, Lulita, Lulu. *See also* Abelard.

 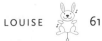

Lourdes The site of a Catholic shrine in southern France, this name has become popularised after singer and actress Madonna chose it for her daughter.

Loveday Originally a name for babies born on a 'loveday', a day reserved especially for settling disputes. Given to boys and girls in the 13th century, but now only to girls. **Variants:** Lovdie, Lowdy, Luveday.

Lucania From the Latin, 'fish, pike'; also an ancient district in southern Italy.

Lucia From the Latin, *lucere*, 'to shine, glitter, be light'. Often given to girls born at daybreak. The 4th-century Sicilian martyr, St Lucy, was a cult in the Middle Ages, spreading the name through Europe. Since her eyes were apparently plucked out, she is patron saint of people with eye diseases. The forms Lucy and Luce gave way to Lucia in the 17th century. **Variants:** Cindy, Lleulu, Lu, Luce, Lucette, Luci, Luciana, Lucie, Lucienne, Lucile, Lucilla, Lucille, Lucina, Lucinda, Lucine, Lucita, Lucky, Lucy, Luz, Luzia, Luzine.

Lucretia In Roman history, the woman who committed suicide after being raped by Tarquinius, sparking off the instant expulsion of the Tarquins from Rome. This episode made the name synonymous with purity and Chastity. **Variants:** Lucrece, Lucrecia, Lucretzia.

Ludella From the Old English, *hludaelf*, 'renowned and clever elf'.

Ludmilla Slavonic, meaning 'beloved by the people'. **Variants:** Ludie, Ludovika.

Lulie From the Middle English, *lullen*, 'to soothe, cause to sleep, dispel fears'.

Luna From the Latin, *luna*, 'moon'. **Variant:** Lunette.

Lupita From the Latin, *lupus*, 'wolf', thus 'a little wolf'. In Roman mythology, the fertility god, Lupercus, was celebrated with an annual fertility festival in Rome. **Variant:** Lupe.

Lydia From the Greek, 'a woman from Lydia'. In the 6th century BC, the kingdom of Lydia covered most of Asia Minor and was ruled by the fabulously rich Croesus. His people were expert merchants and musicians, and possibly invented coinage. **Variants:** Lidia, Lyda, Lydda, Lydie. *See also* Cyrus.

Lynn From the Old English, *hlynna*, 'brook'. Also given to boys. **Variants:** Lin, Linn, Linne, Linnet, Linnette, Lynell, Lynelle, Lynette, Lynne.

Lyris From the Greek, *lura*, 'lyre'. In classical Greece, this harp-like stringed instrument was used to accompany singing and poetry reading.

Lysandra From the Greek, *lysis*, 'free'. Female form of Lysander, an able Spartan general and statesman who lived in the 5th century BC, whose obsession with personal aggrandisement made him thoroughly disliked. *See also* Alexandra.

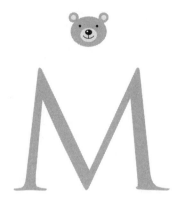

M

Mabel From the Latin, *amabilis*, 'worthy of love'. The name was first used as Amabel and Amabella. Mabel, the shortened form, became a Victorian favourite. Queen Mab is the fairy who delivers dreams to sleeping men. **Variants:** Amabel, Amabella, Mab, Mabb, Mabbit, Mabbot, Mabbs, Mabell, Mabella, Mabelle, Mabilia, Mabilla, Mable, Mably, Mapp, Mapps, Mappin.

Madra Spanish, from the Latin, 'mother'. **Variant:** Madre.

Mae Diminutive form of Margaret made popular following American actress Mae West.

Magdalene From the Hebrew, *miqdal*, 'high tower'. Magdala was the name of a town on the Sea of Galilee in Palestine, hence 'woman from Magdala'. In the Bible, St Mary Magdalene is thought to be both the disciple of Christ (Luke 7) and the harlot who earned forgiveness by washing Christ's feet with her tears (Luke 7). She is patroness of penitents.

The word 'maudlin', meaning tearful, derives from her. **Variants:** Dalenna, Leli, Lena, Lenna, Lina, Lynn, Mada, Madalena, Madeline, Madalynne, Maddalena, Maddie, Maddy, Madeena, Madel, Madelaine, Madeleine, Madelia, Madeline, Madella, Madelle, Madelon, Madelyn, Madge, Madlen, Madli, Madlin, Mady, Mag, Magda, Magdala, Magdalen, Magdalena, Magdaline, Magli, Mai, Mali, Malin, Manda, Marla, Marleen, Marlena, Marlene, Marlie, Marlo, Marlowe, Marlys, Maudlin, Migdana.

Magna Female form of Magnus.

Magnolia In botany, a genus of trees cultivated for their large, pale pink blossoms, named after the French botanist, Pierre Magnol.

Mahala Possibly from the Hebrew, 'barren'; also a Biblical name. Found in Britain occasionally since the 17th century. **Variants:** Mahalah, Mahalia, Mehalia.

Mahina Hawaiian, meaning 'moon'.

Mahira From the Hebrew, 'speed, energy'. From this comes the Arabic word, *mahr*, 'young arab horse'. **Variant:** Mehira.

Mahola From the Hebrew, *mahol*, 'dance'.

Mai A popular Swedish name that derives from the names Margaret and Mary.

Maia In Greek mythology, the fair-haired daughter of Atlas who gave Zeus his favourite illegitimate son, Hermes. In Roman mythology, the incarnation of the Earth Mother to whom Romans offered sacrifice on May Day (May 1). **Variant:** Maya.

Maida From the Old English, *maegden*, 'maiden', meaning a young unmarried girl. *See also* Mary. **Variants:** Maddie, Maddy, Maidel, Maidie, Maidey.

Mairead Irish, from the Old French, *maire*, 'magistrate, judge'.

Mairin Irish form of Mary.

Maisie From the French, *mais*, 'maize'. *See also* Margaret. **Variants:** Maise, Mysie.

Majesta From the Latin, *majestas*, 'greatness, grandeur, dignity'.

Makala Hawaiian, meaning 'myrtle'.

Makani Hawaiian, meaning 'wind'. Also given to boys.

Mala From the French, *mal*, 'ill, wrong, bad'.

Malka From the Arabic, *malaka*, 'queen'. **Variant:** Malkah.

Malvina Another name invented by a poet, this one by James Macpherson (1736–96) as an English form of *maol-mhin*, 'smooth brow'.

Malu Hawaiian, meaning 'peace'. An extended form is **Malulani**, 'beneath peaceful skies'.

Mamie From the French, *m'aimee*, 'my sweetheart'. *See also* Margaret and Mary.

Mangena From the Hebrew, 'song, melody'. **Variant:** Mangina.

Manuela Spanish female form of Emanuel. **Variant:** Emanuella.

Mara From the Hebrew, 'bitter'. Found occasionally since the 17th century. **Variant:** Marah. *See also* Mary, Miriam and Naomi.

Marcella Female form of the prominent Roman family, Marcellus, whose name is derived from Marcus. A widow of the family became a disciple of St Jerome. Found in Britain since the 17th century. The compounds include **Malinda, Marcelinda** and **Melinda. Variants:** Marcela, Marcelle, Marcellina, Marcelline, Marcelyn, Marcha, Marcia, Marcie, Marcile, Marcilen, Marcille, Marcy, Marisella, Marsha, Marshe, Marquita.

Mardell From the Old English, 'meadow near the sea'.

Margaret From the Greek, *margarites*, 'pearl', carrying with it the ancient Persian meaning, 'child of light'. The Persians believed that oysters rose to the water's surface at night to worship the moon and to collect a drop of dew which the moonbeams changed into a pearl. A highly royal and Christian name, which has maintained its popularity, except during the Reformation. The royals include Margaret of Scotland (1045–93), both queen and saint; the 'Maid of Norway' who was Queen of Scotland (1286–90); Margaret of Anjou (1430–82), wife of Henry VI; Margaret Tudor (1489–1541), daughter of Henry VII and wife of James IV of Scotland; Margaret of Valois (1553–1615), daughter of Henry II of France and wife of Henry IV of

France; and the present Queen's sister, Princess Margaret Rose (born 1930), Countess of Snowdon. The saints include the possibly fictitious 3rd-century virgin martyr of Antioch who was a big cult during the Middle Ages. She is patroness of women in childbirth. The compounds include **Margebelle, Marleah**. **The many variants include:** Daisy, Gita, Ghita, Gogo, Greta, Gretal, Gretchen, Gretel, Gretle, Gritty, Madge, Mady, Mae, Maergrethe, Mag, Magge, Maggie, Mago, Maidie, Maiga, Maisie, Mamie, Margalit, Margalith, Margareta, Margarete, Margaretha, Margarethe, Margaretta, Margarette, Margarinda, Margarita, Margat, Marge, Margene, Margerie, Margery, Marget, Marghanita, Margherita, Margiad, Margita, Margo, Margot, Marguerita, Marguerite, Margy, Marjarie, Marjary, Marje, Marjie, Marjorie, Marjory, Marles, Meg, Megan, Mergret, Meta, Midge, Mittie, Mog, Moggy, Molly, Mysie, Peg, Peggy, Polly, Reatha, Reta, Rita. *See also* Daisy and Pearl.

Marigold From the Middle English, *mary-gould*, 'Mary's gold'. In botany, all the species of the genus *Tagetes*, originally from tropical America but now cultivated in Britain for their bright and long-lasting orange and yellow blooms. **Variant:** Marygold.

Marilyn Derived from Mary, meaning 'Mary's line, descendants of Mary'. The actress, Marilyn Monroe (1926 – 62), whose real name was Norma Jean Mortensen, starred in a string of light comedies including *Gentlemen Prefer Blondes* (1953) and *Some Like It Hot* (1959). **Variants:** Maralyn, Marilee, Marilin, Marilynn, Maryln, Marylin, Maryline, Merili.

Marina From the Latin, *marinus*, 'belonging to the sea, produced by the sea'. **Variants:** Mare, Maren, Marena, Maris, Marisa, Marisella, Marissa, Marna, Marne, Marni, Marnina, Marys, Meris, Rina.

Marini Swahili, meaning 'healthy, fresh, pretty'.

Marion A popular folkore figure found in May Day games, morris dancing and, as Maid Marion, the companion of Robin Hood. As Marionette, the name is given to a stringed puppet. *See* Mary.

Marnina From the Hebrew, 'rejoice'. *See also* Marina.

Marquita From the French, *marquise*, 'canopy', used to protect and denote an official. **Variant:** Marquite.

Martha Female form of the Aramaic, *mar*, 'lord'. In the Bible, the sister of Lazarus and Mary and friend of Jesus, who complained to him of her household chores (Luke 10). She is patroness of housewives. Found in Britain since the 18th century. **Variants:** Mardeth, Mardi, Marta, Martelle, Marthe, Marthena, Marti, Martie, Martita, Matty, Merta, Patty.

Martina Female form of Martin. **Variants:** Martella, Martine.

Marva From the Hebrew, 'sage', the sweet-scented, edible herb with healing medicinal properties.

Marvel From the Latin, *mirus*, 'full of wonder', via the Middle English, *marveile*. Thus, a girl who stimulates wonder, astonishment and admiration. **Variant:** Marvella.

Mary English form of the Hebrew name, Miriam, meaning either 'sea of bitterness' or 'child of our wishes'. Carried to Britain by the Crusaders, through the Greek names, Mariam and Mariamne. Mary is first recorded in the Bible, as Miriam, sister of Moses and

Aaron. But the name's popularity comes from the Virgin Mary, mother of Jesus, who inspired an elaborate cult. Sometimes her name was felt to be too sacred to be used directly; see Dolores. But despite this, Mary became the most consistently popular name in Europe, except during the Reformation. A quarter of all Irish girls are baptised Mary today. It has numerous regal associations, too: Mary I (1516–68); Mary II (1662–94); Mary, Queen of Scots (1542–87); Maria Theresa (1717–1780), Queen of Bohemia and Hungary; and her daughter, Marie Antoinette (1755–1793), wife of Louis XVI of France (see Antoinette). Maria is the Latin, French, Italian and Spanish form; Marie the French and Old German; Mair the Welsh; Mairin, Maureen and Moira are all Irish. *See also* Magdalene. The compounds include Maralou, Mariabella, Mariamme, Marian, Mariane, Marianne, Maribel, Maribeth, Marijon, Marijune, Marilee, Marilu, Mariwin, Maryalice, Maryanne, Marybeth, Marylois, Marylou. **The many variants include:** Mae, Maie, Mair, Maire, Mairin, Malia, Mamie, Manette, Manon, Manya, Mara, Maree, Mareea, Mari, Maria, Mariah, Mariam, Mariamne, Marian, Marice, Marie, Mariel, Mariele, Mariene, Mariesa, Mariessa, Marietta, Mariette, Marika, Marion, Mariquilla, Mariquita, Marita, Marya, Masha, Maureen, Maura, Maurine, May, Miliama, Mim, Mimi, Min, Minnie, Mira, Miri, Miriam, Mirit, Mirjana, Mirra, Miryam, Mitzi, Mo, Moira, Moll, Mollie, Molly, Mollye, Morine, Moya, Muire, Polly.

Masada From the Hebrew, 'foundation', implying a strong, supportive character.

Matana From the Hebrew, 'gift'.

Mathilda From the Old High German, *macht*, 'power, strength', and *hiltia*, 'battle', thus 'strong battlemaid'. Introduced to Britain first by William the Conqueror's wife, then by his grand-daughter who was known as Maud. **Variants:** Matelda, Mathilde, Matilda, Matilldis, Matti, Mattie, Matty, Mattye, Matya, Maud, Maude, Maudene, Maudie, Mawde, Metilda, Mold, Patty, Tilda, Tillie, Tilly.

Maud *See* Mathilda.

Maura From the Celtic, 'dark'. Also, an Irish variant of Mary.

Mauve From the French, *mauve*, 'mallow-coloured', from the Latin, *malva*, 'mallow'. In botany, plants belonging to the genus *Malva* have pinkish-blue flowers. **Variant:** Maeve.

Mavis From the Old French, *mauvis*, 'song-thrush'. In use only since the end of the last century. **Variant:** Maeve.

Maxime Female form of Maximilian. **Variants:** Max, Maxi, Maxie, Maxima, Maxencia, Maxine, Maxy.

May From the Latin, *Maius*, 'month of Maia', via the Old French, *mai*. The pagan festivities on May Day celebrate the spring and thus fertility and birth. In botany, a nickname for the hawthorn tree which is coated with pink or white blossoms in May. The compounds include **Maybelle. Variants:** Mae, Mei. *See also* Louise and Maia.

Mazal From the Hebrew, 'star, luck'.

Meave Irish, from *meadhbh*, 'joy'.

Meira Female form of Meir.

Melanie From the Greek, *melas*, 'of black, or dark complexion'. In Greek mythology, Melanion won Atalanta's hand by beating her in a running race. This he did by a clever trick: one by one he dropped the three golden apples given to him by Aphrodite, which

Atalanta paused to pick up. The two 5th-century saints Melania were grand-mother and grand-daughter. Imported from France in the 17th century. **Variants:** Mel, Mela, Melania, Melantha, Melany, Melloney, Melly, Meloney, Milena.

Melody From the Greek, *melos*, 'tune', and *oidia*, 'singing', thus 'choral song', implying one that is pleasingly harmonic and rhythmic. **Variants:** Melina, Melodye, Medosa.

Melina From the Greek, *melos*, 'tune, song'.

Melissa From the Greek, *melissa*, 'bee', implying honey-sweetness. A favourite fairy name for 16th-century Italian poets, and carried to England in the 18th century. **Variants:** Lissa, Lisse, Malissa, Mel, Melesa, Melessa, Melisa, Melisande, Melise, Melisenda, Misha, Missie, Missy.

Melora A compound from the Greek, *melopepon*, 'apple-gourd, melon', and *ora*, 'gold', thus 'golden melon, golden apple'. **Variant:** Melon.

Melosa Spanish, meaning 'sweet as honey, gentle'.

Melvina Female form of Melvin. **Variants:** Malva, Malvinda, Melevine, Melveen, Melvene, Melvine.

Menora From the Hebrew, 'candelabrum'. **Variant:** Menorah.

Meraud A Cornish name, from *mur*, 'the sea'. In use since the 13th century.

Mercy From the Latin, *merces*, 'reward', which later came to imply pity, compassion. With Faith, Hope and Charity, one of the favourite 17th-century Puritan names. **Variants:** Mercedes, Mercia, Mercille.

Meredith See under boys. **Variants:** Bedo, Meridith, Merridie, Merry.

Meri From the Hebrew, 'rebellious'.

Merit From the Latin, *meritus*, 'earned, deserved'. **Variant:** Merritt.

Merle From the Latin, *merulus*, 'blackbird'. Also given to boys. **Variants:** Merla, Merlina, Merline, Merola, Merril, Merrill, Merryl, Meryl, Meryle, Morrell, Murle. *See also* Muriel.

Merlin *See under boys.*

Merrie From the Old English, *mirige*, 'pleasant, festive, jolly'. **Variants:** Marrilee, Merie, Merridee, Merrielle, Merrili, Merris, Merrita, Merry.

Metuka From the Hebrew, *matok*, 'sweet'.

Michaela Female form of Michael. **Variants:** Mia, Mica, Michael, Michal, Michel, Michele, Michelina, Micheline, Michelle, Micky, Miguella, Mikelina.

Miette From the French, 'small sweet thing'.

Migdana From the Hebrew, 'gift'.

Mignon From the Old French, *mignot*, 'delicate, petite'.

Mildred From the Old English, *milde*, 'mild', and *thryth*, 'power'. The 7th-century King Merowald of Mercia, on the Welsh borders, christened his three daughters Milburga, 'gentle defence', Mildgyth, 'gentle gift', and Mildthryth, and they all became saints. As with other medieval names, revived by the Victorians. **Variants:** Mil, Milda, Millie, Milly, Mindy.

Milena From the Old High German, *milo*, 'mild'.

Mili Israeli, meaning 'who is for me'. See also Melissa and Mildred.

Millicent From the German, 'strong worker, determined'. Carried to France as Melisande and Melusine, the name of a well-known fairy in French romance. Millicent was at its most popular at the turn of this century. **Variants:** Meli, Melita, Melleta, Millie, Milly.

Minerva In Roman mythology, goddess of wisdom, invention, the arts and martial strength, the counterpart of the Greek goddess, Athena.

Minna From the Old German, 'love'. **Variants:** Mina, Minda, Mindy, Minee, Minetta, Minette, Minnie, Minny.

Mirabel From the Latin, *mirabilis*, 'marvellous, extraordinary, strange, to be wondered at'. Another medieval name revived by the Victorians. **Variants:** Mirabell, Mirabella, Mirabelle, Mirella.

Miranda From the Latin, *mirandus*, 'astonished, amazed'. Possibly invented by Shakespeare for the heroine of his comedy, *The Tempest* (1611); akin to Mirabel. **Variants:** Marenda, Mira.

Miri English gypsy name, meaning 'mine'.

Miriam The Hebrew form of Mary. In the Bible, Miriam, sister of Moses, led the song and dance of triumph after the crossing of the Red Sea (Exodus 15). Found in Britain since the 17th century.

Misty From the Old English, *mistiq*, 'clouded, obscure'. When used to describe a person, it implies a clouded intellect.

Miyuki Japanese, meaning 'deep snow', a favourite Japanese name, implying peace and silence.

Moana Hawaiian, meaning 'ocean'.

Modesta From the Latin, *modestus*, 'moderate, kind, of gentle disposition'. **Variants:** Modeste, Modestia, Modestine.

Moina From the Celtic, 'gentle, soft'. **Variant:** Moyna.

Moira In Greek mythology, the Moerae, or Fates, overshadowed man's life and were personified as three goddesses: Clotho, spinning the thread of life; Lachesis, a man's fair share of luck in his life; and Atropos, inescapable fate. Also, a form of the Irish Maire, from Mary. **Variants:** Moirae, Moyra, Myra.

Molly *See* Margaret and Mary.

Momi Hawaiian, meaning 'pearl'.

Mona There are seven possible meanings – from the Greek, 'alone'; the Arabic, 'wish'; the Latin, 'advise'; the Old English, *mona*, 'month'; or from three different Irish words meaning 'nun', 'sweet angel' and 'noble'. The 4th-century saint was a model of patience towards her son, the Christian teacher Augustine of Hippo, who later described parenthood in glowing terms. Used in Britain since the end of the last century. **Variants:** Monica, Monique, Monna, Muna.

Montina From the Latin, *mons*, 'mountain'.

Morag From the Gaelic, *mora*, 'the sun'. *See also* Sarah.

Morasha From the Hebrew, 'inheritance'.

Moriah From the Hebrew, 'God is my teacher'. In the Bible, the mountain where Abraham prepared to sacrifice his son, Isaac. **Variants:** Mariah, Morel, Moria.

Morit From the Hebrew, 'teacher'.

DO-IT-YOURSELF NAMES

Every Juliet has Shakespeare to thank. Every Geraldine is a reminder of the disguised love poems written by the Earl of Surrey to the beautiful Lady Elizabeth Fitzgerald. And Percivals might try to live up to the 12th-century French romantic hero who was the first Percival. There is nothing new about making up names. It is easy and fun to do, and increasingly popular. Parents called David and Amanda could name their child Davanda. Two grandmothers' names could be honoured at once, so Janet and Anne might merge as Jananne or Annet. The parents' honeymoon might be remembered – Paris, Florence, or the more unusual Florida, Kashmir, Provence, Eire or Lanka (from Sri Lanka). There is certainly a pair of twins named Fortnum and Mason, and a girl in New York named Hollywood 'because I was made there'.

Morna From the Irish, *muirne*, 'beloved, affection'. **Variants:** Morrow, Myrna.

Morrisa Female form of Morris, from Maurice.

Morwenna Either from *morwaneg*, 'wave of the sea', or akin to the Irish Maureen, from Mary.

Moselle Female form of Moses. **Variant:** Mozelle.

Muriel From the Irish, *muir*, 'sea', and *geal*, 'bright'. Carried to southern England by William the Conqueror's Celts from Brittany. However, it was already well known in northern Britain. After medieval popularity, it was revived last century. **Variants:** Meriel, Merril, Merrill, Merryl, Meryl, Meryle, Miriel, Murial. *See also* Merle.

Musette From the Old French, *muser*, 'to meditate, be absorbed in thought'.

Myfanwy Welsh, meaning 'my treasure, my rare one'. The English form is Fanny. **Variants:** Fanny, Myvanwy.

Myra Probably invented by the poet, Fulke Greville (1554–1628), as a short form of Miranda or Mirabel. He addresses several love-poems to her.

Myrna From the Arabic and Aramaic, 'myrrh'. The strong-scented and highly valued gum-resin of commiphora trees used in preparing perfumes and incense. In the Bible, gold, frankincense ('luxurious incense') and myrrh were the gifts presented to Jesus by the three Magi; *see* Magus. **Variants:** Merna, Mirna.

Myrtle From the Greek, *myrtos*, 'myrtle'. In botany, the genus of shrubs with shiny evergreen leaves and sweet-scented white flowers used for perfumes. In Greek mythology, myrtle was sacred to Venus and therefore a symbol of love. **Variants:** Myrta, Myrtia, Myrtice, Myrtilla.

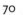

N

Naama From the Hebrew, 'beautiful, pleasant', and the Arabic, 'good fortune'. **Variants:** Naamana, Naamah, Naava, Nama, Nava, Navit.

Nabila From the Arabic, 'noble'. The female form of Nabil.

Nadia Slavonic and Russian, meaning 'hope'; or from the Spanish, 'nothing', derived from the Arabic word, *nazir al-samt*, 'opposite to zenith'. **Variants:** *Nada, Nadie, Nadine, Nadiya, Nado, Nady, Nadya, Natka.*

Nagida From the Hebrew, 'noble, aristocratic woman'.

Naia From the Greek, *naein*, 'to flow'. In Greek mythology, Naiads were the water nymphs who lived in brooks, just as Potamids were nymphs of rivers. They had the gift of prophecy, healed the sick, watched over flowers, fields and flocks and were generally benevolent. They were not immortal – their average life span was 9620 years – but as they lived on Ambrosia they remained young and beautiful throughout their lives. **Variants:** Naiad, Naida, Naiia, Nalda.

Nairne From the Scottish Gaelic, *amhuinn*, 'riverside lime-trees'. Nairn is an area in northeast Scotland. Also given to boys.

Nalani Hawaiian, meaning 'calmness of the skies or heavens'.

Nancy See Hannah and Agnes. The conservative politician, Nancy Astor (1879–1964) married for the second time the immensely rich Waldorf Astor. When he was created a peer in 1919, she stood for his old seat, Plymouth, and was elected the first-ever woman member of the House of Commons. She kept her seat for 26 years. **Variants:** Nan, Nana, Nance, Nancey, Nanci, Nannie, Nanny.

Naomi From the Hebrew, 'charming, delightful'. In the Bible, the mother-in-law of Ruth whose sufferings drove her to want to change her name to Mara, 'bitter' (Ruth 1). A favourite in the 17th century, when it was introduced by the Puritans. **Variants:** Naoma, Naome, Noami, Noemi, Nomi.

Napea From the Latin, *napaeus*, 'from a dell or wooded vale'. In Roman mythology, the Napaeae were the valley-nymphs.

Nara From the Celtic, 'happy', or from the Old English, *nearra*, 'one who is near and dear'.

Narcissa From the Greek, *narke*, 'numbness'. In Greek mythology, Narcissus was the beautiful youth who spurned Echo's love (she then wasted away until only her voice was left), in favour of his own reflection. He then also pined away and was finally transformed into a flower. Hence the general meaning, excessive self-regard and obsession with one's own body. In botany, a genus of bulbs that produce trumpet-shaped white and yellow flowers. A name used since the Renaissance. **Variant:** Narcisse.

Narda From the Greek, *nardos*, 'spikenard'. In botany, an Indian aromatic plant with purple blooms whose ointment was highly prized in the ancient world.

Nasia From the Hebrew, *nes*, 'miracle', and *yah*, 'God', thus 'miracle of God'. **Variant:** Nasya.

Natalie French and German form of the Latin, *natales*, 'birth, origin', and *natalis*, 'birthday, anniversary, festival'. As the most common reference is to Christ's birthday, a name often given to babies born on December 25. The Russian form, Natasha, was popularised by Leo Tolstoy's novel, *War and Peace* (1865–68). **Variants:** Nata, Natala, Natalia, Natalya, Natasha, Nathalie, Tasha, Tashua.

Natania Female form of Nathan. **Variants:** Nataniella, Natanielle, Nathania, Nathaniella, Nathanielle, Netania, Netanya, Nethania.

Nayer From the Persian, 'sunshine'.

Neala Irish female form of Neil. **Variants:** Neila, Neilla, Nelia.

Nebula From the Latin, 'mist, smoke, darkness'.

Nechama Female form of Naham. **Variant:** Nehama.

Nellwyn From the Old English, *wyn*, 'friend', thus, 'friend of Nell', from Eleanor and Helen.

Nema From the Hebrew, 'thread, hair'. **Variant:** Nima.

Neola From the Greek, *neos*, 'young, new'.

Neoma Possibly from the Greek, *neomenia*, 'new moon'.

Nerine In Greek mythology, Nereus is a god of the sea and father of the fifty Nereids, the beautiful sea nymphs of the Mediterranean who attended Neptune, god of the oceans. Thus, in astronomy, a satellite of the planet Neptune. The form Nerissa was given a boost by the witty, spirited and trustworthy character in Shakespeare's comedy, *The Merchant of Venice* (1596). **Variants:** Nerice, Nerissa, Nerita, Nissa.

Nessa From the Old Norse, *nes*, 'headland, promontory'. *See also* Vanessa. **Variant:** Nesha.

Neva From the Old English, *niwe*, *neowe*, 'new', or from the Spanish, *nieve*, 'snow, brilliant white'. **Variants:** Nevada.

Niamh From the name of a sea god in Irish mythology, the name means 'beautiful and bright'.

Nicola Italian female form of Nicholas. Found in medieval Britain. Nicolette, the French form, was known through the disguised captive princess of the medieval romance, *Aucassin et Nicolette*. *See also* Colette. **Variants:** Nicci, Nichelle, Nichole, Nicki, Nickie, Nicky, Nicoletta, Nicolette, Nicoli, Nicolina, Nicoline, Nicolle, Nijole, Nika, Nike, Niki, Nikki.

Nigella The feminine form of the name Nigel.

Nina From the Spanish, 'young girl'. In Assyro-Babylonian mythology, goddess of the oceans; in the Inca mythology, goddess of fire. **Variants:** Nena, Ninetta, Ninette, Ninon, Nina. *See also* Anne.

Nissa From the Hebrew, *nes*, 'sign, emblem'. **Variants:** Nissie, Nissy.

Nitza From the Hebrew, 'flower bud', implying a baby of promise who will later blossom. **Variants:** Nitzana, Nizana.

Nixie From the Old High German, *nihhus*, 'nymph, sprite'. A mythological mermaid, half-woman, half-fish, who could be glimpsed by lovers on nights of the full moon.

Noel French form of Natalie, from the Old French, *nouel*. Also given to boys. **Variants:** Noella, Noelle, Novelia.

Noelani Hawaiian, meaning 'beautiful girl from heaven'.

Nofia From the Hebrew, *nof*, 'panorama', implying the beautiful world created by God. **Variant:** Nophia.

Nokomis North American Indian, meaning 'daughter of the moon'.

Nola Female form of Nolan.

Nona From the Latin, *nonus*, 'ninth', thus suitable for a ninth child, a child born in September or a child born on the ninth day of the month. **Variants:** Noni, Nonie.

Nora Irish form of Honor. *See also* Eleanor.

Norberta From the Old German, *nor beraht*, 'brilliant heroine', or from the Old Norse, 'brilliance of the Njord'. In Norse mythology, Njord was god of the winds and of sailors.

Norma From the Latin, *norma*, 'carpenter's square, pattern', implying keeping to the pattern, unrebellious, peaceful. Popularised by Vincenzo Bellini's successful opera, *Norma* (1831), whose heroine is a princess torn between love and duty.

Norna In Norse mythology, the Nornir (or Norns) were the three fates. Their names were Skuld (the future), Verdandi (the present) and Urd (the past); see also Moira. Norn is also a Norse dialect originally spoken in Orkney and Shetland.

Nova From the Latin, *novus*, 'new, newcomer'. In astronomy, a star that suddenly increases its brightness considerably, returning to its normal state a few weeks, months or years later. **Variant:** Novia.

Noya From the Hebrew, 'decked out by nature, bejewelled'.

Nuala From the Irish Gaelic, *fionnghuala*, 'fair-shouldered'. *See also* Fiona.

Nureen From the Persian and Arabic, *nur*, 'light'. The vast diamond, known as the Koh-i-Nur, 'Mountain of Light', was probably mined at Golconda in India. The Mughal Emperor Babur valued it at 'two and a half day's food for the whole world'. It has sparkled on various rulers' heads and is now part of the British crown jewels kept in the Tower of London and worn for coronations.

 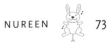

The beautiful and powerful wife of Mughal Emperor Shah Jehan (1569 – 1627) was called Nur Jehan, 'Light of the World'. **Variants:** Nur, Nurah.

Nydia From the Latin, *nidus*, 'nest, dwelling, home'. **Variants:** Neda, Nedda. *See also* Edward.

Nyree An adaptation of the New Zealand Maori name Ngaire meaning 'flaxen', this name was popularised by actress Nyree Dawn Porter. Alternatives include Niree.

Nysa From the Latin, *nisus*, 'goal, aim', or from the Greek, *nissa*, 'beginning, starting point'. **Variants:** Nissa, Nisse, Nissie, Nisy, Nyssa.

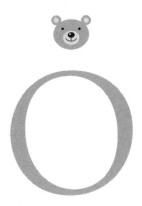

O

Obedience From the Latin, *oboedire*, 'to listen to, submit to'. A Puritan favourite in the 17th century. **Variants:** Beta, O'Bedae.

Obelia From the Greek, *obeliskos*, 'marker, pointer, needle'. An obelisk is a tall, monolithic, tapering shaft of stone erected as a public monument, first used in Egypt.

Octavia From the Latin, *octavus*, 'eight'. In Roman history, the sister (64–11 BC) of Emperor Augustus who married Mark Antony. He later left her for Cleopatra. **Variants:** Octavie, Ottavia, Tavi, Tavia.

Odeda From the Hebrew, 'courageous, strong'.

Odelia From the Greek, *oide*, 'song'. An ode was originally a long poem sung by a chorus at a public festival or as part of a play. Later it became more personal and was often addressed to the object of the poet's admiration and love. Also from the Hebrew, 'God be praised'. **Variants:** Detta, Odelet, Odelia, Odelinda, Odell, Odella, Odetta, Odette, Odilia, Otha, Othelia, Othilia, Othilie, Uta.

Odessa From Homer's epic poem, *The Odyssey*, written in the 8th century BC, which recounts how the god Poseidon frustrated Odysseus's return home to Greece after the fall of Troy–hence the name implies an extended adventurous wandering.

Ofra From the Old English, *offrung*, 'present, gift, sacrifice'.

Ola From the Old Norse, *ala*, 'nourisher, protector', meaning someone experienced and skilled, and also an old person or an ancestor.

Oleander From the Latin, *oliandrum*. An evergreen poisonous tree from the Levant with large red, pink or white flowers. **Variant:** Olinda.

Olga Russian form of the Old Norse name, Helga, 'holy'. The 10th-century saint was

 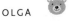

possibly the first Russian Christian baptised in Constantinople who returned to Russia to spread the faith. A name introduced to Britain in the middle of the last century, together with two other Russian names: Sonia, from Sophia, and Vera. **Variants:** Elga, Helga, Olenka, Olia, Ollie, Olly, Olva.

Olivia From the Latin, *oliva*, an evergreen tree cultivated in the Mediterranean, whose bitter fruit is pressed for its valuable oil. Because the trees grow slowly and live for many decades, olive leaves are an ancient symbol of stability and hence of peace – a Greek bride carried an olive garland. An olive wreath was a mark of honour and success. In Christianity, the olive is also a symbol of peace (see Noah). A name found in various forms in Britain since the Middle Ages, and very popular from the Renaissance until the 18th century, when it was probably helped by the character in Shakespeare's comedy, *Twelfth Night* (1601). **Variants:** Liva, Livia, Livvy, Livy, Nola, Nolana, Nollie, Oli, Olia, Oliff, Oliva, Olive, Olivet, Olivette, Ollett, Olli, Olliffe, Olly, Ollye.

Olwyn Welsh, meaning 'white footprint'. In Welsh mythology, a giant's daughter whose hand was won by Prince Culhwch only after he had performed extraordinary tasks. When this Celtic legend was translated in the last century, the name became very popular in Wales and was used occasionally in England. **Variant:** Olwen.

Olympia From the Greek, *Olympos*. In Greek mythology, Olympus was a mountain in north Thessaly, believed to be the abode of the gods and therefore heaven. The Olympic games, held every four years in ancient Greece, were in honour of the supreme god, Olympian Zeus, 'Zeus of Olympus'. **Variants:** Olimpe, Olimpia, Olimpie, Olympias.

Omega From the Greek, *omega*, 'great O'. The last letter of the Greek alphabet, written as a capital O. The name was often given to the last child of a family, since it implies a final deed or word. *See also* Alpha.

Onawa North American Indian, meaning 'wide-awake girl'.

Opal From the Sanskrit, *upalas*, 'precious stone'. A stone resembling quartz whose colours are produced by impurities or by the light catching a tiny crack, creating yellows, reds and the highly prized blue and black gems. **Variants:** Opalina, Opaline.

Ophelia From the Greek, *ophelos*, 'help, succour'. Made popular by the beautiful Ophelia who is driven mad and drowns in Shakespeare's tragedy, *Hamlet* (1602). The play was taken from a 13th-century history of Denmark, so the revived name was part of the fashionable cult of medievalism in the last century. **Variants:** Ofelia, Ofilia, Ophelie.

Ophira From the Hebrew, 'gold'. **Variant:** Ofira.

Oralee From the Hebrew, 'I have light'. **Variants:** Orlee, Orli, Orlit, Orly.

Oriana From the Latin, *oriens*, 'rising sun, morning sun', and thus the orient, or east, where the sun rises. A popular name in old French romances and later used by poets to praise a woman. **Variants:** Oria, Oriande, Oriane, Oriente.

Oriel From the Latin, *aurum*, 'gold', via the Old French, *oriol*; or from the Old German name, Aurildis, a compound of *aus*, 'fire', and *hildi*, 'strife'. A name carried to Britain by the Normans. The compounds include Orabel. **Variants:** Nehora, Ora, Orah, Oralia, Oriole, Orit.

Oriole From the Latin, *oriolus*, 'golden bird'. The name of several species of the *Oriolidae* bird family, whose males have bright yellow and black plumage.

Orion In Greek mythology, a gigantic and very handsome hunter who pursued the seven beautiful daughters of Atlas, called the Pleiades. He was eventually killed by Artemis and transported to the skies where he shines on winter nights. In astronomy, the name of a constellation.

Orla From the Irish Gaelic meaning 'light'. Alternatives include Aurnia, Oralee, Oriel.

Orna From the Latin, *ornare*, 'to adorn', or from the Irish Gaelic, 'pale olive colour'. **Variants:** Ornette, Ornit.

Orpah From the Hebrew, 'fawn', implying young and delicate.

Osma Female form of Osmond.

Osyth The queen and saint (7th century) was the wife of Sighere, King of the East Saxons, and founded a nunnery at St Osyth's in Essex. She then lived there, acquiring great popularity and, later, plenty of legends.

Ottalie Swedish female form of Otto.

Ottilia From the Old German, *othal*, 'fatherland'. **Variants:** Odala, Odette, Odila, Odile, Odilia, Odille, Ottilie, Uta.

Ova From the Latin, *ovum*, 'egg'.

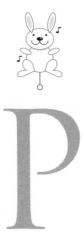

P

Padma Indian name, meaning 'lotus'. The national flower of India, sacred to Hindus. Other Indian names derived from the lotus include Nalina and Arabinda; *see* Lotus.

Page From the Greek, *paidion*, 'child', via the Italian, *paggio*, 'pageboy'. In medieval times, a page was a boy attending a knight as the first stage of his training to become a knight himself.

Pallas From the Greek, *pallas*, 'goddess'. In Greek mythology, Athena, goddess of wisdom, industry and the arts and protectress of heroes, was given the title Pallas Athene.

Palma From the Latin, *palmus*, 'the palm of the hand', and thus 'palm tree', from the shape of its leaves. The large palm frond was a symbol of victory, success or happiness, giving rise to the term 'to carry off the palm'. The Christian crusaders to the Holy Land were known as Palmers because they used to bring home consecrated crosses made of palm leaves. **Variants:** Palmeda, Palmer, Palmyra, Pelmira.

Paloma From the Latin, 'dove'. The bird symbolises peace; *see also* Dove. **Variants:** Palometa, Palomita.

Pamela From the Greek, *pau*, 'all', and *meli*, 'honey'. A name invented by Sir Philip Sidney for his romantic epic, *Arcadia* (1580), in which Pamela and Philoclea are daughters of King Basilius of Arcadia, a never-never pastoral land in a golden age. When Samuel Richardson used it for his successful novel, *Pamela, or a Virtue Rewarded* (1740), it became very fashionable. **Variants:** Pam, Pamelia, Pamelina, Pamella, Pammi, Pammie, Pammy.

Pandora From the Greek, *pan*, 'all', and *doron*, 'gift', thus, 'gifted in everything'. In Greek mythology, Pandora was the first woman, so-called because each god gave her a power that was to bring about the downfall of men. Jupiter's gift was a box, to be opened by her husband. When Epimetheus married her, he opened the box and all the evils flew out into the world. The name therefore implies a present that looks promising but is not.

Panphila From the Greek, *pan*, 'all', and *phila*, 'love', thus 'loving and loved by all'. **Variant:** Panfila.

Pansy From the French, *penser*, 'to think'. In botany, the plants of the genus *Viola*, whose long-lasting blooms have large, velvety petals in shades of blue, red and yellow.

Panthea From the Greek, *pan*, 'all', and *thea*, 'gods', thus someone who honours all the gods and receives their favours. In ancient Rome, the circular Pantheon was built to honour all the gods.

Pascal From the Hebrew, *pesah*, 'to pass over', referring to the Passover or Easter. Suitable for a child born on those festivals. The Paschal lamb is the lamb eaten at the Feast of the Passover. **Variants:** Pascha, Paschal, Pashell.

Patience From the Latin, *pati*, 'to suffer', but today carrying qualities of calm, uncomplaining endurance, tolerance and perseverance – all favourite virtues with the 17th-century Puritans who made the name popular. **Variant:** Patia.

Patricia Female form of Patrick. As a girl's name, it spread through Britain from Scotland where it was first used in the 18th century. In keeping with its aristocratic meaning, Queen Victoria's grand-daughter was Princess Patricia of Connaught, known as Pat, which kept it in vogue. **Variants:** Pat, Patia, Patrice, Patrizia, Patsy, Patti, Patty, Tricia, Trish, Trisha.

Paula Female form of Paul. Pauline was a common Roman name. St Paula (347–440)

came from Rome and founded several convents in Bethlehem, introducing her name to pilgrims who carried it to Europe. **Variants:** Paola, Paolina, Paule, Pauletta, Paulette, Paulina, Pauline, Paulita, Pauly, Pavia, Polly.

Pazia From the Hebrew, *paz*, 'gold'. Also given to boys. **Variants:** Paz, Paza, Pazice, Pazit.

Peace From the Latin, *pax*, 'peace, tranquillity'.

Pearl From the Middle English, *perle*. A smooth and lustrous deposit that forms around a grain of sand in some oysters and other molluscs. Its beauty and value have made it a term of high praise for a woman. Snippets of knowledge are described as pearls of wisdom. As a name, popular since the late 19th century. As the Greek for pearl is *margaretes*, it is sometimes a nickname for Margaret. Also given to boys. **Variants:** Pearla, Pearle, Pearlie, Pearline, Perla, Perle, Perry.

Peke From the Old German, 'shining, glorious'.

Pelagia From the Greek, *pelagos*, 'sea'. Of the several saints of this name, Pelagia of Antioch was a notoriously licentious dancing girl who was converted and went to live on the Mount of Olives. The 4th-century British monk and theologian, Pelagius, rejected theories of predestination and promoted the idea of man's free will to choose to do good or evil.

Pema From the Tibetan meaning 'lotus flower'.

Penelope From the Greek, 'weaver, silent worker'. In Greek mythology, the wife of Odysseus and model of domestic virtues and faithfulness. When her husband was away at war, she kept at bay her many suitors with the promise that she would select one when she had finished her weaving. But each night she continued to weave, until Odysseus returned and slew her admirers. Introduced into Britain during the 16th century, it enjoyed a strong vogue during the 17th. In Ireland, the name was an English translation of Fionnghuala, as was Fenella; *see* Fiona. **Variants:** Pelcha, Pen, Peneli, Penelopa, Pennie, Penny.

Penina From the Hebrew, 'coral, pearl'. **Variants:** Peninah, Peninit.

Pentecost From the Greek, *pentecoste*, 'fiftieth day'. The Christian festival of Whitsuntide, which falls on the seventh Sunday after Easter and commemorates the coming of the Holy Spirit to the twelve Apostles. Given to boys and girls from the 13th to 17th centuries, then rare.

Penthea From the Greek, *penta*, 'five'. A name suitable for the fifth child in a family, or a child born in May or on the fifth day of the month.

Peony From the Greek, *paion*, the ancient Greek hymn of thanksgiving to the gods. In Greek mythology, Paian discovered the peony flower, and Paian Apollo was Apollo's name when he was the gods' physician.

Perdita From the Latin, *perditus*, 'lost'. Invented by Shakespeare for his comedy, *The Winter's Tale* (1611), in which Perdita is an abandoned baby princess found and fostered by a shepherd. As a beautiful shepherdess, she falls in love with the king's son, discovers her identity and lives happily ever after. **Variants:** Purdey, Purdie.

Perfecta From the Latin, *perfectus*, 'perfect, complete'.

Perpetua From the Latin, *perpetualis*, 'constant, universal, everlasting'. A name sometimes given to Catholic children, after the 3rd-century virgin martyr.

Persephone From the Greek, 'dazzling brilliance' or 'she who destroys light'. In Greek mythology, the daughter of Zeus and Demetria who was abducted by Hades, god of the underworld, while gathering flowers. **Variants:** Persephassa, Persephoneia.

Pert From the Latin, *apertus*, 'open, bold'.

Petra Female form of Peter. A tomb discovered in Rome during the Middle Ages led to the belief that St Peter's daughter was called Petronella. She was swiftly made a saint, invoked against fevers and her name became common. **Variants:** Parnall, Parnell, Patch, Pernel, Perri, Perrin, Perrine, Perry, Perryne, Pet, Peta, Petie, Petrina, Petronel, Petronella, Petronia, Petronilla, Petronille, Petty.

Petula From the Latin, *petulans*, 'forward, saucy, impudent'.

Petunia From the French, *petun*, 'tobacco'. In botany, the genus of plants cultivated in tropical America.

Phedre From the Greek, 'shining, light'. **Variants:** Phaedra, Phaidra.

Phemia From the Greek, *pheme*, 'voice, speech'. **Variants:** Phe, Phemie.

Phila From the Greek, *philos*, 'love, loving, dear, beloved'.

Philana From the Greek, *philandros*, 'fond of mankind'. **Variants:** Philene, Philina, Phillina.

Philantha From the Greek, *philos*, 'loving', and *anthanon*, 'flower', thus someone who loves flowers.

Philberta From the Greek, *philos*, 'loving' and the Middle English, *beorht*, 'bright', thus 'glowing with love'.

Philippa From the Greek, *philos*, 'loving', and *hippos*, 'horse', thus someone who loves horses. When Edward III (1312–77) married Philippa of Hainault, she started its fashion in Britain–it was the name of the wife of the poet, Chaucer (1342–1499), who wrote *The Canterbury Tales*. However, it was usually used as Phelip or Phelyp and acquired its feminine ending only recently; *see also* Philip. **Variants:** Felipa, Filipa, Flippa, Pelipa, Phelypp, Phil, Philippine, Philli, Phillippa, Philly, Pine, Pip, Pippa, Pippy.

Philomela From the Greek, *philos*, 'loving', and *melos*, 'song', thus someone who loves singing. In Greek mythology, the gods transformed the Athenian princess, Philomela, into a swallow or nightingale to save her from the lecherous King of Thrace. **Variant:** Filomela.

Philomena *See* Filomena.

Philopena Female form of the German name, Philippchan, meaning 'little Philip', or Philippina. Also the name of a 19th-century adult game in which the two kernels of a freak nut are given to two different people. The next time they meet, the first to greet the other with 'Good morning, Philippine', receives a present from the other.

Philyra From the Greek, *philos*, 'loving', and *lyre*, 'the lyre', thus, someone fond of music. *See also* Filomena.

Phoebe From the Greek, *phoibos*, 'bright, shining'. In Greek mythology, goddess of the moon and counterpart to the Roman goddess, Diana. The male form, Phoebus, was the name given to Apollo when he was god of the sun as well as god of poetry, music and the muses. Used in Britain since the 16th century but never in high fashion. **Variant:** Phebe. *See also* Artemis and Selene.

Phoenix From the Greek, *phoinix*, 'phoenix, purple'. In Greek mythology, the bird of exceptional beauty that consumed itself by fire after 500 years, to be reborn from its ashes–thus a symbol of birth and immortality, of hope after bad times and of beauty. The Egyptian word was Phenice. **Variant:** Phenice.

Phyllis From the Greek, *phyllidis*, 'leafy branch'. In Greek mythology, the maiden who pined away for love until she was transformed into an almond tree, hence a common name in classical pastoral poetry for a country maiden or a sweetheart. After the poet Milton (1608–74) revived it, the name became so popular that it became the nickname for a good waitress, giving it a downmarket character that then put it out of fashion as a given name until the end of the last century. **Variants:** Filide, Philis, Phillida, Phillis, Phyl, Phyliss, Phyllada, Phyllida, Phyllie, Phylliss, Phyllys, Phylys. *See also* Felicia.

Pia From the Latin, *pius*, 'dutiful, careful, faithful'.

Pier French female form of Pierre, from Peter. **Variants:** Pieretta, Pierette, Pierrine.

Piper A modern American girls' name which originally refers to one who plays musical pipes.

Piuta From the Greek, 'poetry'.

Placida From the Latin, *placidus*, 'gentle, peaceful, mild'. **Variant:** Placidia.

 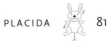

GIRL OR BOY – ONE FOR ALL

Nine months or so of pondering over possible names may have its merits. But having to choose two names knowing that one will be discarded when a girl, or a boy, fails to arrive could strike many expectant parents as unnecessarily hard thinking. The problem is easily solved. With a little tweak, a favourite name can go well for either sex. The father, itching to have a beautiful daughter named Joan Frances Stephanie, can adorn his handsome son with John Francis Stephen – or any of their various forms. The mother, dreaming of a handsome Peter George Nicholas, can swap to pretty girl's versions, perhaps Peta Georgiana Nicolette. An even easier solution for parents is for them to settle for a name that remains exactly the same for girls and boys, such as Adrian, Blair, Carol, Garnet, Lee or Storm.

Pleasance From the Old French, *plaisir*, 'to please, to give pleasure'. Occasionally given to boys. **Variant:** Pleasant.

Plennie From the Latin, *plenus*, 'full up, complete'.

Polly *See* Margaret and Mary.

Pomona From the Latin, *pomum*, 'fruit'. In Roman mythology, the popular goddess of fruit trees courted by the other rural gods and finally seduced by one who approached her in the guise of an old woman.

Poppy From the Latin, *papavar*, 'poppy'. In botany, a tall plant with bright red blooms, whose pale milky juice has narcotic properties.

Pora From the Hebrew, 'fruitful'.

Portia From the Latin, *porcus*, 'hog'. The name of an ancient Roman clan, the Porcii, but brought into use by the heroine of Shakespeare's comedy, *The Merchant of Venice* (1596). She disguises herself as a man and defeats Shylock's demand for a 'pound of flesh' by warning him that he may only take it if he can do so without taking a single drop of blood.

Primavera From the Latin, 'the first green, springtime', implying the re-kindling of life and the birth of new life.

Primrose From the Latin, *primus*, 'first', and *rose*, 'rose', thus 'the earliest rose'. In botany, more than 500 species of primrose in the genus *Primula* grow wild and bloom with pale yellow flowers. Like other flower names, it enjoyed popularity at the turn of this century.

Priscilla From the Latin, *priscus*, 'ancient, old-fashioned, antique, in a strict way', thus

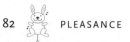

much-loved by the 17th-century Puritans. **Variants:** Cilla, Pris, Prisca, Prissie, Prissy.

Procopia Female form of Procopio.

Prospera Female form of Prospero.

Prudence From the Latin, *prudentia*, 'good sense, discretion, practical judgement'. One of the first abstract virtue names favoured by the Puritans, probably because it had been current since the Middle Ages. **Variants:** Pru, Prud, Prudencia, Prudentia, Prudi, Prudie, Prudy, Prue.

Prunella From the Latin, *prunum*, 'plum', thus 'little plum, plum-coloured'. A name imported from France.

Psyche From the Greek, *psukhe*, 'breath of life, soul'. In classical mythology, a beautiful maiden loved by Eros, god of harmony and sexual love. Despite the jealousies of other women, their love for each other survived and they were finally married on Mount Olympus, symbolising the union of mind and body.

Pulcheria From the Latin, *pulcher*, 'beautiful, fair'.

Pyralis From the Greek, *pyr*, 'fire'. **Variant:** Pyrene.

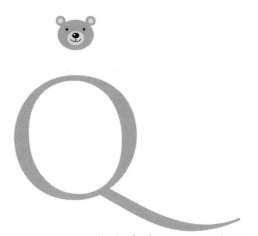

Queenby From the Old English, *cuen*, 'queen', and the Danish, *bye*, 'dwelling place, home', thus 'queen's castle'.

Queenie From the Old English, *cuen*, 'companion, woman, wife, ruler'. Also, the personification of the supreme woman, such as a man's description of his sweetheart as 'queen of my heart' or parents' of their daughter as 'queen of our hearts'. In the epic poem, *Paradise Lost* (1667), Milton says of a queen: 'Grace was in all her steps, heaven in her eye, in every gesture dignity and love.' Popular in the Middle Ages, when the name referred to the Virgin Mary, Queen of Heaven. Later it was used only as a nickname for Regina, but became an independent name again in the last century, when it was also used to refer to Queen Victoria. **Variants:** Quanda, Queena, Quenie, Quinn.

Quella From the Old English, *cwellan*, 'to kill, destroy, pacify'.

Querida Spanish, from the Latin, *quaerere*, 'to ask, enquire, show interest and sympathy'.

Quinta From the Latin, *quinta*, 'fifth'. Like the Greek form Penthea, suitable for the girl's position in the family or for the date, month or year of her birth. Introduced to Britain by the Normans, the name was more popular in Scotland where it doubled as a translation for the Celtic name, Cumhaighe, 'hound of the plain'. **Variants:** Quintilla, Quintina.

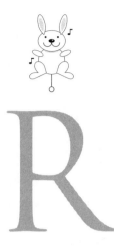

R

Rabia From the Arabic, *rabi*, 'fragrant breeze'.

Rachel From the Hebrew, 'ewe, female sheep', symbol of gentleness and innocence. In the Bible, the wife of Jacob – who laboured seven years to win her hand – and mother of Joseph and Benjamin. After the Reformation, the name was used regularly in Britain. **Variants:** Lahela, Rachael, Rachele, Racheli, Rachelle, Rachie, Rae, Rahel, Rakel, Raquel, Raquela, Ray, Raye, Rochell, Shell, Shelley, Shelly.

Radagund From the Old German, *radi*, 'counsel', and *gundi*, 'war'. St Radagundis was wife of Clothaire I (reigned 556–561), King of the Franks, and is one of the saints named in the full title of Jesus College, Cambridge University.

Raine From the Latin, *regnum*, 'kingly authority, kingship, dominance, influence'. **Variants:** Raina, Rana, Rane, Rayna, Reina, Reine, Reyna.

Raisa From the Yiddish, 'rose'. **Variants:** Raissa, Raizel, Rayzel, Razil.

Ramona Female form of Raymond. **Variants:** Raymonda, Romona.

Ran In Norse mythology, the benevolent goddess of the sea who saved drowning sailors by catching them in her net.

Randa Female form of Randall, from Randolph. **Variant:** Randi.

Rani From the Sanskrit, 'queen'. **Variants:** Rana, Rancie, Ranee, Rania.

Rapa Hawaiian, meaning 'moonbeam'.

Raphaela Female form of Raphael. **Variants:** Rafaela, Rafaele.

Ravital From the Hebrew, 'God is my dew', meaning 'God will provide'.

Rawnie English gypsy name, meaning 'lady'.

Raya From the Hebrew, 'friend'.

Rayna From the Yiddish, 'pure, clean'. **Variant:** Reyna.

 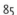

Raz From the Aramaic, 'secret'. Also given to boys. **Variants:** Razi, Razia, Raziah, Raziela, Razille, Razili, Raziye.

Rea From the Greek, 'poppy'; see Poppy.

Reade From the Old English, *raedan*, 'to advise, give counsel'; or from *read*, 'red', implying a bright and fiery character. **Variants:** *Radella, Radinka.*

Rebecca From the Hebrew and Arabic, *ribkah*, 'knotted cord', implying a faithful wife. In the Bible, beautiful wife of Isaac and mother of Jacob and Esau. Like Rachel, the name came into fashion after the Reformation. **Variants:** Becca, Beck, Becka, Beckie, Becky, Bekki, Reba, Rebe, Rebeca, Rebeka, Rebekah, Reva, Rivca, Rivka.

Regina From the Latin, *regina*, 'queen, goddess, noble woman, mistress'; the female form of Rex. In the Middle Ages, the name referred to the Virgin Mary but when it was revived by the Victorians, it probably referred to their queen; see also Queenie. **Variants:** Gina, Queenie, Raina, Rani, Rayna, Reena, Reene, Regan, Reggi, Reggie, Regine, Reina, Rena, Rene, Reyna, Rina.

Reiko Japanese, meaning 'gratitude'. **Variant:** Rei.

Renata From the Hebrew, 'joy, song', and the Arabic, *ranna*, 'sweet melody'. **Variants:** Rene, Renee, Renette, Renita.

Reubena Female of Reuben. **Variant:** Reuvena.

Rexana Female form of Rex; see also Regina. **Variants:** Rex, Rexella.

Rhea From the Greek, 'protectress'. In Greek mythology, the goddess who personified the earth. She was mother of the ruling gods who lived on Olympus and was the Great Mother and author of all being. See also Sylvia.

Rheta From the Greek, 'well-spoken'.

Rhoda From the Greek, *rhodon*, 'rose'; see also Rose. The compounds include **Rhosanna**. **Variants:** Rhode, Rhodeia, Rhodope, Rhody, Rhona, Roda, Rodina, Rona, Rosa, Rose.

Rhonda From the Celtic, 'powerful river'. The two rivers in Wales, Rhondda Fawr and Rhondda Fach, give their names to the surrounding region. **Variants:** Rhondda, Rhonnie, Ronda.

Ria From the Spanish, 'small river'.

Richarda Female form of Richard. **Variants:** Rica, Ricarda, Richanda, Richardyne, Richela, Richenda, Richenza, Richia, Ricka, Ricki, Riki.

Rickma From the Hebrew, 'woven', thus implying the interweaving of the characters of the mother and father in their child. **Variant:** Rikma.

Rilla From the Low German, *rille*, 'small stream, brook'.

Rimona From the Arabic, *rumanah*, 'pomegranate'.

Rishona From the Hebrew, *rishon*, 'first'.

Rita Indian name, meaning 'brave, strong'. **Variants:** Reda, Reeta, Reida, Rheta. *See also* Margeret.

Riva From the Latin, *ripa*, via the Old French, *rive*, 'bank of a stream, seashore'.

River From the Latin, *riparius*, 'someone who frequents river banks', via the Old French, *rivere*, 'river bank, river'. In poetry, the 'river of life' refers to the mixture of ups and downs encountered through life. **Variants:** Rivana.

Roberta Female form of Robert. The compounds include **Robann**. **Variants:** Bobbette, Bobbi, Bobbie, Bobby, Bobbye, Bobina, Bobine,

Bobinette, Rebinah, Robbie, Robena, Robenia, Robin, Robina, Robinette, Robinia, Robyn, Rori, Rory, Rubinah, Ruby, Ruperta.

Rochelle From the Old French, *roche*, 'large stone', thus implying reliability and solidity. **Variants:** Roch, Rochella, Rochette, Shell, Shelley, Shelly.

Roda *See* Rhoda.

Roderica Female form of Roderick. **Variants:** Rori, Rory.

Roisin From the Gaelic Irish meaning 'rose'. Alternatives include Rosheen, Rois, Rosen.

Rolanda Female form of Roland. **Variants:** Ralna, Rolaine, Rolene, Rolleen.

Romelda From the German, 'Roman warrior'; see Romulus. **Variant:** Romilda.

Romia From the Hebrew, 'exalted, high up'. **Variants:** Roma, Romit.

Romola Female form of Romulus. **Variants:** Roma, Romain, Romaine, Romana, Romayne, Romy.

Rona *See* Rhoda.

Ronalda Scottish female form of Reginald. **Variants:** Rona, Roni, Ronl, Ronna, Ronne, Ronnie, Ronsy.

Roni From the Hebrew, 'joy'. **Variants:** Rani, Ranit, Ranita, Renana, Renanit, Ronia, Ronit, Ronli, Ronnit.

Rosabel From the Latin, *rosa*, 'rose', and Belle, thus 'my beautiful rose'. **Variants:** Rosabella, Rosabelle.

Rosalba From the Latin, *rosa*, 'rose', and *alba*, 'white', thus 'white rose'.

Rosalia From the Latin, *rosales escae*, 'feast of roses', the annual Roman festival when tombs were adorned with garlands of roses. The ceremony of hanging the garlands was the *rosalia*. **Variants:** Rosaleen, Rosalie, Rosaline, Rosele, Rozalia.

Rosalind From the Latin, *rosa*, 'rose', and the Spanish, *linda*, 'pretty', thus 'pretty as a rose'. However, the name had arrived in Spain from Germany as the Old High German name, Rosalindis, from *hros*, 'horse', and *lindi*, 'snake', thus 'horse-serpent' – horses were sacred to the early Germanic tribes. The Spanish took the word and gave it the meanings of their own language. It was then carried to Britain by the Normans and soon became widespread. Further popularised by Shakespeare with the heroine of his comedy, *As You Like It* (1599). **Variants:** Ros, Rosaleen, Rosalin, Rosalinda, Rosaline, Rosalyn, Rosalynd, Roseleen, Roselyn, Roz, Rozalin, Rhodalind. *See also* Linda.

Rosamond A similar history to Rosalind. From the Latin, *rosa*, 'rose', and *mundus*, 'world', thus 'rose of the world'; and also from the Old High German name, Hrosmund, from *hros*, 'horse', and *mund*, 'protector', thus 'protector of the horse'. Introduced to Britain by the Normans – the mistress of Henry II (1133–89) was 'Fair Rosamund', whom the queen poisoned in jealousy. **Variants:** Ros, Rosamund, Rosamunda, Rosamunde, Roseaman, Roseman, Rosemunda, Rosomon, Roz, Rozamond.

Rose From the Latin, *rosa*, 'rose, wreath of roses, rose-bush, rose-tree'. In botany, the genus of shrubs and vines whose prickly stems bear multi-coloured and fragrant flowers. The petals and oils are distilled into perfume. The famous lines 'What's in a name? That which we call a rose by any other name would smell as sweet,' come from Shakespeare's tragic romance, *Romeo and Juliet* (1595), when Juliet is speaking of her Romeo, whose name marks him as an enemy of her family. For many poets, the flower and its name are synonymous with love and beauty. In the 13th-century French romance, *Roman de la Rose*, the rose symbolises the beautiful maiden in the tale of courtly love. Rosa of Lima (1586–1617) was the first person born in the Americas to be canonised as a saint. The name may also be related to the Old High German, *hros*, 'horse', the sacred animal; see Rosalind. The compounds include **Roanne, Rohana, Rosabeth, Rosanna, Roseanna, Roseanne, Rosellen, Roselotte, Roselynde, Rosemary, Rozanne. Variants:** Ricki, Roese, Roesia, Rohese, Rois, Rosa, Rosaleen, Roseia, Rosel, Rosella, Roselle, Rosena, Rosetta, Rosette, Rosi, Rosie, Rosina, Rosine, Rosita, Roslyn, Rosy, Royse, Rozalie, Roze, Rozina, Rozy, Ruzena, Zita. *See also* Rhoda.

Rosebud The bud of the Rose flower, full of promise for the opening and blossoming of the flower.

Rosedale From the Latin, *rosa*, 'rose' and the Old English, *dael*, 'broad valley', thus 'valley of roses'.

Rosemary From the Latin, *ros*, 'dew', and *marinus*, 'of the sea', thus 'sea dew'. In botany, an aromatic shrub from southern Europe, with grey-green leaves and pale blue flowers, used in cooking and perfumes. Also a compound of Rose. A name known in Britain in the 18th century but common only in this century. **Variant:** Rosemarie.

Rowena From the Celtic name, Rhonwen, 'slender as a lance, fair'; also the female form of Rowland. Although it was known as early as the 5th century, the name came into popularity with the publication of Sir Walter Scott's *Ivanhoe* (1819).

Roxanna From the Persian, 'dawn, bright light'. **Variants:** Rosana, Roxane, Roxanne, Roxie, Roxine, Roxy.

Royale From the Latin, *rex*, 'king, ruler', via the Middle English, *roial*, meaning anything authorised, founded by, befitting or connected with a king or queen; see also Rex. It also means anything superior in size or quality. **Variant:** Royal.

Ruby From the Latin, *rubeus*, 'red'. A clear deep red precious stone, known as the 'oriental ruby' or 'true ruby' and highly valued; also the deep red colour. **Variants:** Rubetta, Rubette, Rubi, Rubia, Rubina.

Rudelle From the Old High German, *hruod*, 'fame'.

Ruel Female form of Reuel.

Rufina From the Latin, *rufus*, 'red, red-haired'.

Rula From the Latin, *regula*, 'pattern, model, example'.

Rumer English gypsy name, probably from *rom*, 'man', via *romano*, 'gypsy'.

Runa From the Old Norse, *rinna*, 'to flow'.

Ruth From the Hebrew, 'companionship, friendship, beautiful dream'. In the Bible, the loyal and constant daughter-in-law of Naomi. Adopted by the Puritans to symbolise Ruth's purity and sorrow, rather than for its original meaning. **Variants:** Ruthi, Ruthie.

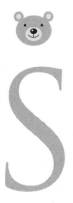

Saada From the Hebrew, 'support, help'.

Saba From the Hebrew, 'old'.

Sabina From the Latin, *Sabini*, 'the Sabines', an ancient Italian people who were conquered and assimilated by the Romans in 290 BC. St Sabina, a 2nd-century Roman martyr, kept the name popular during the Middle Ages. In botany, several species of shrubs and trees including the juniper and red cedar. **Variants:** Sabine, Savina.

Sabra From the Arabic and Hebrew, *sabra*, 'thorny cactus'. A nickname for native-born Israelis whose characters are believed to be outwardly tough and inwardly gentle. **Variants:** Sabrina, Zabra, Zabrina.

Sabrina See Sabra. This name has become popular following the success of television series 'Sabrina the Teenage Witch'.

Sadie From the Old English, *saed*, 'seed'. Like an egg, the seed is the symbol of the promise of life and growth. **Variants:** Sadelle, Sadie, Sady.

Sadira From the Persian, 'lotus plant'; *see also* Lotus.

Saffron From the Arabic, *zafaran*, 'crocus'. In botany, in small bulbous plant which bears purple or white flowers with orange stigmas. The dried stigmas are called saffron, which is highly prized as a strong yellow dye and a spice for cooking.

Sahara From the Arabic, *sahra*, 'desert'. The Sahara Desert, the largest in the world, covers some 9,065,000 square kilometres.

Sakara North American Indian, meaning 'sweet'.

Sakura Japanese, meaning 'cherry blossom'. The Japanese national flower, symbol of wealth and prosperity and also the special flower of March.

Salena From the Latin, *sal*, 'salt, salt water'. Used metaphorically, it means intellectual

  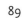

acuteness, cunning, wit and good sense. To say someone is 'the salt of the earth' is to praise qualities of selflessness and common sense. **Variant:** Salina.

Sally *See* Sarah.

Salome Greek, from the Aramaic, *Shalamzion*, or, shortened to Shalamzu, 'peace of Zion'. In the Bible, the niece of King Herod who promised to grant her wish if she danced for him. She chose the head of John the Baptist (Matthew 14) and it was delivered to her on a plate. A name found in Britain since the 17th century. **Variants:** Saloma, Salomi, Shulamit, Shulamith, Shuly. *See also* Zulema.

Samantha From the Aramaic, 'one who listens'. A Biblical name revived in the last century but popular only very recently. **Variants:** Sam, Sammy.

Samara From the Latin, 'seed of the elm'.

Samira From the Arabic, *samar*, 'entertainment', thus entertainer. The female form of Samir.

Samuela Female form of Samuel.

Sancha Spanish, from the Latin, *sanctus*, 'holy, pure'. Introduced into Britain surprisingly early. In the 13th century Richard, Earl of Cornwall, married Sanchia, daughter of the Count of Provence, provoking many English versions of the name. **Variants:** Cynthia, Saint, Sanchia, Sayntes, Sence, Senses.

Sandra *See* Alexandra.

Santa From the Latin, *sanctus*, 'holy, pure'. Santina is the diminutive, for a small person with those qualities. **Variant:** Santina.

Sapphire From the Greek, *sappheiros*, which is possibly from the Sanskrit, *saniprya*, 'precious to the planet Saturn'. A deep blue gemstone made of corundum, and also a deep blue colour. **Variants:** Sapir, Sapira, Sapphira.

Sarah From the Hebrew, *sarah*, 'princess'. It occurs first in the Bible, as Sarai, wife of Abraham and mother of Isaac. St Sara, the legendary handmaid of Mary Magdalene, has a tomb in Provence and is believed by gypsies to have been a gypsy too. Known in Britain since the 12th century, its popularity rose with the vogue for Old Testament names after the Reformation. It has been one of the most common names ever since. Morag is the Scottish Gaelic form. The compounds include **Saran, Sarann, Saranne**. **Variants:** Morag, Sada, Sadella, Sadelle, Sadi, Sadie, Sady, Sadye, Saidee, Sal, Salaidh, Saliee, Sallie, Sally, Sara, Sarai, Sarena, Sarene, Saretta, Sarette, Sari, Sarice, Sarina, Sarine, Sarita, Sayre, Shara, Sharai, Shari, Sher, Sherrie, Socha, Sorale, Soralie, Sorolie, Zara, Zarah, Zaria, Zora, Zorana, Zoreen, Zorene, Zorna.

Saturnia From the Latin, *satus*, 'sowing, planting'. In Roman mythology, Saturn was the most ancient King of Latinum, who was later honoured as god of agriculture and of civilisation in general. The English word, season, also comes from *satus* and is occasionally used as a name.

Saxon Germanic, from the Latin, *saxum*, 'large stone'. The Saxons were a West Germanic people living in north Germany who, with the Jutes and Angles, invaded England in the 5th and 6th centuries. Sasanach and Sasunn are Irish forms. **Variants:** Sasanach, Sasunn, Sass.

Sayo Japanese, meaning 'born at night'.

Scarlet From the Old French, *escarlate*, 'rich, vivid reddish-orange colour'. Popularised in this century by the heroine of Margaret

Mitchell's novel, *Gone With the Wind*, and by the film adaptation (1939). **Variant:** Scarlett.

Scientia From the Latin, 'knowing, expert, skilled'.

Secunda From the Latin, *secundus*, 'the next, the following, the second', thus suitable for a second child.

Seema From the Greek, 'sign, symbol', as in the sign language of semaphore. **Variants:** Sema, Senalda.

Sela From the Hebrew, 'rock'.

Selda From the Old English, *seldan*, 'rare', implying preciousness. **Variant:** Zelda.

Selene From the Greek, *selene*, 'moon'. In Greek mythology, the exceptionally beautiful goddess of the moon, also called Artemis. Each night, as she crossed the skies in her chariot drawn by two white horses, her golden crown illuminated the darkness. When she finished her journey, her brother, Helios, god of the sun, began his. **Variants:** Celena, Celene, Celie, Celina, Celinda, Sela, Selena, Selina, Sillina. *See also* Celeste, Phoebe and Endymion.

Selima From the Arabic, *salim*, 'well-formed, healthy'; also the female form of Solomon. **Variant:** Selimah.

Selma From the Celtic, 'fair', or the Old Norse, 'divinely protected'. **Variants:** Aselma, Zelma.

Semele In Greek mythology, the beautiful mortal with whom the supreme god, Zeus, fell in love. When Zeus' jealous and cunning wife persuaded Semele to ask her lover to appear in his full majestic finery, his dazzling brightness and the accompanying thunder and lightning killed her.

Semiramis In Assyro-Babylonion mythology, the beautiful Assyrian girl who married King Ninus, and founded Babylon. He so loved her that he abdicated in her favour – she quickly had him put to death, but was later slain by her own son. **Variant:** Semiramide.

Septima From the Latin, *septimus*, 'seventh'; thus suitable for a child born in September, the seventh month of the Roman calendar which began in March. **Variant:** Seven.

Seraphina From the Hebrew, *saraf*, 'to burn'. The plural, *seraphim*, means 'celestial beings, each with three pairs of wings'. In the angel hierarchy of the Bible, seraphim are the first of the nine orders and surround the throne of God. A name popularised in the last century. **Variants:** Serafina, Serafine, Seraphine.

Serena From the Latin, *serenus*, 'clear, serene, bright'. **Variants:** Serepta, Sirena.

Shalgia From the Hebrew, 'snow-white'.

Sharman From the Old English, *scearu*, 'cutting, division', implying a person receiving or contributing her fair share or full portion.

Sharon From the Hebrew, *yashar*, 'flat area, plain'. In the Bible, Sharon was an area of Palestine where roses grew in quantity. Also given to boys. **Variants:** Shaaron, Shara, Sharai, Shareen, Shari, Sharma, Sharona, Sharyn.

Sheena *See* Jane.

Sheila Irish, from Cecilia, via the two Old Irish names, Sighile and Sile. **Variants:** Selia, Sheelagh, Sheelah, Sheilah, Sheilla, Shelagh, Shelia, Shelley, Shelli, Shelly, Shiela, Shielah, Sile.

Shifra From the Hebrew, *shefer*, 'beautiful'. **Variants:** Schifra, Shaina, Shaine.

Shimra From the Hebrew, 'to keep safe'. **Variants:** Shimria, Shmrit.

Shira From the Hebrew, 'song'. **Variants:** Shirah, Shiri, Shirlee.

Shirley From the Old English, *scir*, 'shire, county', and *leah*, 'meadow'. In botany, a Shirley Poppy has scarlet or salmon pink flowers and is named after Shirley Vicarage, Croydon, Surrey, where it was first grown. The name was given by Charlotte Brontë to the heroine of her novel *Shirley* (1849) to suggest her independence, since it was then mainly a surname, and thus given as a first name only to men. In the last century the name was mostly found in Yorkshire but in this century it spread across Britain, enjoying a vogue in the 1930s when Shirley Temple rose to child stardom. **Variants:** Sher, Sheree, Sheri, Sherill, Sherline, Sherri, Sherrie, Sherry, Sherye, Sheryl, Shir, Shirl, Shirlee, Shirleen, Shirleight, Shirlene, Shirline.

Shizu Japanese, meaning 'quiet, clear'. A favourite Japanese name. **Variants:** Shizue, Shizuka, Shizuko, Shizuyo.

Shona Female form of the Irish Sean, from John. **Variants:** Shaina, Shaine, Shana, Shanie, Shannon, Shayna, Shayne, Shoni, Shonie.

Sibley From the Middle English, *siblyng*, 'sister or half-sister, brother or half-brother', that is, a child with brothers and sisters who have either one or two parents in common.

Sibyl From the Greek, *sibulla*, 'prophetess, female soothsayer, oracle, wise old woman'. In classical mythology, several women regarded as Sibyls and their prophecies were believed to be inspired by the gods. The most famous was the Sibyl of Cumae who sold a collection of oracles, called the Sibylline Books, to the early Roman king, Tarquin, who consulted them in times of trouble. As some predictions mentioned the coming of Christ, Sibyls were regarded by Christians as acceptable pagans, so when the Normans introduced the name it quickly became widespread. **Variants:** Sevilla, Sib, Sibbie, Sibel, Sibell, Sibett, Sibil, Sibilla, Sibille, Sibley, Sibylla, Sibyllina, Sybella, Sybil, Sybille, Sybyl, Sybylla.

Sidonie Either from the Latin, *sindon*, 'fine cloth', referring to the Sacred Sidon, or Shroud, in which Christ was wrapped, now believed to be preserved at Turin; or from the Hebrew, *tzidon*, 'to lure, entice'. Saida, in Lebanon, was the ancient Phoenician seaport of Sidon, famous for its glassware and purple dyes. Sidonie was the first name of the French writer Colette. **Variants:** Sidney, Sidonia, Sidony.

Sidra From the Latin, *sidus*, 'star, heavenly body' and, in the plural, 'a constellation, the heavens'.

Signa From the Latin, *signum*, 'signal, token, banner, indication', or 'image', as in a sculpture or picture.

Sigrid Female form of Siegfried.

Silver From the Old English, *siolfor*, 'silver, silversmith'. A white metal highly prized as the best metal for conducting heat and electricity, also valued for its malleability, its high polish in jewellery and as a monetary standard for a unit of currency. *See also* Golda.

Silvia *See* Sylvia.

Sima From the Aramaic, 'treasure'.

Simone French female form of Simon. **Variants:** Simeona, Simona, Simonette, Simonne.

Sirena From the Greek, *seiren*, 'to bind, attach', but now meaning 'seductive singing, temptress, warning whistle'. In Greek mythology, the Sirens were malevolent female sea monsters, each one a bird with a woman's head. They lived on the shores of Capri and other places, luring passing sailors to their deaths with their irresistible and bewitching singing. When finally defeated by the musician, Orpheus, one of them threw herself into the sea and was tossed ashore on the very spot where Naples was later founded. **Variants:** Rena, Reena. *See also* Serena.

Sirios From the Greek, *seirios*, 'glowing, burning'. In astronomy, Sirius is the brightest star in the sky and is 8.7 light years away from Earth. Its nickname, Dog Star, derives from its constellation, Canis Major.

Sivia From the Hebrew, *tzia*, 'deer'. **Variant:** Sivya.

Solace From the Latin, *solacium*, 'comfort, relief, a soothing quality'.

Solange From the Latin, *solus*, 'alone, single', also implying best, alone of its class.

Soma From the Greek, 'body'; or from the Sanskrit, an Indian plant whose juice was used to prepare intoxicating drinks consumed in ancient Hindu rituals.

Sona From the Latin, *sonare*, 'to make a noise, resound, cry out, pour forth'.

Sophia From the Greek, *sophia*, 'wisdom'. The huge 6th-century church in Istanbul is dedicated to Hagia Sophia, 'Sacred Wisdom', the Second Person of the Trinity in the Christian Orthodox Church. Introduced to Britain in the 17th century, it became an influential favourite of the 18th-century Hanoverian royal family, then fell right out of favour with the Victorians. **Variants:** Sofia, Sonia, Sonja, Sonni, Sonny, Sonya, Sophie, Sophronia, Sophy, Sunny, Zonya, Zophia.

Sora From the Native American for Songbird. Variations include Sori, Sorree, Sorey, Sorie.

Spangle From the Middle Dutch, *spange*, 'ornament, clasp', via the Middle English, *spangele*, 'small piece of sparkling metal'.

Sparkle From the Old English, *spearca*, 'to glisten and burn, to give a flash of light, to provoke or set in motion'.

Spring From the Old English, *springan*, 'to leap up, explode'. The season of sudden growth of life after winter and thus an image for youth. Also, the source of a river, which in poetical language is the beginning of the river of life.

Stacey Irish form of Anastasia. **Variants:** Stacia, Stacie, Stacy.

Star From the Old English, *steora*, 'star'. In astrology, a heavenly body believed to influence a person's character or future; also associated with excellence and fame – the star pupil, for example, or the star of the show. **Variants:** Starla, Starlit, Starr, Starry.

Stella From the Latin, *stella*, 'star'. As Stella Maris, an invocation of the Virgin Mary, the name is popular with Roman Catholics. However, the simple name Stella was invented by Sir Philip Sidney (1554–86) for his collection of sonnets and songs called *Astrophel and Stella*, inspired by his beloved, Lady Penelope Devereux. A further boost came when Swift (1667–1754) used it as a nickname for Esther Johnson. *See also* Star and Esther.

Stephanie Female form of Stephen. **Variants:** Estephania, Etienette, Stefa, Stefana, Stefania,

MYSTERIOUS MOON, LIFE-GIVING SUN

Almost every language has beautiful names meaning moon and sun. Early peoples often worshipped the moon and sun as gods and made up elaborate stories to explain their daily journeys across the heavens. The Greeks had several moon and sun gods. The beautiful goddesses of the moon included Artemis, Phoebe and Selene. When they had brightened the dark heavens on their nightly journey, Helios, handsome god of the sun, began his, bringing light and energy to the day. Helios was later called Apollo, and was also known as Chrysocomes, Phoebus and Xanthus. And Eos (Dawn), Helios and Selene were all children of Hyperion, yet another god of sunlight. If Greek mythology is too confusing, try Diana (moon), Horus (sun), Ravi (sun) – or just plain Moon and Sunny.

Stefanida, Stefanie, Stefenie, Steffie, Stephanine, Stephenie, Stevana, Stevena.

Storm From the Old English, *storm*, 'tempestuous weather', made up of strong winds with rain, snow, thunder or lightning. **Variants:** Stormie, Stormy.

Sudy From the Old English, *suth*, 'south, southerly wind', the warm wind that brings good weather and nourishes the crops.

Suki Japanese, meaning 'beloved'. *See also* Susan.

Sunny From the Old English, *sunne*, the star that is the basis of the solar system. As the source of heat and light energy, it sustains life on earth. To be sunny is to be bright, energetic and cheerful.

Susan From the Hebrew, *shoshana*, 'lily'. Shushan, in Persia, is the 'city of white lilies'.

In the Bible, it was Susanna who was surprised by the Elders of the Temple while taking a bath. Apart from Shakespeare calling his daughters Susanna and Judith, it was not very common until the 18th century. It kept its high profile under the Victorians, who increasingly used the short form, Susan. The compounds include **Suanne, Suella, Suzanne**. **Variants:** Shoshan, Shoshana, Shoshanah, Shushan, Shushana, Shushanah, Siusan, Sosanna, Su, Sue, Sukey, Suki, Sukie, Susanna, Susannah, Susanne, Susi, Susie, Susy, Suzanne, Suzette, Suzie, Suzy, Zsa Zsa.

Svea From the Swedish, 'south'.

Swana From the Old English, *suan*, 'swan'. One of several large, aquatic birds belonging to the *Cynus* family. In England, all the swans living on the River Thames are owned by the Queen and the cygnets are counted and marked annually on Swan-Upping day. From its regal carriage and associations, 'to swan around' is to behave with an air of superiority and without care.

Sydel Female form of Sydney. **Variants:** Sid, Sidi, Sidne, Sidney, Sydelle, Sydney.

Syke From the Greek, *sukaminos*, 'mulberry tree'. The silk worms that produce the valuable silk yarn live exclusively on a diet of mulberry leaves.

Sylvia From the Latin, *silva*, 'wood, forest'. In Roman mythology, Rhea Silvia was the mother of Romulus and Remus. The rural Roman god Silvanus watched over woods and the Silvanae were his female deities. Thus the name is associated with rural life and, in poetry, is often given to shepherdesses. A popular Renaissance name – Silvia is the sweetheart of one of Shakespeare's *Two Gentlemen of Verona* (1594). **Variants:** Silva, Silvana, Silvano, Silvia, Sylva, Sylvana, Sylverta, Sylvi, Sylvie, Xylia, Xylina, Zilvia.

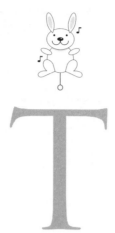

T

Tabitha From the Aramaic, 'gazelle'. In the Bible, the name of a charitable woman looked after by St Peter. A popular Puritan name, falling out of favour with the Victorians. **Variants:** Tabbi, Tabbie, Tabby.

Tacita From the Latin, *tacitum*, 'silent, still, not speaking'. In Roman mythology, the goddess of silence. A popular abstract virtue name for the Puritans. **Variants:** Tace, Tacye.

Taffy Welsh female form of David. **Variants:** Taafe, Tavi, Tavita, Tevita.

Taja From the Arabic, *taj*, 'crown'. Taj-al-Muluk, 'Crown of Kings', was mother of the last Shah of Persia.

Takara Japanese, meaning 'precious object, treasure'.

Tali From the Hebrew, *tal*, 'dew'. **Variants:** Tal, Talia, Talya.

Talia From the Aramaic, 'a lamb'; see also Tali. **Variants:** Tallie, Tally, Talya, Teli, Thalia.

Tallula North American Indian, meaning 'running water'. **Variants:** Tallis, Tallou, Tally, Tallulah.

Talma From the Hebrew, 'small hill'. **Variant:** Talmit.

Talmor From the Arabic, *tal*, 'mound', and *murr*, 'myrrh', thus 'heap of myrrh'. The name implies great preciousness; *see* Myrna.

Talor From the Hebrew, *tal*, 'dew', and *ora*, 'light', thus 'morning dew', implying fresh newness. **Variant:** Talora.

Tamar From the Arabic, *tamr*, 'date palm tree'. The tree is characterised by its height and erectness, and valued for its fruits. By extension, it is associated with perfection. **Variants:** Tamah, Tamara, Tamarah, Tammi, Tammie, Tammy, Temira, Timora, Timi.

Tamarind From the Arabic, *tamr hindi*, 'date from India'. A tropical tree bearing red-striped yellow flowers and producing date fruits.

 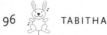

Tamath From the Arabic, *tamasha*, 'to walk around'.

Tamsin *See* Thomasa.

Tangye From the Old Norse, *tangi*, 'sting, point'. Although originally meaning an insect's sting, tang came to mean a sharp prong or pointed knife and hence a sharp, piquant flavour in cooking.

Tania From the Russian, 'fairy queen'. In Shakespeare's comedy, *A Midsummer Night's Dream* (1596), Titania, queen of all the fairy queens and wife of Oberon, is a character taken from the Roman poet, Ovid (43 BC – 18 AD). The accounts of the acts and deeds of St Tatiana, an early Christian martyr, are fabulous, and her identity is so close to two other virgin martyrs, Martina and Priscia, that they are perhaps all the same person. **Variants:** Tanhya, Tanya, Tita, Titania.

Tanith From the Old Irish, *tan*, 'estate'. In Gaelic society, the *tanasiste* was the heir to leadership.

Tao Chinese, meaning 'peach'; *Tao Hua* means 'peach blossom'. The peach is a symbol of longevity and immortality and one of the three sacred Buddhist fruits. The peach tree that bloomed in the mythical garden of the Lady of the West bore its Fruits of Immortality 3000 years later – they were said to have been eaten by the Eight Taoist Immortals.

Tara From the Aramaic, 'to throw, carry'. **Variants:** Tarah, Taryn, Tatiana.

Tasarla English gypsy name, meaning both 'morning' and 'evening'.

Tatum Female form of Tate. **Variants:** Tata, Tate.

Tauba From the German, *taube*, 'dove'. **Variant:** Toby. *See also* Dove.

Tegan From the Celtic, 'doe'.

Tellus From the Latin, *tellus*, 'the earth, the globe, territory'. In ancient Roman mythology, the god Tellumo personified the productive power of the earth. His female partner was Tellus Mater, goddess of fecundity, who both watched over marriage and birth-giving and protected the seeds from the moment they were sown in the soil. After marriage, a bride would offer the goddess a sacrifice before entering her husband's home.

Temima From the Hebrew and Arabic, *tamim*, 'whole, honest'. **Variants:** Tamar, Tamimah.

Temperance From the Latin, *temperantia*, 'moderation, sobriety, discretion, balance'. As with other abstract virtue names, highly popular with the Puritans.

Templa From the Latin, *templum*, 'an open space, a consecrated or sacred place, a sanctuary'.

Terranda From the Latin, *terra*, 'land, soil', and the Greek, *andros*, 'man', thus 'mankind's earth'.

Tertia From the Latin, *tertius*, 'third'. As with Secunda and other numerals, suitable for naming a child according to its position in the family or its date of birth.

Teruma From the Hebrew, 'gift, offering'. **Variant:** Teshura.

Thalassa From the Greek, *thalassa*, 'sea', usually referring to the Mediterranean.

Thalia From the Greek, *thallein*, 'to flourish'. In Greek mythology, the Muse of Comedy, one of the nine muses who presided over music and poetry. Originally nymphs of the springs, they became goddesses and were constant companions to Apollo. Thalia was also one of the Three Graces who spread joy in the hearts of men; *see* Aglaia.

Thana From the Greek, *thanatos*, 'death'. In Greek mythology, Thanatos, god of death, was not sinister and depressing but rather a jolly winged spirit who lived with his brother Hypnos, god of sleep, in the underworld.

Thea From the Greek, *thea*, 'goddess'.

Thekla From the Greek, *thekla*, 'god-famed'. In early Christian stories, the name of the first woman martyr, a convert of St Paul. Revived in the 19th century. **Variants:** Tecla, Tecle.

Thelma Another literary invention, probably from the Greek, *thelema*, 'will'. It was made up by Marie Corelli for the heroine of her successful novel, *Thelma: A Society Novel* (1887). **Variants:** Teli, Telma.

Theodora From the Greek compound, *theos*, 'god', and *doron*, 'gift', thus 'gift of God, divine gift'; female form of Theodore. A name used infrequently since the 17th century. **Variants:** Dora, Fedora, Feodora, Ted, Tedda, Teddi, Teddy, Tedra, Teodora, Thaddea, Thadine, Theda, Thekla, Theo, Theodosia.

Theola From the Greek, 'divine'. **Variant:** Theone.

Theophila From the Greek, *theos*, 'god', and *philos*, 'love', thus 'loved by God'. The name reached its greatest popularity during the 17th century. **Variants:** Offie, Offy, Tesia.

Theresa Probably from the Greek, *therizein*, 'to reap'; alternatively, the Greek may mean 'woman from Therasia', two islands off the coast of Greece. Teresa is the Spanish and Italian form. The first boost for the name came from St Teresa of Avila (1515–82), a Spanish Carmelite nun of intelligence, wit and strong character, who combined an active life of founding 17 strict Carmelite convents with religious contemplation and writing. In 1970 she and St Catherine of Siena were the first women ever to be made doctors of the Church. A more recent Christian is Mother Teresa (born 1910), whose tireless work for the homeless and afflicted she calls simply 'something beautiful for God'. A name carried to England from Spain with the stamp of royalty and Roman Catholicism, but since England was Protestant it was not popular until well after the Reformation, helped first by Maria Theresa (1717–80), Queen of Bohemia and Hungary, and then by another Carmelite nun, the young St Thérèse of Lisieux (1873–97). **Variants:** Resi, Rezi, Tera, Teresa, Terese, Teresina, Teresita, Teressa, Teri, Terri, Terrie, Terrill, Terry, Tess, Tessa, Tessie, Tessy, Thera, Therese, Theresia, Tracey, Tracy, Tresa, Tressa, Tressella, Zita.

Thetis From the Greek, *thetos*, 'dogmatic'. In Greek mythology, one of the beautiful Nereids who was mother of Achilles. *See also* Nerine.

Thirza From the Hebrew, *tirzah*, 'acceptance', or from the name of a city. **Variant:** Thyrza. *See also* Tirza.

Thomasa Female form of Thomas. The female form began to be used in the 14th century and various forms are still popular today. **Variants:** Tamanique, Tamasin, Tamasine, Tami, Tammie, Tammy, Tamsin, Tamzin, Tamzine, Tamzon, Thomasa, Thomasin, Thomasina, Thomasine, Thomasing, Thomassine, Thomson,

Toma, Tomasa, Tomasina, Tomasine, Tommi, Tommianne, Tommy.

Thora From the Norse, 'the thunderer'. In Norse mythology, Thor, also known as Donar, was god of thunder and war, and eldest son of Odin who created the world. He was the most powerful of all gods and the personification of the perfect warrior: noble, simple and always ready to face danger. His name is perpetuated in the day of the week, Thursday, 'Thor's day'. **Variants:** Thodia, Thordis, Tyra.

Thrine From the Greek, 'pure'.

Tiberia From the Latin, *Tiberis*, 'the River Tiber'. A river in central Italy that rises in the Tuscan Apennines and flows some 400 kilometres to empty into the Tyrrhenian Sea at Ostia. On its way it passes through Rome, capital of the Roman Empire and now of Italy.

Tiffany From the Greek, *epiphaneia*, 'manifestation, appearance', thus 'a sudden manifestation of a divine being' or 'a sudden flash of recognition or insight'. The Christian festival of the Epiphany (Twelfth Night) celebrates the revelation of Christ's divinity to the Magi. In French folklore, the word *epiphaneia* became Tifaine and was given to the mother of the Magi; see *Magus*. As a name appropriate for girls and boys born on the Epiphany (January 6), it has been used in Britain since the 13th century. **Variants:** Teffan, Teffany, Thefania, Theophania, Thiphania, Tifaine, Tiffan, Tyffany.

Timothea Female form of Timothy.

Tinkle From the Middle English, *tynclen*, 'the light sound of a small metal bell'. It is especially associated with Christmas bells. The form Tinkerbel was popularised by James Barrie in his play, *Peter Pan: or The Boy Who Would Not Grow Up* (1904), and his later book

of the same story, *Peter and Wendy* (1911), both hugely successful. **Variant:** Tinkabelle, Tinkerbelle.

Tira From the Hebrew, 'enclosure, encampment'.

Tirza From the Hebrew; either 'cypress tree' or 'she will be desirable'. **Variants:** Thirzah, Thyrza.

Tivona From the Hebrew, 'fond of nature'. **Variants:** Tibona, Tiboni, Tivoni.

Toba Female form of Tobias. **Variants:** Tobe, Tobelle, Tobey, Tobi, Tobit, Toby, Tobye, Tova, Tovah, Tove, Tybi, Tybie.

Topaza From the Greek, *topazos*. An aluminium and silicon-based mineral found in granite rocks and polished to be gemstones of shades of blue, yellow and brown.

Tora Japanese, meaning 'tiger'.

Tori Japanese, meaning 'bird'.

Toshi Japanese, meaning 'year'.

Toyah From the Middle English, *toye*, 'amorous sport, dalliance, whims', thus 'one who trifles'.

Tracey *See under boys.*

Tristine Female form of Tristam.

Troth From the Old English, *treowth*, 'truth, pledge, faith'. Another favourite of the 17th-century Puritans.

Tryphena From the Greek, *truphy*, 'daintiness, delicacy'. In the Bible, Tryphena and Tryphosa are both mentioned by St Paul (Romans 16) and both names enjoyed a vogue during the 16th and 17th centuries. Truffeni is the English gypsy derivative. **Variants:** Truffeni, Tryphosa.

 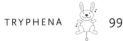

NOAH'S ARK

So many names have animal or bird meanings or associations that a latter-day Noah could probably make a full passenger list for his ark. He would find the fearsome Bernard, Leander, Leonard and Wulfstan; the sly Reynard, Namir the Leopard, and the huge Jumbo. There would be space for Bouvier and for Bowle with his portable house; for Bruno, Chizu, Doe, Dorcas, Felix, Ona, Raleigh, Roswell, Shep, Theodore, Toby (Punch and Judy's dog) and Tzevi. Chanticleer, perched on top of the ark, would crow the morning alarm call. And flying above would be Adler, Calandra, Chilali, Corbet, Falkner, Jay, Malory, Raven and the peace-bringing Columba, Dove and Jonah.

Tuesday From the Old High German, *ziostag*, via the Old English, *Tiwesdaeg*. In Teutonic mythology, Tiw is a son of Odin and brother of Thor. He is a god of war, the counterpart of the Roman god, Mars, and believed by scholars to be related to the Greek god, Zeus.

Turquoise From the Old French, *turqueise*, 'Turkish stone'. A blue or blue-green mineral prized as a precious stone and first found in Turkestan, modern Iran. **Variant:** Turquois.

Twila From the Middle English, *twyle*. A method of weaving that creates diagonal ribs on the finished cloth. **Variant:** Twyla.

Tybal From the Old English, *tiber*, 'holy place, sacrificial spot'. **Variant:** Tyballa.

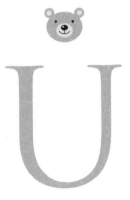

U

Ualani Hawaiian, meaning 'heavenly rain'.

Uda From the Old German, *udo*, 'prosperous'. **Variant:** Udelle.

Ula From the Celtic meaning 'a jewel of the sea'.

Ulalume A name invented by the poet, Edgar Allen Poe, possibly taken from the Latin, 'wailing'.

Ulani Hawaiian, meaning 'bright, light-hearted'.

Ulema From the Arabic, *alim*, 'learned, wise'. **Variant:** Ulima.

Ulla From the Old French, *ouiller*, 'to fill right up'. Ullage is the amount by which a container falls short of being full – hence the name implies making a family complete.

Ulrica Female form of Ulric. **Variants:** Ula, Ulrika, Ulrike.

Ultima From the Latin, *ultima*, 'final, utmost, highest, winner, greatest'. A name denoting supremacy in everything, or a name suitable for a final, ultimate, child.

Ulva From the Old English, *wulf*, 'wolf'. In medieval Europe, a symbol of courage.

Uma Hebrew/Sanskrit name meaning 'the nation' in Hebrew and 'light and peace'. Also the name of a Goddess in Hindu mythology. Recently popularised after American actress Uma Thurman.

Umeko Japanese, meaning 'plum-blossom'. The plum symbolises patience and perseverance.

Una Irish, from the Irish, *uan*, 'lamb', or from the Latin, *una*, 'the very girl' or 'together'. In Spenser's epic poem, *The Faerie Queene* (1596), the poet takes the name to mean 'the oneness of truth' and it is for Una that St George slays the Dragon. This helped the form Unity come into vogue during the 17th century. **Variants:** Oona, Oonagh, Juno, Unity.

Undina From the Latin, *unda*, 'wave, surge, billow'. In Roman mythology, one of the elemental spirits that made up Paracelsus, spirit of the water. She was created without a soul but she could obtain one by marrying a mortal and bearing his child, but this human soul would then have pains and anguishes unknown to deities. **Variant:** Undine.

Uraeus From the Greek, *ouraios*, adapted from the Egyptian word for 'cobra'. In ancient Egypt, the sacred serpent symbolised protection, sovereignty and power and adorned the headress of rulers and gods.

Urania From the Greek, *uranos*, 'heaven'. In Greek mythology, the muse of astronomy, one of the nine muses presiding over music and poetry. Uranus was the earliest supreme god, personification of the sky and heavens. His children were the Titans, whom he hated and kept inside the Earth (see Titus). In astronomy, the plant Uranus, seventh from the sun, was discovered in 1781 and at first named Georgium Sidus in honour of George III.

Urit From the Hebrew, *ohr*, 'light'. **Variants:** Urice, Urith.

Ursula From the Latin, *ursa*, 'she-bear'. In astronomy, the constellation Ursa Major, known as the 'Great Bear', contains the seven stars that make up the Plough, while the stars of Ursa Minor, 'Little Bear', form a ladle. St Ursula has an elaborate and romantic medieval legend surrounding her, but almost no facts. The beautiful English princess escaped marriage by crossing to Europe and visiting Rome with her 11,000 Christian virgin companions. But on their return journey every one of them was martyred by Huns, near Cologne. A popular medieval name, later used by Shakespeare for a gentlewoman in his comedy, *Much Ado About Nothing* (1598). The revival in the last century was a direct response to the heroine of Mrs Craik's bestselling novel, *John Halifax, Gentleman* (1857). **Variants:** Orsa, Orsola, Ursa, Ursala, Ursel, Ursina, Ursine, Ursola, Ursule, Ursulina, Ursuline, Ursy. *See also* Angela.

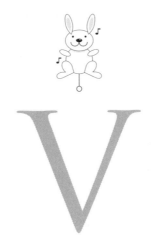

V

Vaino From the Latin, *vanus*, 'empty, unsuccessful, conceited, self-obsessed'. Perhaps because of its meaning, not a very common name.

Valda From the Old Norse, 'ruler, battle heroine'.

Valentine From the Latin, *valens*, 'strong, stout, vigorous, brave, powerful' and also 'hearty, healthy'. The name was spread by the 3rd-century Roman priest, Valentinus, who was martyred on February 13, the day before the pagan festival of Juno, when lots were drawn for lovers. His festival came to be kept on February 14, took on the pagan connotations, and he became patron saint of lovers – valentine cards and other commercial paraphernalia date from the last century. Since the 13th century the name has been given in Britain to either sex, often to a child born on Valentine's Day. **Variants:** Val, Vale, Valeda, Valencia, Valentia, Valentina, Valentino, Valera, Valida, Vallie, Teena, Tina.

Valerie French form of Valentine, from the Latin, *valere*, 'to be strong, healthy'. In ancient Rome, the prominent Valerian family were known for their public service. Introduced from France at the end of the last century. **Variants:** Val, Valaree, Valari, Vale, Valeria, Valery, Valerye, Valora.

Valeska Russian, meaning 'glory, glorious ruler'.

Valonia From the Latin, *balanus*, 'acorn, acorn-like fruit', which included a large type of chestnut and certain kinds of dates. **Variant:** Vallonia.

Vanessa A name invented by Jonathan Swift for his poem, *Cadenus and Vanessa* (1713). The 20-year-old Esther Vanhomrigh was in love with the 43-year-old poet who created her nickname from the first syllable of her surname and a pet form of Esther – Essa. **Variants:** Nessa, Nessi, Nessy, Van, Vania, Vannie, Vanny.

 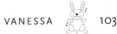

Vania Female form of Ivan.

Vanora From the Celtic, 'white wave'. **Variant:** Vevay.

Varda From the Hebrew and Arabic, *wardah*, 'rose'. **Variants:** Vardia, Vardina, Vardit, Vered.

Vardis Indian name, meaning 'rose'. **Variants:** Varda, Vardia, Vardice, Vardina, Vardit.

Varuna Indian name, the ancient god of the waters whose energy is seen via the shining moon. He is lord of physical and moral order and, together with Mitra, oversees universal order.

Vashti From the Persian, 'beautiful'. In the Bible, wife of King Ahasuerus of Persia.

Veda From the Sanskrit, 'knowledge'. In the pre-Hindu culture of the Indo-Aryans, the holy men compiled religious treatises, called the Vedas.

Vedis From the Singhalese, 'hunter'.

Vega From the Arabic, *al nasr al wagi*, 'the falling vulture', referring to the constellation, Lyra, of which Vega is the brightest star.

Vela From the Latin, *vela*, 'sail', referring to the shape of the constellation, Vela, part of the Milky Way, which is seen in the Southern Hemisphere. **Variant:** Vella.

Velda From the West Germanic, *feld*, 'field, open expanse of land', and thus the further meanings of a field of knowledge, a well-kept playing-field, a range or a field of choice.

Velika Slavic, meaning 'great'.

Velvet From the Latin, *villus*, 'shaggy hair', which came to mean also 'the nap of cloth'. Velvet has a very soft and smooth nap.

Venetia From the Latin, *venia*, 'kindness, mercy, forgiveness'. The Veniti people lived in Venetia in northern Italy, and their main city was Venice. Also an English form of Gwyneth. **Variants:** Venda, Veneta, Venita, Vinetia, Vinita.

Ventura Spanish, meaning 'fortune, good luck'.

Venus From the Latin, 'love, loveliness, beloved, sexual love'. In Roman mythology, supreme goddess of love and counterpart to the Greek Aphrodite, with all her origins and attributes. Although married to Vulcan, god of fire, she had affairs with many other gods including Mercury, by whom she had Cupid, another god of desire and love. As Venus Genetrix, 'who has given birth', she was also a symbol of marriage and motherhood. In astronomy, the second planet from the sun, Earth being the fourth. **Variants:** Venita, Vinita, Vin, Vinnie, Vinny.

Vera From the Russian, *viera*, 'faith'. A favourite Russian Christian name, introduced to Britain in the mid-19th century. *See also* Olga.

Verdi From the Latin, *virere*, 'to be green', usually referring to the verdant, lush and healthy vegetation of springtime. **Variants:** Verda, Verne, Vernee, Vernie, Vernique, Vernita, Vernona, Virida, Viridis.

Verena From the Latin, *veritas*, 'truth, reality, the truth of nature, integrity'. **Variants:** Vera, Veradis, Vere, Verene, Verina, Verine, Verinka, Verita, Verity, Verla, Verna, Verochka, Veronica, Virna.

Veronica From the Latin, *veraiconica*, 'true image'. According to the Christian legend,

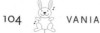

the woman who wiped Christ's face when he was carrying the cross up to Calvary and who then discovered Christ's image on the piece of cloth. With this miracle, she became patron saint of photographers. A name first popularised in France, carried to Scotland in the 17th century and to England in the 19th. Sometimes confused with Berenice. **Variants:** Ronni, Ronnie, Vera, Veronika, Veronike, Veronique, Vonnie, Vonny.

Vespera From the Greek, *hesperos*, 'evening'. Vesper is the evening star and a vesper is the evening bell which summons the faithful to vespers, evening prayers.

Vesta In Roman mythology, goddess of the hearth, counterpart to the Greek Hestia, with all her symbolism. In the Temple of Vesta in ancient Rome the virgin priestesses, known as the Vestal Virgins, tended the sacred fire. In astronomy, the third largest asteroid of the solar system.

Vevila From the Celtic, 'harmonious'.

Victoria From the Latin, 'victorious'. Queen Victoria (1819–1901) reigned from 1837 until her death. During her reign Britain was immensely powerful and the British empire expanded rapidly; she became Empress of India in 1877. Her personal qualities of sense of duty, self-improvement and strict morals were highly influential and characterised the age named after her. Equally influential was the example of a huge family–four sons and five daughters–and the names of her children: Victoria, Albert Edward, Alice, Alfred, Helena (see Helen), Louise, Arthur, Leopold and Beatrice. The south-eastern state of Australia, the capitals of British Columbia in Canada and of Hong Kong, the largest lake in Africa, the waterfalls on the Zambezi river, a

railway station, a pigeon, a planet, a variety of plum and the highest military decoration are all named after her. **Variants:** Vici, Vick, Vicki, Vickie, Vicky, Victoire, Victorine, Vika, Viki, Vikie, Vikki, Vikkie, Viktorija, Vita, Vitoria, Vittoria, Viqui.

Vila From the Latin, *villa*, 'country house, farm'.

Vincentia Female form of Vincent. **Variant:** Vinnette.

Vinia From the Latin, *vinum*, 'wine, grapes'.

Viola Italian, from the Old Provençal, *violar*, 'to play the viol', a four-stringed musical instrument slightly larger than a violin. A viola da gamba, or viol, was very popular during the 16th and 17th centuries. A name popularised by the heroine of Shakespeare's comedy, *Twelfth Night* (1601). *See also* Violet.

Violet From the Latin, *viola*, 'violet or stock, gilly flower'. In botany, a genus of low-growing plants with purple-blue, or sometimes yellow or white, blossoms. The flower gives its name to the deep purple colour. The name was found in the Middle Ages, symbolising modesty, and was thus a flower name in use long before the flower vogue of the turn of this century. **Variants:** Vi, Viola, Violante, Violeta, Violetta, Violette, Voleta, Voletta, Yolanda, Yolane. *See also* Eolande.

Virgilia Female form of Virgil.

Virginia Probably from the Latin, *virginius*, 'manly race', rather than *virginitas*, 'maiden-hood, virginity', although the name has absorbed both meanings. The name of a Roman maiden of the 5th century BC whose father stabbed her to death to save her from the amorous clutches of one of the unpopular city officials. He then raised a revolt in the

 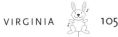

forum and a more paternalistic government replaced the one overthrown. In America, Virginia was named by Sir Walter Raleigh in 1584 after Elizabeth I (1533–1603), who was known as the 'Virgin Queen'. Although popular in France during the 18th century, the name caught on in Britain only towards the end of the last century, probably due to the hugely successful romance, *Paul et Virginie* (1878), by Bernardin de Saint-Pierre. **Variants:** Ginnie, Ginny, Virgie, Virginie.

Vita From the Latin, 'life, living, mankind, a lifetime'. **Variant:** Vida. *See also* Victoria.

Vivien From the Latin, *vivus*, 'alive, possessing life'. Found in England by the Middle Ages and mostly given to boys. When Tennyson published his poem, *Vivien and Merlin* (1859), based on an Arthurian romance, the witty enchantress-heroine revived and popularised the name for girls; see also Arthur and Merlin. **Variants:** Bibiana, Fithian, Vevay, Viv, Viveca, Vivevca, Vivi, Vivian, Viviana, Vivie, Vivienne, Vyvyan.

Volante Italian, from the Latin, *volare*, 'to fly'.

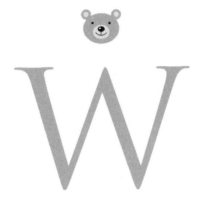

W

Wacil From the Old English, *wac*, 'slothful, weak, mean'.

Wahalla From the Old Norse, *valr*, 'those killed in battle', and *holl*, 'hall', thus 'hall of immortality'. In Norse mythology, the place where the souls of slain warrior heroes were received and enshrined by Odin, god of war, intelligence and law. Here, too, the warrior soul collected all his wordly possessions that had been burnt with his body on the funeral pyre. **Variants:** Valhalla, Walhalla.

Wahkuna North American Indian, from *warnhu*, 'wood of arrows'.

Waikiki Hawaiian, meaning 'spring of water, gushing water', carrying the symbolism of the nourishing water of life.

Wakenda From the Old Norse, *vakna*, 'wake up, rouse to activity, stir up'.

Walburga The 8th-century English saint was abbess of the double monastery of Heidenheim and then strangely became part of the German legend surrounding May 1, the night of witchcraft known as Walpurgisnacht.

Walda Female form of Walter.

Wallis From the Old Norse, *val*, 'choice, selection'; from the Old English, *weallan*, 'to boil, gush forth'; or from the Old English, *wall*, 'defence, fortification, rampart'. It was for love of Mrs Wallis Simpson that Edward VIII forfeited his throne. Also a female form of Wallace. **Variants:** Wallie, Wally.

Wanda From the Old Norse, *wandur* and *vondr*, 'a straight, slender stick, a young shoot'. As a carved ebony or silver rod, it is a sign of office, such as in the Church, a royal household or halls of justice. The phrase 'a wave of the wand' implies actions of magic, speed and skill beyond human ability, such as magicians, witches and gods perform. **Variants:** Vanda, Vandis, Vona, Vonda, Wanaka, Wandie, Wandis, Wandy, Wenda, Wendeline, Wendi, Wendy, Wendye.

Wannetta From the Old English, *wann*, 'dark, gloomy', but now implying a pale complexion. **Variant:** Wanette.

Wapeka From the Old Norse, *vapn*, 'weapon, instrument for self-defence and protection'.

Warrene Female form of Warren. **Variants:** Warnette, Waurene.

Wasila From the Middle English, *waes haeil*, or *wassayl*, 'be in good health', the old version of 'cheers' when drinking someone's health. Also, the liquor used to drink people's health, especially the spiced ale traditionally swilled amid the revelry on Twelfth Night (January 6) and New Year's Eve – hence the term wassailers for people singing carols and songs.

Welcome From the Old English, *wil*, 'desire, pleasure', and *cuma*, 'arrival', thus 'someone who gives pleasure by their arrival'. Also given to boys.

Wenda From the Gaelic, *gwen*, 'fair', or from the Old Norse, *venda*, 'to change course, to travel, to move forward'. **Variants:** Vendelin, Wendeline, Wendey, Wendi, Wendy. *See also* Gwendolen and Winifred.

Wendy A name invented by the children's novelist and playwright, James Barrie (1860–1937) by his child friend, Margaret. It was probably evolved from her pronunciation of the word 'friend' as 'fwend'. Widespread after the success of Barrie's play, *Peter Pan: or The Boy Who Would Not Grow Up* (1904); *see* Tinkle. *See also* Gwendolen, Gwyneth and Wanda. **Variant:** Wanda.

Wenona From the Old High German, *wunja*, via the Old English, *wynn*, 'provider of joy and bliss' as well as 'being joyful and blissfully happy'. **Variants:** Wenonah, Winona, Wynona.

Werburgh Like Walburga, one of the several 8th-century English saint abbesses, this time a princess. Her shrine at Chester was a place of pilgrimage until its destruction during the Reformation. The other abbess-saints include St Cuthburga and St Cyneburga.

Whaley From the Old English, *hwael*, 'big fish' and, by extension, anything large. The slang words 'whacker' and 'whopper' come from this.

Whitney From the old English term meaning 'one from the white island', Whitney became increasingly popular after American singer Whitney Houston.

Wilda Female form of Willoughby. **Variant:** Willow.

Wilfreda Female form of Wilfred.

Wilhelmina Female form of William. As a girl's name, introduced to Britain from Germany or Holland during the 18th century. **Variants:** Bill, Billy, Guglielma, Guillelmine, Guillema, Guillemette, Helma, Mimi, Mina, Minna, Minnette, Vilhelmina, Vilma, Vilna, Wileen, Wilhelma, Wilhelmine, Willa, Willabelle, Willamae, Willamina, Willandra, Willene, Willeta, Willetta, Willette, Willi, Willy, Wilma, Wilmena, Wilmet, Wilmette, Wylma.

Willow From the English name of a tree that grows near water.

Wilona From the Old English, *wil*, 'desire, pleasure', thus 'desired or wished for'.

Winema North American Indian, meaning 'woman chief'.

Winifred From the Old English, *wine*, 'friend', and *frithu*, 'peace', thus 'friend of peace' or 'gentle friend', or the English form of the Welsh name, Gwenfrewi, meaning either 'white wave' or 'blessed reconciliation'. St Winifred, also called Gwenfrewi, was a wonder of medicine, according to her legend. When her head was chopped off by a repulsed suitor, the ground opened up to swallow him while her uncle, St Bueno, put her head back on and she lived a good life as a nun until the end of her days. In addition, the water that sprang from where her head had fallen possessed medicinal curing powers, spreading the saint's cult to England by the 12th century, although the name was not used much until the 16th. **Variants:** Freda, Freddi, Freddie, Freddy, Fredi, Guinever, Gwenevere, Gwenfrewi, Gwinevere, One, Oona, Usa, Vinnette, Wenefreda, Win, Winefred, Winnie, Winnifred, Winny, Wyn, Wynelle, Wynette, Wynne. *See also* Gwendolen and Gwyneth.

Winona North American Indian, meaning 'first-born daughter'. **Variants:** Wenona, Wenonoah, Winnie, Winonah. *See also* Wenona as popularised by actress Winona Ryder.

Woodren Female form of Woodrow.

 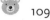

X

Xanthe From the Greek, *xanthos*, 'yellow'. Xanthous is a yellowish-brown colour, so a person with a xanthocroid complexion is fair. Thus a name suitable for a fair girl. **Variant:** Xantha.

Xanthippe From the Greek, *xanthos*, 'yellow', and *hippos*, 'horse', thus 'yellow horse'. The name of the long-suffering wife of the somewhat eccentric Greek philosopher, Socrates (469–399 BC), although she was supposed to have given him a hard time with her scolding and shrewish behaviour.

Xaviera Female form of Xavier. **Variant:** Xavier.

Xenia From the Greek, *xenos*, 'stranger, guest' and also 'hospitable person'. In botany, xenogamy is cross-pollination between plants. A xenophobe is someone who dislikes strangers and foreigners and their cultures. **Variants:** Cena, Xena, Xene, Ximena, Xiomara, Zena, Zenia.

Ximenia In botany, the genus of tropical herbs and trees, named after the Spanish missionary, Ximenes. Chimene, the French form, was the heroine of Corneille's play, *Le Cid* (1636). **Variants:** Chimene, Ximena.

Xylophila From the Greek, *xulon*, 'wood', and *philia*, 'love', thus 'someone who loves woods and forests'. In art, xylography is wood-block printing; in music, a xylophone is a percussion instrument made of wooden bars of decreasing length. **Variant:** Xylona.

OLIVER TWIST ASKS FOR MORE

Names are often invented or given fresh popularity by writers. Just as Geraldine was made up for a love poem, so Percival was created for a romantic hero and Lorna for R. D. Blackmore's successful novel, *Lorna Doone*. Vanbrugh probably invented Amanda, Sir Philip Sidney created Pamela, and Jonathan Swift made up Vanessa. The vivid characters in the highly successful novels of Sir Walter Scott promoted Ellen, Fergus, Flora and Waverley. The same is true for the equally vibrant Dorrit, Oliver and Pip of Charles Dickens. More recently, Ian Fleming's handsome and smooth James Bond has surely produced some namesakes.

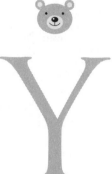

Y

Yakira From the Hebrew, 'precious'.

Yardena Female form of Yarden and Jordan.

Yarkona From the Hebrew, *yarok*, 'green'. A bird with yellow-green plumage that spends summers in Israel and winters in Egypt.

Yasu Japanese, meaning 'peaceful'.

Yatva From the Hebrew, *tov*, 'good'.

Yedida From the Hebrew, 'dear friend'. **Variant:** Yedidah.

Yehiela Female form of Jehiel, from Jedaiah. **Variant:** Yehiella.

Yeira From the Hebrew, *ohr*, 'light'.

Yelena From the Latin, 'lily blossom'. **Variants:** Lenusya, Liolya. *See also* Helen.

Yemina Female form of Benjamin.

Yepa North American Indian, meaning 'snow maiden'.

Yeshisha From the Hebrew, 'old'.

Yigaala Female form of Yigal. **Variant:** Yigala.

Yoi Japanese, meaning 'born in the evening'.

Yoko Japanese, meaning 'positive, female'. In Japanese philosophy, Yo and In lay dormant in an egg until it split into heaven and earth.

Yolanda From the Latin, 'modest'; a form of Eolande; or, the most likely, from Violante, from Viola. **Variants:** Eolande, Iolanthe, Iolende, Jolande, Joleicia, Jolenta, Olinda, Yolande, Yolane, Yolanthe.

Yona Female form of Jonah. **Variant:** Yonina.

Yoshi Japanese, meaning 'good, respectful'. Also given to boys. **Variant:** Yoshiko.

Yovela From the Hebrew, *yobhel*, 'ram's horn', because that was used to proclaim a special anniversary, via the Latin, *jubilaeus*, 'the year of jubilee, a joyful time of celebration'. *See also* Jubal.

Yuki Japanese, meaning 'snow, lucky'. **Variants:** Yukie, Yukiko.

Yulan Chinese, from *yu lan*, 'jade orchid', a type of magnolia tree cultivated for its large, cup-shaped fragrant white flowers.

Yullis From the Old Norse, *jol*, a heathen festival lasting 12 days, adapted as the Old English, *geola*, and then *yule* and *yule-tide*. Or from the Old Norse, *ylir*, the calendar month starting about half-way through November, later called *giuli* in Old English.

Yvonne Female form of the French name, Yves, from John. Its popularity has increased in this century. **Variants:** Evona, Evonne, Ivetta, Yevette, Yve, Yvette.

Note: many names beginning with Y can also begin with J.

Z

Zada Syrian, meaning 'lucky one'.

Zahara From the Swahili, 'flower'.

Zaida From the Arabic, 'good fortune, growth'.

Zara From the Arabic, 'dawn'. **Variant:** Zarah. *See also* Sarah.

Zariza From the Hebrew, 'industrious'. **Variant:** Zeriza.

Zaza From the Hebrew, 'movement'. **Variant:** Zazu.

Zea From the Latin, *zea*, 'a grain' or 'a variety of rosemary'.

Zehava From the Hebrew, *zahav*, 'gold, brilliantly bright'. **Variants:** Zehara, Zehari, Zehavi, Zehavit, Zehuva, Zohar, Zoheret.

Zehira From the Hebrew, 'protected'.

Zelia From the Hebrew, *zelus*, 'zealous, ardent'. **Variants:** Zele, Zelie, Zelina.

Zena From the Persian, *zan*, 'woman'. **Variant:** Zenia.

Zenda From the Persian, *zend*, 'sacred'.

Zenobia See Seema. Name of the Queen of Palmyra, who became regent for her son after her husband, Odenathus, died in 267 AD. Under her, the empire grew to include Syria, Egypt and part of Asia Minor until defeat and capture by the Romans in 272 AD. **Variants:** Zena, Zenaida, Zenda, Zenia, Zenna, Zenobie, Zinaida.

Zephira From the Hebrew, 'morning'.

Zephyr From the Greek, *zephuros*, 'the west wind'. In Greek mythology, Zephyr (or Zephyros), god of the west wind, was benign son of Eos, goddess of dawn, and brought soft, gentle winds.

Zeta From the Hebrew, *zevit*, 'olive'. **Variants:** Zayit, Zetana, Zetta.

Zeva Female form of Zev.

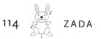

Zevida From the Hebrew, *zeved*, 'gift'. **Variants:** Zevuda.

Zevula Female form of Zebulun.

Zia From the Hebrew, 'to tremble'.

Zila From the Hebrew, *tzel*, 'shade'. Found in Britain since the Reformation. A favourite English gypsy name. **Variants:** Zila, Zilla, Zillah, Zilli.

Zilpah From the Hebrew, 'dripping, sprinkling'.

Zimra From the Hebrew, *zemer*, 'branch' or 'song of praise'. **Variants:** Zamoka, Zamora, Zemira, Zemora, Zimria, Zimriah.

Zinnia In botany, the genus of tropical plants from the USA, now cultivated in Britain for their brightly coloured blooms. They are named after the German botanist and physician, Johann Gottfried Zinn (1727–59). **Variants:** Zeena, Zina.

Ziona Female form of Zion. **Variant:** Zeona.

Zippora From the Hebrew, *tzipor*, 'bird'. In the Bible, the wife of Moses. **Variants:** Cipora, Zipporah.

Zita See Theresa. Also a Spanish name, meaning 'little rose', and a French name, meaning 'bedroom' – the French St Zita is patron saint of domestic servants.

Ziva From the Hebrew, 'to shine out brightly'. **Variant:** Zivit.

Zoe *See* Eve. Zoe was the Greek translation of the Hebrew, *hawwah*, first used when the Alexandrian Jews translated the Bible. It was immediately popular as a Christian name, having none of the sacred immunity of Mary, but it has been used in Britain only since the last century.

Zola *See under boys.*

Zona From the Greek, 'girdle, belt'.

Zora *See* Sarah. Also, from the Slavonic, 'dawn'. **Variants:** Zarya, Zohra, Zorah, Zorana, Zoreen, Zoreene, Zorene, Zorina, Zorine, Zorna.

Zsa Zsa Hungarian form of Susan. **Variant:** Zsusanna.

Zuleika From the Arabic, 'pretty, fair girl'. In the Bible, the name of Potiphar's wife. Max Beerbohm's satire, *Zuleika Dobson: or An Oxford Love Story* was published in 1911; *see* Maximilian.

Zulema From the Arabic name, Suleima, 'peace'. **Variants:** Zuelia, Zuleika. *See also* Salome.

YOUR BABY'S HOROSCOPE

by Penny Thornton DF ASTROLS

To attain accurate and individual personal characteristics through astrology, the entire horoscope – including all the planets, the Moon and the Ascending sign – needs to be judged. The Sun-sign is only a small, although very important, part of the whole birth-chart. A child who does not greatly resemble his or her Sun-sign may well have *only* the sun in that sign, while the remainder of the chart presents a radically different picture. Also, many astrologers consider that the Moon and the Ascending sign are far more indicative of a child's nature, and that the Sun-sign potential does not develop until adolescence.

Some of the words associated with the 'elements' of the zodiac signs have passed into our everyday language. The airy character is communicative, and associated with thoughts and concepts; while the fiery person is spontaneous, enthusiastic and impulsive. If a child's Sun sign is of the earth group, he will be practical and organised, whereas the watery person has characteristics that are emotional, intuitive and sensitive. The 'quality' of a sign is equally important. Fixed and mutable mean, as they imply, characteristics such as resistance to change, and adaptability. The 'cardinal' element is less well-known – a child born under signs in this group will show great self-motivation and will always seek to take the initiative throughout his life.

Aries *March 20 – April 20*
Element *Fire* Quality *Cardinal*
Ignoring your Aries youngster is going to be difficult. Master and Miss Aries like to be noticed; second place is not for them. Even from the pram the Aries babe has a commanding presence and an insistent personality. Provided everything is to his satisfaction, he'll beam and gurgle contentedly; but delay his feed, his walk, his bath, or

forget to serve Marmite soldiers with his egg, and he'll provide a startling rendition of a miniature distressed whale.

Aries babies usually reach their milestones early–pioneers to a lamb. They can't wait to talk to you and find their independent way around the world. But as in adult life, they tend to up-end themselves all too easily and put their foot in their mouth a little too often.

Master and Miss Aries are frequently the adventurous sort: they seem drawn, like magnets, to the most difficult and dangerous route to their goals. Arians also love anything new, and tend to throw themselves headlong into experiences–sometimes quite literally.

Aries children rarely move in mysterious ways. They are frank, open, affectionate, loyal and trusting. They wear their hearts on their sleeves, and are easily crushed and deflated. Their less laudable traits include arrogance, selfishness, inconsideration and insubordination.

Some little Arians put all their energies into mental pursuits, for this sign is renowned for its quickness and brightness, while others forge ahead in more physical or creative areas. They tend to be ambitious and competitive, and most make extremely bad losers.

Sometimes the Aries child *appears* reticent, even shy, but by adolescence almost all will show the forceful, assertive qualities of this sign. Of one thing you can be sure, life with an Aries child will never be dull.

Taurus *April 20–May 21*
Element *Earth* Quality *Fixed*
The Taurean infant is usually one of the most placid, contented and amenable in the Zodiac. That is, unless you have one of the really stubborn sort. This sign is noted both for its peaceful, accommodating nature *and* its stoic resistance. Try to get your Taurean child to do something against his will, and you'll need the strength of an all-in wrestler and the patience of Job. This infant knows what's best for him, and unless you intend to go prematurely grey, acquiescence is usually the better part of valour.

The best way to a little Taurean's heart is through his tummy. Indeed, the baby Bull can become quite a gourmet as he grows up. Sometimes a sweet tooth, combined with the Taurean aversion to strenuous activity, can make him on the chubby side.

Taurean children are enormously sensual, and many are artistically gifted; most, at the very least, love painting, singing and dancing. The baby Taurean will love to be cuddled and cosseted, and the more secure he feels the better. Taureans, young and old, tend to find change extremely threatening. Your little Taurus is far happier in family surroundings, safe in his normal routine and, unless there are many airy or fiery planets in his chart, he will need considerable coercion to adapt to a new order.

Reliability, gentleness and sensitivity are Taurus' strengths; intractability, possessiveness and rigidity are its more negative features.

Master and Miss Taurus are not the Zodiac's trailblazers. The Bull likes to take his time. He may appear a little slow to grasp new concepts, but once he understands something, he rarely forgets it. He is fundamentally a practical, sensible sort and, as he grows older, almost always responds to good commonsense.

Introverted or extroverted, your little Bull knows where he's going in life, and no matter how sweetly or gently it's done, the Taurean will make sure that nobody – not even you – stands in his way.

Gemini *May 21 – June 21*
Element *Air* Quality *Mutable*

Some books maintain that young babies sleep for 23 hours out of 24; unfortunately, few Geminian babies seem to have read any of them. These Mercurial mites are curious about the world from the moment they emerge from the womb. They don't like to miss a thing (a habit they never grow out of) and care little about the time of day or night when it comes to their favourite pastime – socialising.

From their first days, Geminian babies need toys to stimulate their minds, and plenty of trips in the pram or car to satisfy their need for movement and changing vistas. Master or Miss Gemini will probably be an early talker and start walking as soon as strength permits. Most will drive you to distraction with endless questions, but also reward you with their comical remarks and quaint assumptions.

Geminian youngsters are easily bored. Unless there is plenty to interest and amuse them they become naughty and obstreperous. Since they hate to lose out on activity of any sort, many of them push themselves into frenetic overdrive at times. Until they are able to work off their apparently inexhaustible supply of energy and their need for constant stimulation in playgroups or school, your time will be spent carting them off to zoos, amusement parks and the like.

The Geminian child is often highly intelligent. He learns quickly but, since his concentration span tends to be short and his mind easily diverted, he sometimes fails to maximise his intellectual abilities.

Manual dexterity, mental and physical agility, mimicry and humour are all good Gemini traits; unreliability, mendacity and superficiality are its less desirable features.

Whether you have one of the more familiar bubbly, ubiquitous Geminians, or one of the introverted sort, his quicksilver mind will continually fascinate and enchant you.

Cancer *June 21 – July 22*
Element *Water* Quality *Cardinal*

Mother is the most important and special person in the world to the Cancerian, whether he's 3 months old or 93. He'll never forget the feelings of security and sensuality he experienced in his mother's arms, especially at the breast. As a child, the Cancerian tends to mother his siblings, and when he grows up, he often marries and starts a family early.

This sign is one of the most sensitive and impressionable in the Zodiac. Both male and female Crabs need an enormous amount of love and physical closeness to become confident and secure outside the family. Most are exceedingly loving, helpful and keen to please, but sometimes they can be appallingly clingy and whingey. They have huge emotional ups and downs – one moment they are sunny, sweet and outgoing and the next moody, sullen and remote. Many Cancerian children have artistic abilities, and they are at their best using their rich imaginations to read and make up stories.

Cancerians, young and old, are often avid collectors. Whether it's photographs, old bus tickets, stamps or antiques, the Cancerian can be relied upon to hoard them away in a secret, secure place along with all his other memorabilia. Crabs also have memories like proverbial elephants, and always remember where they've buried the hatchet!

Compassion, feeling, responsiveness, tenacity and determination are Cancer's strengths; defensiveness, secretiveness and meanness are its weaknesses.

Despite their sensitivity, Cancerian little boys and girls can be ambitious and masterful. Success matters to them tremendously. Rather than fail at a task, they'll often avoid it completely. They also hate to be ridiculed – to the extent that some of them can't take a joke about themselves at all.

Cancerians' struggle for independence is a hard one, and no matter how far they wander in life, home is where they secretly yearn to be.

Leo *July 22 – August 23*
Element *Fire* Quality *Fixed*

Leo children are the Zodiac's greatest actors and entertainers. Centre-stage in the limelight is their natural habitat, and woe betide any other contenders for the leading role – inside or outside the family.

Little Leos are full of smiles and engaging coquetry, but if they cannot get their way, or your undivided attention, they'll scream, shout and throw a show-stopping drama instead. These children are full of personality and enthusiasm, and most are enormously difficult to suppress or subdue. Sometimes they show off unbearably, but often their precocious talent to amuse is outstanding.

Master and Miss Leo enjoy play and activity far more than quiet and studiousness; they are highly creative individuals and in their element when building extraordinary constructions out of cardboard boxes and pipe cleaners, or liberally splashing paint on a giant mural. Many display literary talents at a remarkably early age.

The Leo infant is a natural leader, although sometimes he is a little over-zealous with his authority. Even the shyer type of Leo can be very bossy. Sometimes they lose a few friends by being over-pushy and self-important, but children born under this sign rarely suffer from loneliness.

Generosity, decisiveness and honour are Leo's qualities; pride, dogmatism and obstinacy are its faults.

Leos, both children and adults, tend to hold a rather high opinion of themselves. When they cannot win at games or shine in their endeavours, they become truculent and rebellious. Most also take a keen interest in their appearance, and love wearing new clothes – the brighter the colours the better.

A quiet moment may be difficult to find with your Leo child, but his sunny personality and warmhearted nature will spread enormous fun and happiness throughout your life.

Virgo *August 23 – September 23*
Element *Earth* Quality *Mutable*

Virgos often suffer in silence – but *ask* their opinion about anything, and you'll be subjected to a full and precise analysis, liberally laced with criticism. Even baby Virgos can make you feel guilty if you've forgotten their favourite mittens or failed to mash their banana finely enough. This perfectionist sign rarely makes a song and dance about its needs, but it's wise to remember that 'silence hath a mighty sound'.

Bright and inquisitive, industrious and thorough, the Virgoan infant is never far from the hub of activity. These considerate children are often very helpful, hoovering the carpet with their musical push toys, or cleaning the loo with Daddy's toothbrush! Their highly intelligent minds need plenty of stimulation, which is why as babies they are often fractious and restless. These are the children best suited to educational toys, and also the ones who insist that you never change so much as a single word in their night-time story.

Virgos of all ages tend to worry excessively; they also prefer to hold their emotions in check and rarely voice their doubts and fears. (Parents of a Virgo child will soon learn to spot major distress by any obsessive behaviour.) Organisation and routine is a must for them – little Virgos believe that there is a right place for everything. Although this is one of the shyer signs, these children often have a talent for acting which, combined with their helpful, considerate natures, makes them popular companions.

On the plus side, Virgos are dependable, dutiful, sensible and painstaking; conversely they can be carping, shrewish, neurotic and negative.

Although, as children, Master and Miss Virgo may have you running round in ever-decreasing circles, rest assured that they will do exactly the same for you when you're drawing your old-age pension.

Libra *September 23 – October 23*
Element *Air* Quality *Cardinal*

Libran babies can be some of the prettiest and most pleasing in the Zodiac. Almost all come into the world equipped with the knowledge that smiles and gurgles (later charm and flattery) will get them everywhere in life. This sign is extremely harmonious and obliging and, unless there are many stressful factors in the birth-chart, Libran infants are rarely difficult or unmanageable.

Making up their minds always presents a problem for Librans of any age. Never give Master or Miss Libra a choice – you'll go grey watching them decide which jumper looks best, or which nursery rhyme they want. What often makes their dilemma worse is that they're also trying to please you!

Libran children are sensitive souls. Most hate crowded places, loud noises and unpleasant surroundings. They also dislike sticky fingers, and cannot remain in a mess for long. Quarrelling adults or a severe reprimand upsets them deeply although, as they grow older, they seem all too keen to argue each and every point, and will play the devil's advocate. Despite their personable, easy-going natures, Libran children are nevertheless ambitious and competitive. Even those who are not academically gifted usually excel in some other area of life.

Master and Miss Libra usually enjoy artistic pursuits, especially music and dancing; most seem to have natural grace and an in-built sense of balance and style. However, they can be on the lazy side, and it's frequently the Libran infant who places walking last on his list of priorities, although he may well be a precocious communicator.

The ability to mediate, to decide fairly and to use diplomacy and tact are Libra's attributes; argumentativeness, superficiality and social climbing are its drawbacks.

Although tempting, 'to spare the rod and spoil the child' is not always the best policy with little Librans. Underneath their delicate and charming exteriors, they're really quite tough.

Scorpio *October 23 – November 22*
Element *Water* Quality *Fixed*

As far as Scorpio children go, 'When they're good, they're very, very good, but when they're bad ...' This is a sign of radical extremes; like the Cancerian, it's all smiles one minute and emotional torrents the next. From birth, this little individual seems convinced that life is a battleground, so he has come well prepared – he has a stainless steel backbone and the sort of willpower that moves mountains – or, at least, you.

Master and Miss Scorpio are acutely aware of, and responsive to, their mothers' emotional states, which is why the more inexperienced, first-time mother frequently finds her Scorpio baby difficult to manage. But be warned; these small Scorpios are physically and psychologically extremely strong, and will manipulate you mercilessly if given the chance.

Scorpio infants require Jumbo-sized helpings of love and security. Like any child they need rules and discipline, but the Scorpio toddler in a tantrum will calm down far quicker with a big hug than a smack – he's probably terrified by the power of his own anger, and doesn't need yours as well.

Routine and the familiar are important for little Scorpios; they become deeply attached to those they love, from their families to their moth-eaten comforters. Sudden change or the loss of a beloved possession can devastate them completely. Scorpio infants are also immensely loyal, and can be relied upon to keep a secret or protect a friend, even if they themselves suffer in the process.

Scorpios of any age hate to be pushed or rushed into anything, and their progress is always improved by praise and encouragement rather than criticism or threats. Once they feel confident in their abilities, they can soar.

Determination, single-mindedness, resourcefulness and tenacity are Scorpio's strengths; manipulation, vengefulness and obstinacy are its faults.

Although your little Scorpio extremist may give you a few sleepless nights, with plenty of love and understanding he'll make the sort of indelible mark on life of which you can be proud.

Sagittarius *November 22 – December 21*
Element *Fire* Quality *Mutable*

Sagittarian babies are the family's most special Christmas present. They arrive when the Christmas shopping is at or near its peak, just in time for all the celebrations. It is clearly no cosmic coincidence that these are the Zodiac's jolliest and most extravagant souls.

The Sagittarian child wants to be everyone's pal, and does his best to amuse all of the people all of the time. He learns to smile and chuckle early, and treats feeding and changing time as a fun and games period. However, despite their cheeky grins, December babies can be wearing on their parents, with their restless natures and inconsiderate ways.

The Sagittarian asserts his independence from the moment he can crawl. First, the allure of the next-door neighbour's garden beckons and, before you know it, it's Katmandu! Sadly, the parents of Sagittarian boys and girls come poor seconds to their hobbies, friends and their wanderlust.

Like the Geminian, this infant needs plenty of variety in his life – he loves socialising and visiting distant relations and friends. Unless he has one of the gentler, more passive signs on the Ascendant, he'll treat sleep as an unwanted interruption to his hectic schedule – only closing his eyes when he (and you) are thoroughly exhausted.

Sometimes these children are exceedingly bright, but often their impatience to move on to the next item means they fail to retain all they've learned. Also, with their slap-dash, happy-go-lucky natures, they often appear irresponsible to others.

Master and Miss Sagittarius always seem to be in a hurry; they rarely have time to button their coats or do up their shoe-laces; consequently, with their eyes permanently gazing into the distance, they tend to be rather accident-prone.

Optimism, honesty, geniality and broad-mindedness are Sagittarius' strengths; over-enthusiasm, rudeness and inconsideration are its weaknesses.

Make the most of your little Sagittarian's childhood, because as an adult he or she will drop in and out of your life with the irregularity of a London bus!

Capricorn *December 21 – January 20*
Element *Earth* Quality *Cardinal*
Life is a serious business to Capricorn. Even the new-born Goat seems to have a worldly-wise expression on his face and, as a child, he seems older than his years and more serious than his friends.

This child has an uncanny knack of making you feel inadequate at times. He's not the sort to throw noisy tantrums when he can't get his way – he'll simply refuse to budge from his position. There's also no point in trying to jolly him out of a sulk – you'll end up feeling frustrated and faintly ridiculous. Even the smallest Capricorns get a perverted pleasure out of feeling hard-done-by.

Master and Miss Capricorn adapt well to routine. They are very practical, efficient and organised children. Capricorn infants will line up their toys neatly, and place their carefully constructed lego space-ships (made exactly according to the instructions) out of reach of their younger siblings.

Capricorn children like to do well at school. They hardly ever work in fits and starts – they plod determinedly up the academic mountain, accepting the odd failure and obstacle as par for the course. They make excellent prefects and form captains – leadership and responsibility are second nature to them. Sometimes they can be rather autocratic, a tendency that, unfortunately, increases with age.

Don't be misled by their stalwart personalities; underneath their capable exteriors they're exceedingly sensitive and need plenty of affection and encouragement. They are tremendously loyal to their loved ones and prefer one or two special friends to a great many acquaintances.

Capricorns are renowned for their reliability, consistency, coolness and sense of honour; they can also be ruthless, callous, rigid and cold.

Your Capricorn child thinks the world of his family. While he may be a trifle stingy with gifts on mother's and father's day, he'll *always* be there when you need him.

Aquarius *January 20 – February 18*
Element *Air* Quality *Fixed*
Aquarian youngsters are some of the most unusual and unpredictable in the Zodiac. It's no use expecting your little Aquarian to feed regularly every four hours, or think, because he adored buttered carrots on Monday, that

he'll feel the same way about them on Tuesday. Also, despite his wonderful smiles and twinkling eyes, he's as stubborn as a mule! Even the Aquarian infant, who is more compliant and docile, will eventually demonstrate some remarkably quirky behaviour.

Aquarians of all ages are friendly, gregarious individuals; as babies they love new surroundings and novel experiences and, later, they enjoy packing their bags to stay with friends.

Master and Miss Aquarius tend to fall into two categories – the rigid conservative or the radical progressive. The more serious Aquarian can be disciplined and reasoned with, all will be accommodating to his family. The renegade Aquarian chomps at the bit for independence as soon as he can toddle, and goes his own sweet way whether you like it or not. Both types, however, have extraordinary charm and are rarely short of friends or champions.

The Aquarian tends to develop in fits and starts; some weeks soaring ahead, others lagging forlornly behind. Master and Miss Aquarius sometimes have genius abilities that at first go unrecognised. They apply themselves in unorthodox ways and are easily bored. Often they have great difficulty in responding to a rigid teaching system and thus appear to do poorly at school. Almost all of them are inventive and creative and many love performing – on stage and off. By and large they tend to prefer mental games to physical ones and usually make reluctant sportsmen.

Altruism, determination, honesty and brilliance are Aquarius' strengths; obstinacy, wilfulness, selfishness and detachment are its weaknesses.

Life with your Aquarian child can be a magical mystery tour. Don't worry if he seems to be the only one out of step – he's usually the sort of duckling that will turn into a swan.

Pisces *February 18 – March 20*
Element *Water* Quality *Mutable*

Pisces youngsters seem full of wisdom and understanding right from the cradle. Although on the surface they can be placid and malleable, it's worth remembering that there are turbulent depths to this passive and gentle sign.

The Pisces toddler is as slippery as the proverbial fish. If you're not continually watching him, he'll disappear into an inaccessible hole, then dissolve into copious tears because he feels frightened and abandoned. He'll hate to make you angry, especially if you shout at him, but since he can't resist temptation, he often lands himself in trouble.

Pisces children are extremely sensitive and intuitive. They have huge stores of sympathy and compassion, and are often to be found comforting their friends or ministering to their pets and the neighbourhood animals. They prefer to hide away from the harsh realities of life, and need a hefty push to launch them out into the world, whether it's their first day at school, or their first job.

Pisces is also a highly imaginative sign. Many of these children appear to live in a permanent fantasy land, often with an imaginary friend. Even when very young, they are captivated by the sound of a story and later become adept at making up a few of their own! An artistic streak can be found in many Pisceans, and almost all take a delight in wielding a paint brush or putting on ballet shoes. At school they are often more at home in the art room than the science lab.

Master and Miss Pisces tend to be dreamy and forgetful. Many find learning the alphabet and reciting their tables super-human tasks, but later on will experience no trouble at all in writing brilliant essays and understanding algebra and geometry. Firm, but gentle, direction is essential for Pisces girls and boys.

Pisces' attributes include self-sacrifice, patience, sensitivity and artistic talent; self-deception, fecklessness and a tendency to martyrdom are its more negative traits.

You may find yourself mopping up after a little Piscean in more ways than one, but with their enchanting smiles and loving ways, you're not very likely to mind.

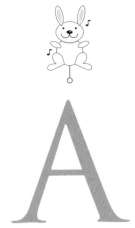

Aaron Several meanings are possible for this name, all from the Hebrew: 'sing', 'shine', 'teach' or 'mountain'; alternatively, from the Arabic, 'messenger'. In the Bible, the original High Priest of the Hebrews and older brother of Moses (Exodus 28). His rod blossomed and produced almonds (Numbers 17), giving the nick-name Aaron's Rod to *Verbascum thapsus*, a plant with clusters of yellow flowers. Another plant, Aaron's Beard, has yellow flowers and is also known as Rose of Sharon or St John's Wort. **Variants:** Aharon, Ahron, Arend, Ari, Arnie, Arny, Aron, Haroun, Ron, Ronnie, Ronny.

Abba From the Aramaic, *abba*, 'father', which also became the Hebrew word. An honorific title in some Eastern churches. The French *abbaie*, 'monastery, convent, abbey church', developed from *abba*, as did the Latin, *abbas*, 'abbot', the superior or father of a monastery. **Variants:** Aba, Abad, Abbas, Abbe, Abbey, Abbie, Abboid, Abbot, Abbott, Abby, Abott.

Abdul From the Arabic, *abd*, 'servant', and Allah, thus 'servant of Allah'. Allah, whose name *al-Ilah* means 'the god', is the Supreme Being in the Muslim faith. **Variants:** Ab, Abdal, Abdel, Abdullah, Del. *See* Ali.

Abel Possibly from the Hebrew, *ablu*, 'son'. In the Bible, the second son of Adam and Eve who was slain by his brother, Cain (Genesis 4). Popularised as a monastic name in medieval England, it was widespread by the 13th century. It was revived in the 17th century, with Ben Jonson's comedy *The Alchemist* (1610), in which Abel Drugger, nicknamed Nab, is one of the alchemist's victims. **Variants:** Abelard, Abeles, Abell, Abelot, Abi, Able, Hevel, Nab.

Abelard From the Middle English, 'guardian of the abbey larder'. The French philosopher and theologian, Peter Abelard (1079–1142) married one of his followers, Heloïse, but only after their child was born. The wrath of

Heloïse's family led them to arrange Abelard's castration. The lovers turned monk and nun and devoted the rest of their days to God. **Variants:** Ab, Abbey, Abby.

Abid From the Arabic, *abd*, 'servant'. **Variants:** Abdi, Abdiel.

Abir See Abira under girls. **Variants:** Abira, Amoz, Amzi, Azaz, Aziz, Aziza.

Abishai From the Hebrew, 'my father's gift', implying a gift from God. In the Bible, a grandson of Jesse and therefore one of Christ's ancestors. **Variant:** Abisha.

Abishur From the Hebrew, 'my father's glance, look', implying God's strength and support at all times.

Abner From the Hebrew, 'father of light'. In the Bible, a cousin of Saul and commander of his army. Like other Old Testament biblical names, it enjoyed popularity after the Reformation. **Variants:** Ab, Abbey, Abby, Avner, Eb, Ebbie, Ebner.

Abraham From the Hebrew, 'eternal father of the cosmos'. In the Bible, the first patriarch and progenitor of the Hebrews and father of Isaac (Genesis 11–25). His name was originally Abram, meaning 'exalted and mighty father'. The 'ah' was added after he accepted the idea of a single God rather than many; the Hebrew 'H' was a symbol for God, and it was the Jewish custom to alter a name to mark a great occasion. Although at first considered disrespectful to God if used as a name, it later became highly favoured amongst Jews. A few early Eastern Christians took up the form Abram and carried it to northern Europe where it became popular with the Puritans. In Britain, the full-length name was used after the Reformation, when Old Testament bibli-cal names came into vogue. It received a strong boost from the twice-elected President of the United States of America, Abraham Lincoln (1809–65), nicknamed 'Abe', who fought against slavery and led the north in the American Civil War. **Variants:** Ab, Abe, Abi, Abie, Abrahamo, Abrahan, Abram, Abramo, Abran, Ali Baba, Avraham, Avram, Avrom, Avrum, Bram, Habreham, Ham, Ibrahim.

Absalom From the Hebrew, 'father of peace'. In the Bible, King David's favourite son, who rebelled against his father and was finally killed (2 Samuel 13–18). A popular name during the Middle Ages, but not since. **Variant:** Absolom.

Acayib Turkish, meaning 'wonderful and strange'.

Ace From the Latin, *as*, 'a unit', via the German, *azzo*, hence the dice or card with the value of one unit, which is the winning one. To say that someone 'holds all the aces' is to say that they have everything going for them. **Variants:** Acelet, Acelin, Acey, Acie, Asce, Asselin, Azzo, Ezzelin.

Achilles In Greek mythology, the son of Peleus and the sea-nymph Thetis, who grew strong on the marrowbones of bears and the entrails of lions. As recounted by Homer in the epic poem, *The Iliad* (8th century BC), this valiant warrior-hero fought at the siege of Troy where he killed the legendary Hector with a single blow, before Apollo (some say Paris) shot an arrow into his only vulnerable spot, his heel. Hence the term 'Achilles heel' for a tiny weakness in something otherwise very strong. A name found more in Germany and France than in Britain. **Variants:** Achille, Achilleus.

FROM STATUS TO SILLINESS

While Kendrick, Leonard, Reginald and Xerxes are kingly names in a subtle way, other names give status more directly. There are Count (Basie), Duke (Ellington), Duchess, Earl and Lord for aspirants to nobility, and even Queenie, Princess and Prince for seekers after blue blood. At the other end of the scale are the fun, celebratory names: Aliza, Bubbles, Hilary, Holly, Jubilee, Yullis or, for champagne and longevity, the full-blown Methuselah. At the far end of the silliness scale lie some up-to-the-minute names, often new forms of old favourites. Dallas comes from Dale, Humpty from Humphrey, Lazer from Lazarus, Luscious from Lucius, and Telly from Theodore or Terence. But it might be best to avoid Nappy, a form of Napoleon.

Ackley From the Middle English, *akern*, 'acorn', and *ley*, 'meadow', thus 'meadow of oak trees'. **Variant:** Ackerley.

Acton From the Old English, *ac*, 'oak', and *tun*, 'village', thus 'village with oak trees'. Occasionally given to girls.

Adair From the Scottish Gaelic, *athdara*, 'from the oak-tree ford'.

Adalric From the German, *adal*, 'noble', and *richi*, 'ruler, power', thus 'noble ruler' **Variant:** Adelric.

Adam From the Hebrew, *adamah*, 'earth'. In the Bible, the first man, created by God after he had made the world (Genesis 2). God gave Adam the Garden of Eden and, while he slept, created woman. Thus Adam and Eve are the source of mankind. The name was used by Christians from the 7th century, when it was found in Ireland. St Adamnan (c. 628–704),

abbot of Iona and a peace-loving and humble man, was distantly related to St Columba and wrote his biography. The name enjoyed popularity among the poorer people in northern England in the Middle Ages, where Adam Bell was the Robin Hood figure. It moved south to be used by Shakespeare for a servant in his comedy, *As You Like It* (1599), but was then hardly used until the post-Reformation vogue for Old Testament biblical names. **Variants:** Ad, Adamo, Adams, Adamson, Adan, Adao, Addie, Addison, Addos, Addoson, Adekin, Adinet, Adom, Edie, Edom.

Adar From the Hebrew, *adhar*, 'dark and cloudy', referring to the sixth month in the Hebrew calendar, or from a different Hebrew word, meaning 'noble, fire, eminent, exalted'. **Variants:** Addar, Addi, Addie, Adin, Adino, Adir, Adna, Ard, Arda.

Ader From the Hebrew, 'a flock'.

Adler From the German, *adlar*, 'eagle'.

Adolph From the Old German, *athal*, 'noble', and *wolfa*, 'wolf', thus 'noble wolf', a trusted and brave guard of home and family. As Aethelwulf, the name is found in England in the 11th century. It was latinised by German royal families, and then both Adolph and Adolphus were carried to Britain by the 18th-century Hanoverian kings. **Variants:** Ad, Adolf, Adolfo, Adolphe, Adolpho, Adolphus, Aethelwulf, Dolf, Dolph, Dolphus, Dolly.

Adon From the Phoenician, *adon*, 'lord', via the Hebrew, *adonai*, 'belonging to my master or lord'. In Judaism, an alternative word for God.

Adonis From the Phoenician, *adon*, 'lord', via the Greek, where it became associated with the epitome of male physical beauty. In Greek mythology, Adonis was the gorgeous young god of agriculture, born from a tree into which his mother had transformed herself. Two principal legends surround him. In one, the goddesses Aphrodite and Persephone compete for his charms until the great god Zeus declares he will live with each of them for six months of the year. In the other, Aphrodite, loving him deeply, forsees tragedy in his passion for hunting and, sure enough, a wild boar or bear kills him. The annual Adonia, the most beautiful and lavish of all Phoenician festivals, marked his death with processions, wax images, dances and singing.

Adrian See Hadrian, and Adrian under girls. Under the Romans, Adrian and Hadrian were interchangeable. Later, two Christian saints helped to spread the form Adrian. The first was a high-ranking Roman officer who was converted to Christianity and was then martyred with his wife, Natalia, in about the year 304. The second was African-born (died 710), twice refused invitations to become Archbishop of Canterbury but became abbot of SS Peter and Paul, Canterbury where his scholarship and administration helped create an exceptional monastic school. When Nicholas Breakspear (died 1159) became the first and only English pope, he chose the name and became Adrian IV. **Variants:** Ade, Adriano, Adrianus, Adrien, Arne.

Adriel From the Hebrew, 'God is my majesty' or 'one of God's congregation'.

Aegir In Norse mythology, god of the sea.

Aelfric From the Old English, 'elf-rule', implying wise and clever rule.

Aeneas In classical mythology, the son of Anchises and Aphrodite, whose adventures after the sack of Troy and before settling in Italy and founding Rome are recounted by Virgil (70–19 BC) in his epic poem, *The Aeneid*. A name found in Scotland and Ireland as Aonghus or Angus, as well as in its original form. **Variants:** Angus, Aonghus, Eneas, Enne, Oenghus, Oengus. *See also* Lavinia.

Aggrey From the Latin, *ager*, 'land, field, open country'.

Ahab From the Hebrew, 'father's brother', that is, uncle.

Ahearn From the Irish Gaelic, *eachthighearn*, 'lord of the horses, owner of horses'. **Variants:** Aherin, Ahern, Aherne, Hearn, Hearne.

Ahmed From the Arabic, 'most highly adored'. **Variant:** Ahmad. *See* Mohammed.

Ahren From the Old German, 'eagle'.

Aidan From the Latin, *adjuvare*, 'to help', via the Middle English, *eyden* and *aiden*, or from the Irish Gaelic, *aodhan*, 'little fiery one'. The Irish St Aidan (c. 600–51) was sent as a missionary to Northumbria in 635 where he founded and became bishop of the monastery at Lindisfarne, which became an important cultural, educational and missionary training centre. **Variant:** Eden.

Aiken From the Old English, *ac*, 'oak', and *en*, 'made of', thus 'made of oak', implying strength and solidity. In northern England, the name can also mean 'little Adam', and is given to a child to imply that he is the image of his father. **Variants:** Aickin, Aikin.

Ain Scottish, meaning 'own, belonging to oneself'. Also given to girls.

Ainsley Scottish, from *ain*, 'own', and the Middle English *leye*, 'field, open country, meadow', thus 'my meadow or land'.

Ajani Nigerian name meaning 'the victor'.

Akira Japanese name meaning 'intelligent'.

Aladdin From the Arabic, 'height of faith'. One of the heroes of the ancient Arabian tales, *Ala Laylah wa Laylah*, 'A Thousand and One Nights', which the princess Scheherezade recounted nightly to her Persian king and husband, thereby saving her threatened life because he was always curious for the next instalment. Finally, he grew to love her so much that he allowed her to live. In the tales, Aladdin can rub his magic lamp and ring to summon up two genies who will fulfil his wildest desires.

Alan From the Celtic, possibly meaning 'harmony, peace', or from the Gaelic, 'bright, fair, handsome'. A name used first by the French, as Alain, then introduced to Britain by the Normans – it was the name of two members of William I's court, the Count of Brittany and the Earl of Richmond. A name consistently popular in Scotland. **Variants:** Ailin, Al, Alain, Alair, Aland, Alano, Alanus, Alawn, Alein, Alena, Aleyn, Aleyne, Allan, Allayne, Allen, Alleyn, Allwyn, Allyn, Alun, Alyn.

Alard A shortening of the Old German name, Adalhard, from *athal*, 'noble', and *hardu*, 'hard', thus 'tough and resilient, noble'. Aethelheard, an English version, was Archbishop of Canterbury (died 805). The shorter form was probably brought over by the Normans. **Variants:** Aderlard, Adlard, Aethelheard, Alart, Allard.

Alaric From the Old German, *ala*, 'all', and *ric*, 'ruler', thus 'ruler over all'. Of the several medieval kings with this name, Alaric I (370–410) was the king of the Visigoths who plundered Greece in 395 and triumphantly captured Rome in 410. The name became popular during the 19th-century medieval revival. **Variants:** Alarick, Alarico, Alarik, Rich, Rick, Ricky, Ulric, Ulrich.

Alastair The old Gaelic form of Alexander. **Variants:** Alasdair, Alastor, Alistair, Alister.

Alban *See* Albina *under girls*. Meaning 'white', it is suitable for boys with blond hair or complexion. The British saint (3rd century) was a Romano-Briton living in Verulanium, now St Albans, who gave shelter to persecuted Christians before being beheaded himself to become the first British martyr. The abbey of St Alban rose on the site of his martyrdom and was later one of the greatest in Britain. However, this did not popularise the name much until the last century, when the Tractarians favoured it because of its associations with early Christianity. **Variants:** Alba,

 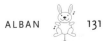

Alben, Albin, Albino, Albion, Alboin, Alva, Alvah, Alvan, Alvin, Alwin, Alwyn, Aubin, Auburn, Elva, Elvin, Elvis. *See also* Alwyn.

Alberic From the Middle High German, *alp*, 'elf', and *richi*, 'powerful', thus 'clever and wise ruler'. Carried to Britain by the Normans, as Alberi and Auberi. In Norse mythology, Alberich is the all-powerful king of the dwarfs, revived to popularity by Richard Wagner's opera, *The Ring of the Nibelung* (1876), in which Alberich is the Nibelung of the title and the first possessor of the magic Ring. **Variants:** Aelfric, Alberi, Alberich, Auberi, Auberon, Aubrey, Avery, Oberon.

Albert From the Old High German name, Adelbrecht, from *adal*, 'noble' and *beraht*, 'bright', thus 'noble and illustrious'. Although an old name, known first as Aethelbert and then Ethelbert, it was altered by Norman influence to Albert and then remained almost forgotten until the last century, though it survived in the north and in Scotland as Halbert. It was then reintroduced when Prince Albert of Saxe-Coburg–Gotha (1819–61) married Queen Victoria in 1840 and became Prince Consort. A major influence on her rule, he promoted the importance of family life and worked obsessively hard as a patron of the arts, education, sciences, industry and agriculture. **Variants:** Al, Adalbert, Adel, Adelbert, Adell, Ailbert, Al, Albe, Alberti, Albertino, Alberto, Albertus, Albrecht, Albie, Aubert, Bert, Bertel, Bertie, Berty, Del, Delbert, Elbert, Elbie, Elvert, Ethelbert, Hab, Halbert, Hobbie, Imbert, Olbracht, Ulbricht. *See also* Alberta *under girls*.

Alcander From the Greek, *alkinoe*, 'strong-minded'.

Alcot From the Old English, *ald*, 'old', and *cot*, 'modest house', thus 'old cottage'. **Variant:** Alcott.

Alcuin Although the origin is unknown, the name was popularised by the English scholar and theologian (735–804) who became adviser to Emperor Charles the Great, known as Charlemagne, and was part of his enlightened court which revived classical learning and brought about the Carolingian Renaissance.

Aldous From the Germanic name, Aldo, from *ald*, 'old', implying the wisdom, maturity and superiority of age. Found in Britain since the 13th century, particularly in East Anglia. **Variants:** Aldan, Alden, Aldin, Aldis, Aldivin, Aldo, Aldon, Aldous, Aldos, Aldren, Aldus, Ealder, Elden, Elder, Eldon, Eldor, Eltis, Elton.

Aldred From the Old English name, Ealdred, *eald*, 'old, wise', and *raed*, 'advice', implying wise advice gained from experience. At its most popular in medieval Britain, but still used occasionally. **Variants:** Dred, Eldred.

Aldrich From the Old High German, *alt*, 'old', and *richi*, 'powerful', thus 'old and wise ruler'. **Variants:** Aldric, Audric, Eldric.

Aldwin From the Old English, *ald*, 'old, wise', and *winne*, 'friend', thus 'wise and reliable friend'. Like Aldred, at its most popular before the Tudor period. **Variants:** Aldan, Alden, Aldin, Edwin.

Aleron From the Latin, *alarius*, 'on the wing' (*ala* was the 'wing' of an army), hence an ally in battle.

Alexander From the Greek, 'man's defender and protector'. In Greek mythology, an honorific title given to Paris for saving his father's cattle herdsmen. In reality, the name of King Alaksandus is written on a Hittite clay tablet dated 1300 BC. This old and quality name has been popular for well over 3000 years, periodically boosted by famous, successful and often royal bearers of it. Most important was Alexander the Great (356–323 BC), King of Macedonia, who conquered most of Asia Minor, Syria, Egypt, Babylon and Persia in just four years during his twenties. Macedonian kings were, traditionally, called alternately Alexander and Philip. Others include Alexander Nevsky (1220–63), Russian military hero, politician and saint; Pope Alexander VI (1431–1503), enormously wealthy, powerful and ambitious, who is supposed to have said, 'God gave us the Papacy; let us enjoy it'; and Alexander II (1818–81), the ablest and most liberal Tsar of Russia. The name is especially popular in Scotland, where it was introduced from Hungary by Queen Margaret for her son. He later became the first of three Alexanders to be kings of Scotland in the 13th century. **Variants:** Al, Alasdair, Alastair, Alaster, Alec, Aleck, Aleister, Alejandro, Alejo, Alek, Aleksander, Aleksandr, Aleksei, Alesaunder, Alessander, Alessandro, Alex, Alexandre, Alexis, Alexius, Alic, Alick, Alika, Alisander, Alisandre, Alisaunder, Alistair, Alister, Alix, Alizaunder, Allesandro, Allistair, Allister, Allistir, Allix, Altie, Alysanyr, Alysaundre, Eck, Eckie, Elexander, Ellick, Elshender, Elysandre, Sacha, Sander, Sanders, Sandey, Sandor, Sandro, Sandy, Sasha, Saunder, Saunders, Saundra, Sawney, Sender, Zander.

Alfred From the Old English, *aelf*, 'elf', and *raed*, 'advice', thus 'man of intelligent and wise judgement and counsel'. First fashionable in Britain under the exceptional Alfred the Great (849–99), King of Wessex (which stretched roughly from Sussex to Devon). He drove out the Danes, strengthened the army and defences and built Britain's first navy, as well as drawing up a legal code and stimulating learning and culture. Such variants as Alured evolved because Anglo-Saxons often wrote a 'v' or 'u' for an 'f'. The name went out of favour during the 16th century, to be revived in the 18th. The Swedish chemist and philanthropist, Alfred Nobel (1833–96), who invented dynamite and developed nitro-glycerin as a high explosive, was so appalled at what his inventions led to in war that he initiated the Nobel prizes, funded with his fortune. **Variants:** Aelfric, Ailfrid, Al, Alf, Alfeo, Alfie, Alfredo, Alfric, Alfrick, Alfrid, Alfris, Alfy, Allie, Alured, Auveray, Avere, Avery, Elfrid, Fred, Freddie, Freddy.

Alger From the Old English, *aelf*, 'elf', and *gar*, 'spear', thus 'clever and quick-witted warrior'. **Variants:** Aelgar, Algar, Algor, Elgar, Eylgar.

Algernon From the French, *aux gernons*, 'with a moustache'. According to the tale, the nickname given to an 11th-century Count of Boulogne, whose real name was Eustace, to avoid confusion with his father, also Eustace, who was known as *à l'oeil*, with the eye'. Introduced into Britain when the 5th Earl of Northumberland was named Henry Algernon Percy, later known as Algernon the Magnificent after his extravagant display with Henry VIII (1491–1547) at the Field of the Cloth of Gold. But the widespread popularity of the name dates from last century. **Variants:** Al, Alger, Algie, Algy, Alick.

Ali From the Arabic, *Allah*, from *al-Ilah*, 'the god', the Supreme Being in the Muslim faith. This shortened form was the name of Mohammed's cousin and son-in-law

(c. 600–61) who was one of the first converts to Islam and became the Fourth Calif. In the ancient Arabic tales, *A Thousand and One Nights*, Ali Baba is the poor woodcutter who enters the treasure-filled cave of the forty thieves by saying 'open sesame'.

Alim From the Arabic, 'wise, learned'. **Variant:** Alem.

Allison 'Son of Alice'; *see* Alice *under girls*. **Variants:** Al, Alison.

Almarine *See* Alma *under girls*.

Almeric From the Old German, *amal*, 'work', and *richi*, 'powerful, ruler', thus 'hard-working ruler'. Carried to Britain by the Normans. **Variants:** Amaury, Ameri, Amery.

Alon From the Hebrew, 'oak tree'. **Variant:** Allon.

Aloysius *See* Louis.

Alpha *See under girls*.

Alphege From the Old English, 'elf-high', implying the legendary great intelligence and quick wits of an elf. The English saint (954–1012), also known as Aefheah, was Bishop of Winchester and Archbishop of Canterbury before being taken hostage by the Danes and killed by them at Greenwich.

Alpheius In Greek mythology, the hunter who fell deeply in love at first sight with the sea-nymph Arethusa. He transformed himself into a river in order to pursue his beloved who had changed into a stream. Finally he joined her and their waters mingled. **Variant:** Alpheias.

Alphonse From the Old High German, *adal*, 'noble', and *funsa*, 'ready, apt'. Popularised in Spain by Alphonsine the Wise, King of Castile and inventor of the astronomical tables named after him. **Variants:** Al, Alf, Alfie, Alffonso, Alfons, Alfonse, Alfonso, Alfonsus, Alfonzo, Allon, Alon, Alonso, Alonza, Alonzo, Alphonsine, Alphonso, Alphonsus, Fons, Fonsie, Fonz, Fonzie, Lon, Lonas, Lonnie, Lonny, Lonsdale, Lonzo.

Alpin From the Latin, *alpes*, 'high mountains'. *See also* Alban.

Alroy A short form of the Irish Gaelic, *giollaru-aidh*, 'red-haired youth'.

Alter From the Old High German, *alter*, 'elder, senior', often implying someone in political, religious or social authority.

Alto *See* Alta *under girls*. **Variants:** Altie, Altus.

Alton From the Old English, *ald*, 'old', and *tun*, 'village, enclosed space', thus 'old town'.

Aluph From the Hebrew, *aluph*, 'leader, prince, head, chief'.

Alvah From the Hebrew, *alva*, 'injustice'. **Variants:** Alva, Alvan.

Alvis From the Old Norse, *alwiss*, 'wise'. In Norse mythology, the dwarf who demanded the hand of the mighty god Thor's daughter.

Alwyn *See* Alvina *under girls*. **Variants:** Al, Aloin, Aluin, Aluino, Alvan, Alvie, Alvin, Alvy, Alwin, Aylwin, Elwin.

Amadeus Male form of Amadis; see Amabel. The most famous bearer of the name is the Austrian child prodigy and composer, Wolfgang Amadeus Mozart (1756–91). **Variants:** Amadis, Amado.

Amadore From the Latin, *amartio*, 'love', and the Greek, *doron*, 'gift', thus 'gift of love'. The legend of the hermit, St Amadour, recounts his founding the shrine of our Lady of

Rocamadour in France. When an actual tomb was found there in the 12th century, his story was elaborated to make him both a servant of the Virgin Mary and husband of St Veronica. **Variants:** Amadis, Amado, Amando.

Amal *See* Amalia *under girls.*

Amand *See* Amanda *under girls.*

Ambert From the Old High German, *beraht*, 'shining, bright, illustrious'.

Ambrose *See* Ambrosia *under girls*. The saint (334–40) from Trier practised law before becoming Bishop of Milan in 374, chosen by the citizens although he was not even baptised. The prestigious city of Milan was the administrative capital of the western part of the Roman empire and also a major centre for new converts to Christianity. Ambrose was deeply involved in both politics and religious instruction. His teaching was very practical and, with Augustine, Jerome and Gregory the Great, he is considered to be one of the four great Latin teachers of Christianity. A name highly popular in medieval Britain through Ambrosius Aurelianus, a historical character on whom King Arthur is perhaps based. **Variants:** Ambie, Ambros, Ambrosio, Ambrosius, Ambroys, Amby, Brose, Emrys.

Amfrid From the Old German name, Anafrid, from *ano*, 'ancestor', and *frithu*, 'peace'. Carried to Britain by the Normans.

Ami From the Hebrew, 'my people'; or from the French, 'friend' (see Amy under girls). The extended names Amiel and Amiram mean 'God of my people' and 'my people is praised'. **Variants:** Amiel, Amiram.

Amin From the Arabic and Hebrew, 'truth, certainty, affirmation'. To say 'amen' after a statement, prayer or wish is to re-affirm

belief in the truth of the words. In the Bible, Ammon was one of King David's sons. **Variants:** Amen, Ammon, Amnon, Amon.

Amir From the Arabic, 'prince'; *see also* Amira *under girls*. **Variant:** Emir.

Amitai *See* Amita *under girls*. **Variant:** Amitan.

Amory From the Latin, *amor*, 'love', thus 'loving person'. **Variants:** Amati, Amery, Ames, Amias, Amice, Amiot, Amyas, Embry, Emory, Imray, Imrie. *See also* Almeric.

Amos From the Hebrew, 'troubled, weighed down'. In the Bible, the book containing the prophecies of Amos, a prophet of the 8th century BC.

Amr From the Arabic, 'life', or from the Hebrew, 'mighty nation'. **Variants:** Amiram, Umar. *See also* Omar.

Anan From the Hebrew, 'cloud'.

Anastasius *See* Anastasia *under girls*. **Variants:** Anastagio, Anastase, Anastasio, Atanasio, Stas, Stasi.

Anatole From the Greek, 'rising sun'. Anatolia is the part of Turkey that lies in Asia, and has a history of trading and meeting between East and West since ancient times. Gradually conquered by the Ottoman Turks during the 14th and 15th centuries, it remained part of their empire until Turkey became a republic in 1923. **Variants:** Anatol, Anatolio, Anatoly, Antal.

Ancel From the Old German, *ansi*, 'god'. Taken up by the Normans, it evolved first into Ancelin and Ancelot, and then into Lancelot. **Variants:** Ancelin, Ancelot, Ansela, Ansell, Ansellus, Ansila.

 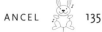

Ancher From the Greek, *ankura*, 'anchor', implying reliability, and both physical and psychological stability.

Andrew From the Greek, *andreios*, 'manly'. In the Bible, a Galilean fisherman who was the first to be called by Christ to become one of the twelve Apostles; the brother of Simon, later called Peter. The accounts of St Andrew's later life have little or no factual basis, not even the claim that he was martyred on an X-shaped cross. He is patron saint of Scotland (relics were carried to the city named after him), and 637 churches in England alone are dedicated to him. Among other saints bearing the same name are St Andrew of Crete (c. 660–740), known for his preaching, poetry and hymns; Andrew Avellino (1521–1608), a zealous Italian missionary; and Andrew Fournet (1752–1834), who helped establish the congregation of the Daughters of the Cross. Andrew is one of the most consistently popular names in Britain. During the Tudor period, it acquired comic associations: a Merry Andrew was a quack doctor's attendant and humourist at a fairground, and Sir Andrew Aguecheek is the ridiculous figure in Shakespeare's *Twelfth Night* (1601). **Variants:** Anderewe, Anders, Andersen, Anderson, Andie, Andonis, Andor, Andre, Andrea, Andreas, Andrei, Andrej, Andres, Andreu, Andrewes, Andrey, Andronicus, Andros, Andvari, Andy, Bandi, Dandi, Dandie, Dandy, Drew, Dries, Drud, Drugi, Tandy.

Aneurin Welsh, derived either from Honor, or from the Welsh, *an*, 'all', and *eur*, 'gold', thus 'pure gold'. An old name, known since the 7th century and still current today. The politician Aneurin Bevan (1897–1960), known as Nye, was Minister for Health from 1945 to 1951 and instrumental in setting up the National Health Service. **Variants:** Aneirin, Nye.

Angel *See* Angela *under girls*. The name of Tess' husband in Thomas Hardy's novel, *Tess of the D'Urbevilles* (1891), who notably fails to live up to his name. **Variants:** Angell, Angelo, Angelos, Angie.

Angelico *See* Angelica *under girls*.

Angus From the Gaelic name, Aonghus, 'unique choice'. This has remained an almost exclusively Scottish name, its use in Scotland dating from at least the 3rd century BC. According to legend, Aonghus Turimleach was one of three Irish brothers who invaded Scotland and gave his name to the people and to the breed of fine cattle. They brought with them the Stone of Destiny, the 'Stone of Scone', which is now in the Coronation Chair in Westminster Abbey. In Celtic mythology, Angus Og was the son of the Dagda, father of all and the lord of perfect knowledge. As one of the chieftain-gods, Angus used supernatural powers and the four magical treasures – the Dagda's cauldron, a spear, a sword and a stone – to maintain the well-being and increase the prosperity of mankind. **Variants:** Ennis, Gus. *See also* Aeneas.

Anselm From the Old German, *ansi*, 'god', and *helma*, 'helmet', thus 'helmet of God', implying God's protection throughout life. A name popular in Lombardy where St Anselm (1033–1109) was born; he later brought the name to Britain when he became Archbishop of Canterbury. **Variants:** Ancel, Ancelm, Ansel, Ansell.

Anson 'son of Anne'. **Variants:** Ansonia, Hanson. *See* Anne.

Anthony From the Greek, 'flourishing', and possibly also from the Latin, 'priceless'. One

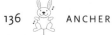

of the most distinguished of several Roman emperors bearing the name was Antoninus (86–161) who succeeded Hadrian in 138–his integrity, dedication and mildly progressive policy earned him the title Pius. It was during his rule, in 142, that the 58-kilometre long Antonine Wall was built from the Firth of Forth to the Clyde in Scotland, marking the northern boundary of the Roman Empire. Another Roman, Antonius Marcus, known as Mark Antony (83–30 BC), emerged from a dissipated youth to become both soldier and statesman and one of the ruling triumvirate after Caesar's assassination. His good looks, strength and affability led to popularity, success and a long affair with the beautiful Queen Cleopatra of Egypt until his death by suicide after defeat in battle, followed by her own suicide. Among the saints who influenced the name's use are Anthony of Egypt (251–356), who forswore wealth to become a hermit in the desert and is regarded as the founder of Christian monasticism, and Anthony of Padua (1195–1231), follower of St Francis, biblical scholar and exceptional preacher, who is associated with various miracles at Padua and is the patron saint of lost property. It was these two who made the name so popular in Britain from the 12th century onwards. The 'h' was added in the 16th century, and the nickname Tony was widespread by the 17th. **Variants:** Antal, Antoine, Anton, Antone, Antoni, Antonin, Antonina, Antonio, Antonius, Antony, Tonetto, Toney, Toni, Tonio, Tony.

Anwar From the Arabic, 'light'.

Apollo Possibly from the Greek, 'to repel, destroy'. In Greek mythology, son of the supreme Zeus and Leto, and twin brother of Artemis. He was god of the sun and light, whose other names included Phoebus, 'the brilliant', Xanthus, 'the fair', and Chrysocomes, 'golden locks'. Since he made the crops ripen, he was therefore a pastoral god, as well as protector of sheep and a god of prophecy, building, navigation, founding towns, music (especially song and the lyre), and destroyer of crop pests. Reared on sweet Ambrosia, he grew handsome, graceful and strong, chose Delphi as his home, was a superb archer and player on the lyre, presided over his retinue of the nine Muses of poetry and music and, naturally, had numerous affairs. Thus, an Apollo is a man of considerable physical beauty, charm and talent. **Variants:** Apollinaire, Apollinaris, Apollonian.

Ara From the Latin, *ara*, 'altar, monument'.

Aram From the Assyrian, *aramu*, 'high up'. The biblical name for ancient Syria.

Archibald From the Germanic name, Ercanbald, 'very bold'. It seems to have entered England through the East Anglian royal family, one of whom became Erkenwald, Bishop of London, in the 7th century, but its usual form came from Scotland where it has been a consistent favourite with the Campbell and Douglas clans. When James VI of Scotland (1566–1625) became James I of England, he brought with him to London the jester, Archie Armstrong; the name's comic overtones have continued to be associated with fictional aristocratic characters. **Variants:** Arch, Archaimbaud, Archambault, Archer, Archibaldo, Archie, Archy, Arkady, Arky, Ercanbald, Erkenwald, Gillespie.

Arden From the Latin, *ardere*, 'to be on fire, ablaze, sparkle, glitter, dazzle', especially with eagerness, enthusiasm, passion or love.

 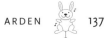

In Shakespeare's comedy, *As You Like It* (1599), the Forest of Arden is the setting for several twists and turns of romance and passion. **Variants:** Ard, Arda, Ardie, Ardin, Ardy.

Ardon From the Hebrew, 'bronze'.

Argus From the Greek, 'bright-eyed, highly observant'. In Greek mythology, the giant with a hundred eyes, whom Hera, jealous wife of Zeus, employed to guard Zeus' mistress, Io. However, Zeus won the day by ordering Hermes to charm the giant into sleep by playing his flute, then chop off his head. The defeated Hera distributed his eyes in the tail feathers of her favourite bird, the peacock.

Ariel In Hebrew, one of the names for God. In the Bible, a name for Jerusalem, city of David. The name was promoted by the rebel angel in Milton's epic poem, *Paradise Lost* (1667), and by the witty and clever spirit who serves Prospero in Shakespeare's comedy, *The Tempest* (1611). **Variants:** Arel, Areli, Ari, Arie, Ario, Ary, Arye, Aryeh, Aryell.

Arion *See* Aria *under girls.* **Variant:** Ario.

Aristo From the Greek, *aristos,* 'best'. Aristophanes (488–387 BC), poet and dramatist, was the greatest Greek writer of satirical comedy. Aristotle (384–322 BC), one of the most influential of the Greek philosophers, studied under Plato, taught Alexander the Great and set up the Lyceum school in Athens. **Variants:** Ari, Aristophanes, Aristotle.

Arjuna In Indian mythology, the prince-hero of the Hindu epic poem, *The Mahabharata.* Before the great battle in the passage known as the *Bhagavad Gita*, Arjuna's charioteer, the god Krishna in disguise, expounds to him the whole nature of existence, God and how to worship God.

Arles From the Hebrew, 'pledge, promise'. **Variants:** Arland, Arlee, Arleigh, Arlen, Arley, Arlie, Arlin, Arliss, Arlo, Arlyn.

Arlo From the Old English, 'fortified hill'.

Armand French form of Herman. **Variants:** Arman, Armando, Armine, Armino. *See also* Arnold.

Armon From the Hebrew, 'castle, palace'. **Variant:** Armoni.

Arnold From the Old German name, Arinwald, from *arin*, 'eagle', and *vald*, 'power'. Popular Teutonic tribal chieftain name, which became more generally widespread in northern Europe up to the 16th century. Introduced to Britain by the Normans as Arnaud or Aunaut, it evolved via Ernald and Ernaldus into Arnold. It fell out of use after the 17th century, to be revived in the 19th and 20th. **Variants:** Ahrens, Ahrent, Arend, Armand, Armant, Arn, Arnald, Arnall, Arnaud, Arnaut, Arndt, Arnell, Arne, Arness, Arnet, Arnett, Arney, Arnie, Arno, Arnoldo, Arnoll, Arnolt, Arnot, Arnott, Arny, Ernald, Ernaldus.

Arsen From the Greek, *arsenikos,* 'strong, virile'.

Artemis *See under girls.* **Variants:** Artemas, Artemus, Artimus, Artis.

Arthur There are four theories about the origin of this popular name. From the Gaelic, *art*, 'rock'; from the Celtic, *artos*, 'bear'; from the Norse, 'follower of Thor', god of war, or, finally, from the Roman family name, Artorius. It was the name of the semi-legendary 6th-century British king, whose huge popularity in Britain and France during

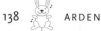

TIDY SETS

N ow that parents have the chance of controlling how many children they wish to have and perhaps when to have them, names that make up a tidy set may come back into fashion; there are even theories claiming to offer the secrets of how to ensure a daughter or son. There are many ways of making up a set of names. One obvious one is the Three Graces of Greek mythology. They spread joy in the hearts of men and presided over the new life of spring and the rich harvest of autumn, so they have much to recommend them. And their names would suit the current fashion for the unusual: Aglaia, Euphrosyne and Thalia.

The Christian Puritans of the 17th century found a triad of simpler abstract virtue names: Faith, Hope and Charity. Names that keep to a theme might include Amadeus, Richard and Robert, after the composers Mozart, Wagner and Schumann, or Bella and Calista, both meaning 'beautiful'. Or perhaps the two Norse gods, Woden and Thor, who gave their names to Wednesday and Thursday. But it might be going a bit too far to follow the example of one Nigerian house-boy, who named his seven children Monday to Sunday.

---

the 10th century stimulated countless elaborate tales of his victories in battle, his court at Camelot (thought to be in Somerset), his Round Table (to prevent quarrels about superiority), his beautiful queen Guinevere who was loved by Lancelot, and the Quest of the Holy Grail. The name lapsed after the 14th century, but was revived when the Arthurian legends and their associated names became part of the Victorian vogue for medievalism, helped particularly by Tennyson's poems, especially *The Idylls of the King* (1859) which sold 10,000 copies in the first week of publication. The popular hero, Arthur Wellesley, 1st Duke of Wellington (1769–1852), who defeated Napoleon at Waterloo (1815), also boosted the name to the extent that Queen Victoria's youngest son was named Arthur after Wellington, who was his godfather. **Variants:** Acur, Ard, Art, Artair, Arth, Arthgen, Artie, Artis, Artor, Artro, Artuir, Artur, Arturo, Artus, Arty, Azer, Azor, Azur, MacArther.

Arva *See under girls.* **Variants:** Arvada, Arval.

Arvid From the Old English, *winne*, 'friend'. **Variants:** Arv, Arvad, Arve, Arvin, Arvy.

 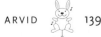

Asa From the Hebrew, 'healer or physician'. In Japanese the same word means 'born in the morning' and is given to boys and girls.

Asaph From the Hebrew, 'to gather'.

Asgard From the Old Norse, *ass*, 'god', and *garth*, 'hall, courtyard'. In Norse mythology, the heavenly abode of the gods and of slain heroes. It was believed that the gods built this paradise themselves, each with his own divine palace modelled on the German farms of the lesser nobility. Between Asgard and Earth was a bridge, the rainbow.

Ash From the Old English, *aesc*, 'ash tree', a wood valued for its durability and flexibility. Hence Ashley, 'a field of ash trees'. **Variants:** Ascanius, Ashbey, Ashby, Ashford, Ashley, Ashly, Haskel, Haskell, Huxley.

Asher From the Hebrew, 'fortunate, happy'. In the Bible, a son of Jacob and head of one of the twelve tribes of Israel to which he gave his name (Genesis 49). **Variants:** Aser, Asser.

Astley From the Greek, *aster*, 'star', and the Old English, *leah*, 'meadow', thus 'starlit field'.

Athelstan From the Old English name, Aethelstan, from *aethel*, 'noble', and *stan*, 'stone', thus 'noble and reliable'. A popular early medieval name, borne by a king of Wessex (925–40), but hardly used after the Norman Conquest.

Athene Male form of Athena. **Variant:** Athens.

Atlas In Greek mythology, the giant Titan whose punishment for rebelling against the gods was to carry the world upon his shoulders, hence the name of the lofty Atlas Mountains in north-west Africa, which then gave their name to the Atlantic Sea and thus to the legendary island of Atlantis. Because early maps depicted the world upheld by Atlas, the name is given to a collection of maps.

Attica The region of ancient Greece that surrounds Athens. Attic was the ancient Greek dialect of Athens, and implies a character of style that is pure, simple and elegant.

Atticus See Attica. This variation has been popularised by the character Atticus Finch in Harper Lee's Pulitzer prize-winning novel *To Kill a Mockingbird*.

Attila From the Greek, *atta*, 'father'–a respectful term for an older person. A popular Gothic name, borne by Attila the Hun (died 453), the notorious Barbarian enemy of the Romans, who persistently and successfully attacked the empire from the east, forcing back the Roman frontier. **Variants:** Atli, Atoy, Attilio.

Aubrey See Alberic.

Augustus From the Latin, 'majestic, venerable, worthy of honour'. The first Roman emperor, Octavius Caesar (63 BC–14 AD), grand-nephew of Julius Caesar and his adopted son, gave himself this honorific surname after he had attained undivided authority. His successors then followed suit, making the name equivalent to the title 'His Imperial Majesty'. The golden age of Latin literature, when Horace, Livy and Ovid lived, was called Augustan, and so was a similar literary flourishing in 18th-century England. The name is also the origin of that of the eighth month of the year. Augustus began to be used again as a name in the 16th century, when German princes were emulating everything Roman. Their descendants, the Hanoverian kings, carried it to Britain, where two early Christian saints also boosted its popularity. Augustine of Hippo (354–430) was a follower of St Ambrose and one of the four great Latin doctors of Christianity. Augustine of Canterbury (died 605), a Benedictine missionary sent by Pope Gregory I to Britain in 597, brought Christianity to southern England, converted King Ethelbert of Kent, and became the first Archbishop of Canterbury. **Variants:** Agostin, Agostinho, Agostino, Agosto, Aguistin, Agustin, Augie, August, Augustin, Augustine, Augustino, Augusto, Augy, Austen, Austin, Gus, Gussie, Gustus.

Aurelius From the Latin, *aureolus*, 'gold coin, gilded, golden, splendid, brilliant, beautiful'. Marcus Aurelius (121–80) was an emperor and philosopher, whose huge equestrian statue still stands on the Capitoline Hill in Rome. A later emperor, Aurelianus (215–275), checked the Barbarian attacks on the Roman Empire in a series of victorious battles. **Variants:** Aurea, Aurek, Aurel, Aurelio, Aurelo, Aury.

Austin Derived from the Latin August meaning 'exalted' or 'majestic'.

Averell *See* Averil *under girls.* **Variants:** Averil, Averill.

Avi From the Hebrew, *abi* or *avi*, 'my father', implying God; the various expanded forms can be spelt with a 'b' or a 'v'. They include Avidan, 'God of wisdom and justice'; Avidor, 'father of the generation'; Aviel, 'God is my father'; Avigdor, 'paternal protector'; Avinoam, 'father of delight'; and Avital, 'father of dew'. **Variants:** Abi, Av, Avodal.

Avitus *See* Avis *under girls.*

Avlar From the German, 'elf-army', implying speediness and intelligence.

Axel From the Germanic, *aiks*, 'oak', thus 'small oak tree', implying the potential to become strong and dependable. **Variant:** Aksel.

Aylmer From the Old English, Aethelmaer, 'noble and famous'. **Variants:** Ailemar, Athel, Eilemar, Elmer.

Azaria From the Hebrew, 'God is my help'. In the Bible, a king of Judah. A name favoured by the 17th-century Puritans. Also given to girls. **Variants:** Azariah, Azriel.

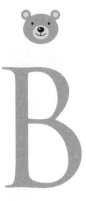

B

Bacchus In classical mythology, god of wine and pleasure, called Dionysius by earlier Greeks. From at least the 5th century BC, the festival in honour of the god, the Bacchanalia, was an excuse for drunken revelry and riotous enjoyment. Men would join the Bacchae (the female followers of the god) to sing and dance through the cities and countryside. The hooliganism became so bad that in 186 BC Bacchus worship was outlawed, though it was revived later as a mystery religion.

Badiah Meaning 'astonishing' 'amazing' or 'orignal creation'.

Bailey From the Middle English, *baile*, 'the outer wall of a castle'. **Variants:** Bail, Bailey, Bailie, Baily. *See also* Barnham.

Bal English gypsy name, derived from the Sanskrit, *bala*, 'hair', and given to a child born with a good head of hair.

Balder In Norse mythology, son of the god Oden and the goddess Frigg. Of exceptional wisdom and radiant beauty, he was god of peace and light and loved by all his fellow gods. Indeed, the whole world took a vow never to harm him, except for one person – Loki, who hated him, and killed him with a branch of mistletoe. When Balder's brother petitioned the goddess of Hel, the kingdom of the dead, she promised to release Balder from death on the condition that every person on earth wept for him – and everyone did, except for Loki. **Variants:** Baldewin, Baldwin, Ball, Baudoin.

Baldric From the Old German name, Baldarich, from *balda*, 'bold', and *richi*, 'power, ruler', thus 'bold ruler'. Widespread in medieval Britain after its introduction by the Normans. **Variants:** Baldri, Baudrey, Baudri.

Baldwin From the Old German name, Baldawin, from *balda*, 'bold', and *wini*, 'friend', thus 'courageous friend'. Carried to

Britain from Flanders during the Middle Ages. **Variants:** Baldawin, Baudoin, Bawden, Bealdwine, Boden, Bodkin, Bowden.

Balfour From the Old English, *bal*, 'hill', and *feorr*, 'distant, remote', thus 'distant hill'.

Balint Hungarian, meaning 'strong and healthy'. **Variant:** Baline.

Ballard From the Latin, *ballare*, 'to dance', via the Provençal, *balada*. A ballad is a narrative and usually romantic poem or song, often from the folk tradition, that is recited to music.

Balthasar From the Hebrew, *Belshazar*, and later the Greek, *Baltasar*, 'May Bel [God] protect the king'. A royal name given by St Augustine to one of the three Magi who brought gifts to the baby Jesus – the other two were Caspar and Melchior. All three names were used in Britain during the Middle Ages. **Variant:** Belshazzer. *See also* Magus.

Bancroft From the Middle English *ben*, 'bean', and *croft*, 'small field, smallholding', thus 'bean field'. **Variant:** Banfield.

Baptist From the Greek, *baptein*, 'to dip'. Baptism is a ceremony of dipping people in water, or sprinkling them with water, to symbolise cleansing and initiation. Within the Christian church, it symbolises spiritual regeneration and the cleansing of original sin, and is the occasion when a person receives Christian names and is admitted into Christianity. In the Bible, St John the Baptist (died c. 29), the son of Elizabeth and the last prophet to foretell the coming of Christ, performed the first baptisms, including that of Christ himself, before being thrown into prison and later beheaded at the request of Herod's niece, Salome. He is the patron saint of tailors, missionaries and of several cities,

including Florence. In Britain the name of Baptist has been used only since the Reformation. Compounds include **Gianbattista** and **Jean-Baptiste**. **Variants:** Baptista, Baptiste.

Barak From the Hebrew, 'flash of light'.

Barber From the Latin, *barba*, 'beard', thus a barber. An old occupational name now found more often as a surname than a first name. In the USA, a 'barbershop quartet' is usually male-voice singing in close four-part harmony. **Variant:** Barbour.

Bard From the Gaelic, *bard*, and the Welsh, *bardd*, the ancient Celtic singing poets who lived at court or travelled the country learning, composing and reciting long poems about the history and legends of their land. The name can also describe a more recent important poet, but the term 'The Bard' is reserved for Shakespeare. **Variant:** Baird.

Barden From the Middle English, *barrlig*, 'barley', and the Scottish, *denne*, 'small wooded dell', thus 'a small valley where barley grows'. **Variants:** Bardon, Borden.

Bardolf From the Old High German, *beraht*, 'bright', and *wulfa*, 'wolf', implying strength. Carried to Britain by the Normans and quite popular until brought into disrepute by the low-life character who haunts taverns with Falstaff in Shakespeare's history plays, *King Henry IV* (1597) and *The Life of Henry V* (1599), and in his comedy, *The Merry Wives of Windsor* (1597). **Variants:** Bardell, Bardolph.

Barker From the Old English, *beorce*, 'birch', thus someone who logs birch trees. Like Barber, an old occupational name. Barksdale would therefore mean a broad valley of birch trees. **Variants:** Barksdale, Birk.

Barnabas From the Aramaic, 'son of exhortation'. In the Bible, a Cypriot Jew who became a disciple of Paul and, although not one of the Twelve, an unofficial Apostle. He was later a missionary in Antioch and took Christianity to Cyprus. A name used in Britain from the 13th century and later modified to Barnaby, a version boosted by the simple and innocent messenger in Dickens' novel, *Barnaby Rudge* (1841). **Variants:** Barn, Barnaba, Barnabe, Barnaby, Barney, Barnie, Barny, Burnaby.

Barnum From the Old English, *beren*, 'barley house, store house'. The American showman, Phineas Taylor Barnum (1810–91), was the first to popularise 'freak shows'–his exhibits included the Siamese twins, Chang and Eng. In 1881 he finally merged his fine circus with that of his great rival, J. A. Bailey.

Baron From the medieval Latin, *baron*, 'man, warrior'. Originally, a feudal tenant directly responsible to the king or ruler; today, the lowest rank of nobility in Great Britain. The name is also given colloquially to anyone with enormous commercial or industrial power, such as a 'press baron' or an 'oil baron'. **Variant:** Barron.

Barry From the Old Celtic name, Bearrach, 'spear, good marksman'. The name of several early Irish Christians including one hermit after whom Barry Island is named. Also, a Welsh patronymic, 'Ap-Harry', from Harry (*see* Harold and Henry). Although confined to Ireland until the last century, it has since become widespread in Britain. **Variants:** Barett, Bari, Barnard, Barnett, Barri, Barrie, Barrington, Barris, Barrymore.

Bartholomew From the Aramaic name, Bar Talmai, from *bar*, 'son', and Talmai. In the Bible, one of the Apostles about whom almost nothing is written but it is possible that he spread the Gospel to Lycaonia, India and Armenia, where he was martyred. (A later saint, Bartholomea (1807–33), was noted for her determination and selflessness, and helped found the Sisters of Charity of Lovere in Lombardy, designed to teach the young and nurse the sick.) The name was widespread after introduction by the Normans–165 churches in England were dedicated to the saint – and it received another boost after the founding of St Bartholomew's hospital in London by Rahere, a court jester to Henry I who was cured of illness after having a vision of the saint. The king helped Rahere and also gave permission for an annual fair to raise money for the hospital–a tradition upheld until the last century when it was suppressed for rowdiness. **Variants:** Bardo, Barholomee, Bart, Bartel, Bartelot, Barth, Bartholomaus, Bartholomieu, Bartle, Bartlemey, Bartlett, Bartley, Bartold, Bartolo, Bartolome, Barton, Bat, Batcock, Bate, Batkin, Batly, Batty, Bertel, Meo, Mewes, Tholy, Tolly, Tolomieu, Tolomey.

Barush From the Hebrew, 'blessed'. In the Bible, the companion and secretary of the prophet Jeremiah. A name popular in Britain since Tudor times, especially in the Midlands.

Basil From the Greek, *basilon*, 'royal'. St Basil the Great (330–97) came from a remarkable Christian family: his grandmother, father, mother, elder sister and two younger brothers are all saints. As Bishop of Caesarea in Cappadocia, he possibly wrote *The Liturgy of St Basil*, which is still used in the Eastern Orthodox Church. In his defence of Christian persecution, he joined his brother, St Gregory of Nyssa, and St Gregory of Nazianzus to become one of the Cappadocian fathers. He certainly encouraged the name's use in Byzantium, even by the emperors, and the Crusaders carried it back to Britain where it later rose to popularity in the last century under the influence of the Tractarians. **Variants:** Basie, Basile, Basilie, Basilio, Basilius, Basine, Baz.

Bavol English gypsy name, meaning 'wind, air'. **Variant:** Beval.

Baxter From the Old English term meaning 'a baker'.

Bayard From the Latin, *badius*, via the Old French, *bai*, 'reddish-brown colour', especially a horse of this colour, hence the word Baylor for a horse-trainer. In medieval legend, Charlemagne reputedly gave Rinaldo a horse called Bayard who possessed magical powers. A later Bayard (1476–1524) was a French soldier renowned for his chivalry and fearlessness.

Baye From an African word meaning 'straightforward'.

Beasley From the Old English, *pise*, 'peas', and *lea*, 'meadow', thus 'field of peas'. **Variants:** Beals, Peasley.

Beattie *See* Beatrice *under girls*. **Variant:** Beeson.

Beau From the French, 'beautiful, handsome'; the male form of Belle. A nickname for a girl's sweetheart, or less appealing, a name popularised by George Bryan Brummell (1778–1840). His highly fashionable, dandyish and outrageous dress earned him the nickname 'Beau', later applied to any man obsessed by fine clothes and social etiquette.

Beaumont From the French, *beau*, 'beautiful', and *mont*, 'mountain', thus 'beautiful mountain'.

Beauregard From the French, *beau*, 'beautiful', and *regard*, 'opinion', thus 'held in high regard'. **Variants:** Beau, Bo.

Beck From the Old Norse, *bekkr*, 'small brook, stream'. A word and name found mostly in northern England.

Bede From the Middle English, *bede*, 'prayer'. St Bede (673–735), better known as the Venerable Bede, became a Benedictine monk and priest at the monastery of Wearmouth in Northumbria. He was both historian and theologian, the first known writer of English prose, one of the most influential writers of his time in Western Europe and author of *The History of the English Church and People*. In 1899 Pope Leo XIII made him the first English Doctor of the Church. **Variant:** Bedivere.

Bedir Turkish, meaning 'full moon'.

Belden From the Latin, *bellus*, 'beautiful', and the Middle English, *den*, 'small room' or, in Scottish, 'small wooded dell', thus 'a small place of beauty'.

Bell From the Latin, *bellus*, 'beautiful, handsome, charming, neat, agreeable'. The extended form Bellamy means 'beautiful friend' and Belton, 'beautiful town'. **Variants:** Bel, Bellamy, Bellini, Belton.

Belveder From the Italian, *bello*, 'beautiful, fine, handsome', and *vedere*, 'to see, observe', thus both 'beautiful to look at' and 'a vantage point for a fine view'. **Variant:** Belvedere, Belvidere.

Bemus From the late Latin, *bema*, 'platform'. In religious architecture, the sanctuary or area around the altar in an Eastern Orthodox church or the platform from which services are conducted in a synagogue. **Variant:** Bimah.

Ben From the Scottish Gaelic, *beann*, 'peak, height, mountain' (as in Ben Nevis, the highest mountain in Great Britain); or from the Middle English, *ben* or *binne*, which in Scotland means 'parlour' or 'house', or from the Hebrew, *ben*, 'son'. **Variants:** Benn, Bennie, Benny, Benroy, Benson, Benton. *See also* Benedict and Benjamin.

Benedict From the Latin, *benedicere*, 'to bless, speak well of, praise'. In Christianity, benediction is a blessing or invocation of divine blessing, usually at the end of a service. The Italian monk, St Benedict (480–547), is the father of western monasticism. After studying in Rome and living as a hermit in Subiaco, he established the first Benedictine monastery in 529 at Monte Cassino. Here he formulated his influential monastic *Rule of St Benedict*, which emphasised discipline and respect for fellow men and their individual capabilities, but which he hoped would be 'neither harsh nor rigorous'. Among the other saints of the same name was Benedict of Aniane (750–821), who founded the Benedictine monastery at Corbière and became virtually the supreme abbot of all the monasteries in Charlemagne's empire. After heading the council of abbots at Aachen in 817, he issued a code of regulations to reform, systematise and centralise the monasteries which had lasting effect. Before him, the English St Benedict Biscop (628–90) travelled twice to Rome before founding and running the monasteries at Wearmouth and Jarrow. He equipped them with relics, glaziers, masons and even singers from Rome, as well as two excellent libraries used by Bede. These saints and 15 popes called Benedict encouraged the name's use; it was given a new meaning by Shakespeare through his character Benedick in the comedy, *Much Ado About Nothing* (1598–9), who is a firm bachelor until he reluctantly woos and marries Beatrice. The liqueur, Benedictine, is named after the Benedictine abbey at Fécamp where it is made. **Variants:** Banet, Banko, Barrie, Barry, Baruch, Ben, Benayt, Bendix, Benedetto, Benedicto, Benes, Benet, Benett, Beneyt, Benigno, Benito, Beniton, Bennet, Bennett, Benny, Benoit, Bento, Berachya, Bettino, Betto, Boruch, Dix, Dixie.

Ben-Gurion From the Hebrew, *ben*, 'son', and *gurion*, 'lion', thus 'son of the lion'. Other compounds include **Ben-Ami, Ben-Burion, Ben-Hur** and **Ben-Zvi**.

Benjamin From the Hebrew, *ben*, 'son', and *yamin*, 'right hand', thus 'son of my right hand', implying strength and good fortune. In the Bible, the youngest and favourite of Jacob's 12 sons, from whom one of the tribes of Israel was descended. His mother, Rachel, who died when he was born, called him Benoni, 'son of sorrow', which was altered by Jacob to Benjamin (Genesis 35). In Britain, the name became popular among Jews in the Middle Ages, spreading to Christians in the 16th century when Old Testament names were in vogue and when the dramatist Ben Jonson (1572–1637) lived. Benjamin Disraeli (1804–81), grandson of a Venetian Jew, was converted to Christianity and embarked on a political career; as an MP, he pushed through the Reform Bill (1867) and then became Prime Minister in 1868 and again in 1874. It was Disraeli who established the Conservative Party as a political group upholding monarchy, empire and the Anglican Church. But the name then fell out of favour, until it was revived recently. It is the nickname for the clock tower of the Houses of Parliament, after Sir Benjamin Hall who was Commissioner of Works. The British composer Edward Benjamin Britten (1913–76) wrote song-cycles and operas, including *Peter Grimes* (1945) and *Death in Venice* (1973). **Variants:** Bannerjee, Ben, Benji, Benjie, Benjy, Benmajee, Bennie, Benno, Benny, Berihert, Yemin.

Bentley Possibly from the Old English, *beon*, 'to exist, become'. **Variant:** Bently.

Beowulf The hero of the epic narrative poem composed in Old English during the 8th century. The action is set in Norse lands where Beowulf, a valiant and strong young man, rids King Hrothgar of the fearsome monster Grendel and his mother who live on human flesh. He later reigns as king for 50 years before being mortally wounded while killing a dragon.

Ber From the Old Norse, *bua*, 'to dwell', via the later German word, 'boundary line'. **Variants:** Berlin, Berlyn.

Berg From the German, 'mountain, fortified hill'; also from the earlier Old Norse, *borg*, 'fortified hill, castle'. **Variants:** Bergen, Berger, Bergin, Borg, Borje, Bourke, Burke.

Bergren Swedish, meaning 'mountain stream'.

Beriah From the Hebrew *boneh*, 'creature'.

Berkeley From the Old English, *beorce*, 'birch tree', and *lea*, 'meadow, grassland', thus 'field where birch trees grow'. **Variants:** Barcley, Berkley, Berkly.

Bern From the Old English and Old High German, *beren*, 'to support or carry with suc-

cess, exercise power, hold office, tolerate'; also from the Old High German, *bero*, and the Old Norse, *bjorn*, both meaning 'a bear'. **Variants:** Barnes, Bear, Berna, Berne, Berno. *See also* Bernard.

Bernard From the Old High German name, Berinhard, from *bero*, 'bear', and *hart*, 'brave, stern', thus 'bold as a bear'. Bears were the largest and strongest animals in northern Europe and considered sacred. The name was imported into Britain as Beornheard by the Anglo-Saxons, then as Bernard and Barnard by the Normans. It fell out of favour in the 17th century, to be revived by the Victorians. The French St Bernard of Clairvaux (1090–1153), abbot and theologian, was one of six brilliant sons of a Burgundian noble and contributed significantly to the reform and expansion of the Cistercian order of monasticism. He established the monastery at Clairvaux which soon had 68 daughter-houses, including Rievaulx in England and Mellifond in Ireland. He was noted for his charity and his attacks on the luxurious lifestyle of his fellow clergy. Among the other saints of the same name is Bernard of Montjoux (c. 996–1081), who cleared the passes over the Alps and has two of them named after him, the Little and the Great St Bernard; he is patron saint of mountaineers. More recently, the name's use has been encouraged by Thomas John Barnardo (1845–1905), known as Dr Barnardo, who devoted his life to the protection and education of orphans and destitute children and founded his first homes in Stepney, east London, in 1867. **Variants:** Banet, Baretta, Barnard, Barnet, Barnett, Barney, Barny, Barr, Barre, Barret, Barrett, Bear, Benno, Bern, Bernadin, Bernardo,

Bernarr, Bernd, Berndt, Bernhard, Bernhardi, Bernhardt, Berni, Bernie, Bernis, Bernt, Bjarne, Bjorn, Bjorne, Levar.

Berry From the Old English, *berige*, 'berry', a fleshy fruit that contains the seeds of the next plant, implying flourishing life in the next generation.

Bersh English gypsy name, meaning 'one year'. **Variant:** Besh.

Berthold *See* Bertha *under girls*. **Variants:** Bert, Bertell, Bertie, Bertil, Bertin, Bertol, Bertold, Bertole, Bertolt, Berton, Labert.

Bertram From the Old German name, Berahtraben, from *beraht*, 'bright, shining', and *hraben*, 'raven', thus 'bright raven'. In Norse mythology, the sacred bird belonging to the supreme god, Odin. The name Bertrand really means 'bright shield', but merged with Bertram early on. The philosopher, Bertrand Russell (1872–1970), born into the nobility, became a prominent pacifist, the doyen of British philosophy and was awarded the Nobel prize for literature in 1950. **Variants:** Bert, Berteram, Bertie, Bertran, Bertrand, Bertrando, Bertrem.

Berwin From the Old English, *beren*, 'to support, have power, hold office', and *winne*, 'friend', thus 'supportive and influential friend'.

Beryl *See under girls.*

Bethel *See under girls.*

Beverley *See under girls.* **Variant:** Beverly.

Bevis From the Latin, *bos*, 'ox', via the Old French, *boef* and *buef*, 'bull' or 'meat of an ox, bull or cow'; also the Welsh patronymic of Evan. Another Norman imported name that was popular throughout the Middle Ages, to

be revived by Richard Jefferies' novel, *Bevis: The Story of a Boy* (1882). **Variants:** Bevan, Bevin, Bivian, Bix, Buell.

Bezalel From the Hebrew, 'under God's protection and shadow'. In the Bible, the skilled man who built the tabernacle for Moses.

Bin *See* Binnie *under girls.* **Variants:** Bing, Bingham, Binnie.

Bingo A sailor's slang word for 'brandy', made up by combining 'brandy' with the 'sting', or kick, that the spirit gives, and then adding the 'o' to give it a musical sound.

Bion From the Greek, *bios*, 'life, way of life'.

Birch From the Old English *beorce*, 'birch'. **Variants:** Birk, Burch.

Bishop From the Greek, *episkopos*, 'overseer, superintendent', meaning overseer of a person's spirit. A rank in the Christian Church or a chief priest. Also, a name for mulled wine or port.

Blair *See under girls.*

Blake From the Old Norse, *bleikr*, 'shining, white', via the Old English, *blac*, 'pale, wan'. **Variants:** Blanchard, Blanco.

Blandon From the Latin, *blandus*, 'with a smooth tongue', implying flattery, charm, persuasion and seduction. **Variants:** Bland, Blanton.

Blase From the Greek, *blaisus*, 'stammering, lisping, hesitating in speech'.

Blaze From the Old English, *blaese*, 'torch, flaming fire', implying a brilliant burst of fire, emotion, activity or excitement. The bishop, St Blaise, supposedly martyred early in the 4th century, was a popular cult in 8th-century Europe and acquired numerous legends about

THE IMPACT OF RELIGION

Christianity has made a great contribution to popular British names. Matthew, John, Peter, Ann and other Gospel figures arrived in Britain with the first missionaries. Then came the saints, their monasteries, their dramatic martyrdoms and their elaborate cults. They popularised Benedict, Christopher, Clare, Columba, Francis, Gregory, Helen, Margaret, Patrick, and many more. The Reformation put popish names out of fashion but inspired a new interest in Old Testament names. This was when Adam, Daniel, Eve, Joseph, Sarah, Tobias, and many other Hebrew names were introduced. The Puritans loved abstract virtue names, not just Faith, Hope and Charity, but also names with moral associations, such as Penelope.

---

his healing miracles on humans and animals; he is still invoked today against throat diseases. The cult of another 4th-century martyr saint, Blasius, was especially strong during the Middle Ages, because he was patron saint of wool-workers. Also given to girls. **Variants:** Biagio, Blaise, Blaisot, Blas, Blase, Blasien, Blasius, Blayze, Braz, Vlass.

Blythe From the Old English, *blithe*, 'joyful, frivolous, carefree'. **Variant:** Bligh.

Boaz From the Hebrew, 'strength, swiftness'. In the Bible, the wealthy second husband of Ruth, whom he first spotted labouring in his fields (Ruth 2).

Bodi Hungarian, meaning 'may God protect the king'.

Bogart From the Gaelic, *bog*, 'soft', via *bogach*, 'soft ground, marsh, swamp', implying slowness, being hindered. Popularised recently as a first name by the surnames of two dashing actors: Humphrey DeForest Bogart (1899–1957), and Dirk Bogarde (Derek Niven van den Bogaerde, 1921–1999). **Variants:** Bo, Bogey, Bogie.

Boleslav Polish, meaning 'prepared for war'. **Variant:** Bolivar.

Bonamy From the French, *bon* and *ami*, 'good friend, pal, mate'. **Variants:** Bonaro, Boni, Bunn.

Bonaventure From the Italian, *buono*, 'good', and *avventura*, 'adventure', thus 'good fortune, lucky'. The Italian scholar, monk and saint (1221–74) became such a successful leader of the Franciscan order that he is considered a second founder after St Francis of Assisi. Emphasising simplicity of faith, his works on theology, philosophy and mysticism were highly influential, leading him to be declared a doctor of the church. **Variant:** Bonaventura.

Bond From the Old Norse, *band*, 'to bind, fasten together', implying close union and trust. **Variants:** Bondie, Bondon, Bondy.

Boniface From the Latin, *bonifacies*, 'with a handsome face'. A name associated with several notable Christians who popularised its use. St Boniface of Crediton (c. 675–754), known as the 'Apostle of Germany', was teacher and preacher, wrote the first Latin grammar in English, and was a highly successful missionary in Germany and Holland, where he was finally martyred in old age. Boniface I (418–22) was the first of several popes who took the name. Although found in Britain in the 13th century, the name fell out of use after the Reformation and, under the influence of George Farquhar's play *The Beaux' Stratagem* (1707), became the type name for an inn-keeper. **Variants:** Boneface, Boni, Bonyface, Facio, Fazio.

Booker From the Old English, *boc*, 'written document, book', probably derived from *boka*, 'beech tree', since ancient runes were written on tablets of beechwood. Until the advent of printing, books were considered extremely valuable, because of the time it took to copy the script, their elaborate decoration and the knowledge they contained. **Variant:** Boog.

Boone From the Old Norse, *bon*, 'a blessing, a favour granted'; or from the Latin, *bonus*, 'good', meaning a jolly and affable companion. **Variants:** Bone, Boonie, Boony.

Booth From the Old Norse, *both*, 'dwelling'. A name made popular by William Booth (1829–1912), a minister in the New Methodist Church before he devoted his life to evangelical work. He established the East London Revival Society which in 1878 became the Salvation Army. **Variants:** Boot, Boote, Boothe, Bootie, Boothy.

Bor English gypsy name, meaning 'hedge'.

Borden From the Old French, *borde*, 'cot, small farm' (the same word also acquired the meaning 'brothel').

Boris Russian, from the Slavonic, *borotj*, 'to fight'. One of the few Russian names to become widespread in Britain. The Russian Christian brother princes, Boris and Gleb, were murdered in 1015 by their eldest brother, Svyatopolk, to consolidate his position. Instantly regarded as saints, their festival (July 24) is still observed in Russia. The hero of Moussorgsky's opera, *Boris Godunov* (1874 and 1928), was the son-in-law of Ivan the Terrible and Tsar of Russia from 1598 to 1605. The actor Boris Karloff (1887–1969), who played the monster in the 1931 film of Mary Shelley's novel *Frankenstein* (1818), was born William Pratt.

Bors From the Germanic, *borz*, 'to borrow, to become indebted to someone, to protect'. In Arthurian legend, a nephew of Sir Lancelot and Knight of the Round Table.

Bosley From the Middle English, *bosk* and *buck*, 'bush, underwood', and *leve*, 'meadow', thus 'a large thicket'. **Variants:** Boston, Boswell, Bosworth.

Botan Japanese, meaning 'peony'. In Japan, the flower for the month of June.

Bourne From the Old French, *borne*, 'limit, boundary', implying the ultimate destination or goal. In the south of England, the name also means 'small stream'. **Variant:** Bourn.

Bouvier From the Latin, *bos*, 'ox, bull cow'.

Bowle English gypsy name, meaning 'snail'.

Boyd From the Celtic, 'yellow, yellow-haired'. **Variants:** Bow, Bowen, Bowie.

Braden From the Old English, *brad*, 'to broaden, make spacious, widen, be plain-spoken', and also 'to be tolerant, to have a broad range of opinion and interests'. The compounds include **Broderick**. **Variants:** Brad, Bradford, Bradleigh, Bradley, Brady, Broadus, Ford, Lee, Leigh.

Brage In Norse mythology, son of the supreme Odin and god of poetry and of skalds, the ancient Scandinavian Bards. He was famed for his wisdom and eloquent speech and entertained and amused the other gods by telling stories at their feasts. **Variants:** Braggo, Bragi.

Brand From the Middle English, *brand*, 'flaming torch, fire, sword', with the later meaning of a personal mark brandished onto flesh or printed onto a box to denote ownership or maker. **Variants:** Brandi, Brandon, Brandt, Brant, Brent.

Bray From the Old French, *braire*, 'to cry out, make a loud and harsh noise'.

Brendan The Irish St Brendan the Voyager (486–578) founded the monastery at Clonfert in Galway, but the hugely popular 10th-century tale, *Brendan's Voyage*, has less credibility. Translated into several languages, it spread his fame throughout Europe as a monk who, among other adventures, sailed to the Land of Promise in the Atlantic. In Celtic mythology, Bendegeit Bran, 'Bran the Blessed', was a god of enormous strength and size, who possessed supernatural powers and was a harpist and poet; his cauldron could bring the dead back to life. The legend of Brennan of the Moor, an Irish Robin Hood figure, further popularised the name. It remains a favourite in Ireland. **Variants:** Bramwell, Bran, Brand, Brandon, Brant, Breandan, Brenain, Brend, Brenden, Brendin, Brendon, Brennan, Brondan.

Brett From the Old French, *Briton*, via the Celtic, *Breton*, 'a person from Brittany, the Celtic language of Brittany', the area of north-west France. **Variants:** Bret, Brit, Briton, Britton.

Brevard From the Latin, *brevis*, 'short, little, concise'.

Brewster From the Old English, *breowan*, 'to brew and make ale'. Like Barber, an old occupational name.

Brian From the Greek, *briaros*, 'strong', via the Celtic name, Briareus; or from the Irish, *bre*, 'hill'. In Greek mythology, the world began when Ghea, goddess of earth, appeared out of Chaos. She created Uranus, god of sky and stars and by him gave birth to the Titans, the Cyclops and three monsters: Briareus, Cottus and Gyges. These were known as the Centimanes because each had a hundred unbeatable arms and fifty heads. The name Brian was popular in Brittany but more so in Ireland where the hero warrior-king Brian Boru (926–1014) finally drove the Norse armies out of Ireland at the battle of Clontarf in 1014. The name was carried to England by the Normans where it was popular until the 16th century, to be revived in the 19th. **Variants:** Briano, Briant, Brianus, Briar, Brareus, Brien, Brienus, Brion, Brior, Briunal, Bryan, Bryant, Bryon.

Brice A patronymic, meaning 'son of Rice', from the Old High German, *richi*, 'powerful, wealthy, ruler'. The French St Brice (died 444), one of St Martin of Tours' clergy, was highly revered in medieval Britain, thus spreading the name. **Variant:** Brick, Bristol, Bryce. *See also* Richard.

 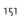

WISHFUL NAMING

Catherine might preserve the purity of a daughter and Nicholas ensure victory for a son. Wishful naming opens up a host of possibilities. The openly ambitious would find Dione or Gilbert just right; the fashion-conscious might choose Miles. There is Jubal for a musical family; Edmund or Stanislav for actors; Joshua or Raphael for painters; Inigo, John or Wyatt for architects. Geologists might ponder over Hutton, and journalists over the Harmsworth brothers, Albert and Harold. Francis and Sinbad are sailors' names, but Harley is best kept for the bookish librarian. Charles, Geoffrey, Walter and William might be on a writer's short list. Committed pacifists should avoid Louis and go for Romain or Pablo, from Paul. And vegetarians will find namesakes in St David, George Bernard Shaw, Leo Tolstoy, Leonardo da Vinci and Percy Bysshe Shelley.

Brigham From the Old Italian, *brigare*, 'to contend, fight'. A light-armed foot-soldier or a bandit or highway-robber. The Romans called the most northern and powerful people in Britain the Brigantes, whose power was shattered when Cerialis was Roman legate to Britain, from 71 to 74. **Variant:** Brigman.

Brindley From the Old Norse, *brandre*, 'piece of burning wood', which came to mean the reddish-browns and grey colours of burning wood. **Variant:** Brinley.

Brishan English gypsy name, given to a child born while it is raining.

Brock From the Old English, *broc*, 'badger', which derives from the same Gaelic word, or from the Celtic, *broch*. The traditional name given to a badger in folk and children's stories. **Variants:** Badger, Braxton.

Bromley From the Middle English, *brom*, 'broom', a shrub with yellow blossoms, and *leye*, 'meadow'. **Variants:** Bram, Bromwell.

Bronte From the Greek, *bronte*, 'thunder'. Although used as a first name, it is best known as the surname of the three novelists and poets who were daughters of an Anglo-Irish clergyman who changed his name from Brunty: Charlotte (1816–55), Emily (1818–48) and Anne (1820–49).

Brook *See under girls.* **Variants:** Brooke, Brooks.

Brooklyn The name of a district in New York City and the name given to the son of English footballer, David Beckham.

Brown From the Old English, *brun*, 'brown', the colour of a bear and probably from the same root word. *See also* Bernard and Bruno.

Bruce From the French name, Brieuse, 'woods, copse', the name of a Norman feudal lord and his village and castle outside Cherbourg. A member of the family arrived in Britain with William the Conqueror. The name was anglicised, and one of the descendants living in Scotland was Robert the Bruce (1274–1329) who seized the Scottish crown in 1306 and won Scotland's independence from England at the battle of Bannockburn in 1314, ratified 14 years later. As a first name, it gained ground only in the last century and is still found mostly in Scottish families. **Variants:** Brucey, Brucie, Bruis.

Bruno From the German, *brun*, 'brown'. The traditional name for a bear in folk and children's stories. Popular since the time of St Bruno of Cologne (1033–1101), a nobleman who founded the Carthusian order of monks near Grenoble in 1084. **Variants:** Brewis, Bronson, Browse, Bruin, Bruns, Labron, Lebron. *See also* Bernard.

Brutus From the Latin, *brutus*, 'heavy, irrational, stupid, unreasonable'. The Roman soldier and statesman, Marcus Junius Brutus (85–42BC), was party to the assassination of Caesar and later committed suicide at the battle of Philippi against Mark Antony and his allies.

Bubbles Name given to Bhawani Singh, son of the wealthy and powerful Indian Ruler of Jaipur, because so much champagne was drunk to celebrate his birth in 1931. He was the first male heir born to a ruling Maharaja of Jaipur for two generations.

Buck From the Old English, *buc*, 'stag', and *bucca*, 'he-goat', today meaning a 'male deer'. The term buck describes a young man with the animal's qualities of robustness and high spirits. **Variants:** Buckner, Bucky.

Burgess From the late Latin, *burgus*, 'fortified place'. A freeman of an English borough or town and, formerly, the name for a Member of Parliament who represented a borough, university or town. **Variant:** Burgiss.

Burley From the Old French, *bourre*, 'coarse wool', meaning a knot in yarn or cloth as well as a knot in wood. **Variants:** Burl, Burle, Burleigh.

Burns Scottish, from the Old English, *burn*, 'stream, fountain'. A name doubtless encouraged by the Scottish poet, Robert Burns (1759–96), who was so popular that the Scots dedicate an annual feast to him on his birthday, January 25, of haggis, turnip and whisky. **Variants:** Burnell, Burnham, Burnis.

Burr From the Middle English, *burre*, 'rough edge'. **Variants:** Burbank, Burrell, Burris, Burton.

Byrd From the Middle English, *bryd*, 'young bird'. Man's laborious attempts to imitate a bird's effortless power of flight led to the phrase of admiration, 'like a bird', meaning 'with ease'. **Variants:** Bird, Birdie, Burdette.

Byron From the Old English, *byre*, 'stall, hut, cottage', or from the Middle English, *bere*, 'bear' (see Bernard). Although used as a first name, it is always associated with the Scottish poet, Lord George Gorden Byron (1788–1824), who inherited a barony at 10 years old and became a leader of the British Romantic Movement. His poem, *Childe Harold's Pilgrimage* (1812), made him the most highly sought-after celebrity in London before he fell into equally deep disfavour and spent the rest of his life abroad. **Variants:** Biron, Buiron, Byram, Byrom.

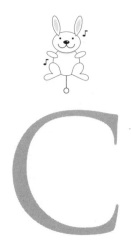

C

Cadmus In Greek mythology, the founder of Thebes on a site to which he was guided by a cow on the advice of the oracle of Delphi. When he killed a local monster, the goddess Athene told him to pluck out its teeth and sow them in the ground. From these sprang the Spartan warriors who immediately fought each other, but the five survivors became the ancestors of Thebes. Cadmus also discovered how to cast metal, invented the alphabet, was the divine legislator and married the beautiful Harmonia, daughter of Aphrodite. **Variants:** Cadmus, Cadwallader, Cadwell, Cal, Caldwell.

Cadoc The 6th-century Welsh saint was certainly an important missionary and possibly the founder of Nant Carfan monastery near Cardiff. His popular cult in Britain and Brittany led to some imaginative legends, including his being carried on a cloud to become a bishop in Italy.

Cadwallader From the Welsh, *cad*, 'battle', and *gwaladr*, 'leader'. A name found in Wales since the 7th century or earlier, both as first name and surname. **Variants:** Cadwaladar, Cadwalader, Cadwalladr. *See also* Cadmus.

Caesar Several theories, all from the Latin. From *caesaries*, 'dark and beautiful hair'; *caesariatus*, 'long hair, hairy'; *caedere*, 'to cut up', or from *caesius*, 'blue-grey colour'. The general, statesman and writer, Gaius Julius Caesar (100–44 BC), gave the name its associations of power and leadership. He invaded Britain in 55 BC and became a popular hero; crushed his rival, Pompey, and installed Cleopatra as Queen of Egypt while having an affair with her. With his people's approval, he became the first emperor of the Roman Empire in 46 BC, but was murdered on the Ides of March (March 15), 44 BC. Among his many reforms were the introduction of public libraries and the Julian calendar, later corrected to the one used now, the Gregorian.

After the emperor Hadrian, 'Caesar' became the honorific title of the junior emperor, while the senior emperor was titled 'Augustus'. Kaiser and Tsar are the German and Russian versions. A Caesarian operation to deliver a baby derives from the meaning, 'to cut up'; Caesar was allegedly born that way. The energetic bishop and preacher, St Caesarius of Arles (470–543), founded the first convent of women at Arles in Gaul. As a classical name, it was favoured during the Renaissance and was possibly introduced to Britain by Queen Elizabeth I's Venetian physician, Cesare Adelmare (1558–1636). **Variants:** Casar, Cesar, Cesare, Kaiser, Tsar.

Cahil Turkish, meaning 'young, naive'.

Cajetan The Italian saint, also called Gaetano (1480–1547), was a prominent Roman Catholic reformer and helped found the first congregation of clerks regular, the Theatines, who emphasised the study of the Bible. He also set up a series of charitable, non-profit-making shops in Naples.

Calchas In Greek mythology, the seer who foretold that Achilles would conquer Troy, thus a name implying wisdom and foresight.

Caleb From the Arabic, *qhaleb*, 'brave, victorious'; or from the Hebrew, 'bold, impetuous'. In the Bible, the leader of the Israelites after the death of Moses who, with Joshua, was permitted to enter the Promised Land (Numbers 14). Popularised after the Reformation, the name fell out of favour in this century, except in Scotland. **Variants:** Cal, Cale.

Callis From the Latin, *calix*, 'cup, goblet', especially one used in ceremonies of ritual or religion.

Calvert From the Old English, *cealf*, 'calf', thus 'herdsman, cowherd'. **Variant:** Calbert.

Calvin From the Latin, *calvus*, 'bald'. The doctrines of the French Protestant reformer and theologian, John Calvin (1509–64), were highly influential and became the basis of Presbyterianism as well as stimulating the Calvinist movement. They emphasised that truth is to be found in the Scriptures above all, that God is all-powerful and that man is sinful and needs a rigid moral code. **Variants:** Caiv, Cal, Vin, Vinnie, Vinny.

Camden From the Scottish Gaelic, 'winding valley'.

Cameron From the Celtic, 'bent nose'. A favourite Scottish name, possibly helped by two Scots: the scholar and theologian, John Cameron (1597–1625), whose doctrine was passive obedience; and the preacher, Richard Cameron (died 1680), who gave rise to the Cameronian movement, or Reformed Presbyterians. **Variant:** Cam.

Camillus See Camilla under girls. St Camillus (1550–1614) was a reformed gambler who, appalled at nursing standards, set up proper homes and hospitals in Naples, founded the order of the Servants of the Sick, and sent nurses to the battlefield. He is patron saint of the sick and of nurses. **Variant:** Camillo.

Camlo English gypsy name, meaning 'lovely, amiable'.

Campbell A compound from the Latin, *campus*, 'open field, even and flat place, plain', and *bellus*, 'beautiful' (*see* Bell); or from the Celtic, *cam beul*, 'curved mouth'. A favourite first name in Scottish families and the surname of one of the ancient and illustrious

Scottish clans which was given a barony in 1445 and whose descendants include the dukes of Argyll and Cawdor. **Variants:** Cam, Camp, Campie, Campy.

Candide *See* Candace *under girls.*

Canice The Irish saint (died 600), also known as Cainnech and Kenneth, spread the Gospel in Scotland before accompanying St Columba on his mission to the Picts and then returning to Ireland to found Aghaboe monastery at Ossory.

Canute *See* Knute. **Variant:** Cnut.

Cappi English gypsy name, meaning 'good fortune, profit'.

Caradoc From the Welsh name, Caradawg, 'amiable'. Popular in Wales ever since the 1st century, when the brave chieftain fought against the Romans and gave his name to Ceredigion, or Cardigan, in Wales. The Irish form is Carthac. **Variants:** Caractacus, Caradawg, Caratacos, Carthac, Carthage. *See also* Cedric.

Carden From the Old French, *carder*, 'to card, comb out', the process wool is put through before it is spun.

Carew From the Latin, *carus*, 'precious, beloved and loving'; or from *carruca*, 'four-wheeled state or travelling coach'.

Carmel *See* Carma *under girls*; but the name has significance for Roman Catholics as well as for Jews. St Louis built a church and convent on Mount Carmel, 'garden mountain', in Palestine, and dedicated it to the Blessed Virgin Mary. **Variants:** Carmeli, Carmelo, Carmen, Carmi, Carmiel, Carmine, Karmel, Karmeli, Karmi, Karmiel.

Carmen *See under girls.* **Variants:** Carman, Carmine.

Carol *See* Charles.

Carr From the Old Norse, *kjarr-myrr*, 'marsh ground, moor, boggy ground', or in Northumberland dialect, *carr*, 'rock, especially coastal rocks'. Hence Carvel, 'house by the marsh or rocks'. **Variants:** Carson, Carsten, Carvel, Carvell, Karr, Kerr, Kerry, Kerwin.

Carter From the Old Norse, *kartr*, 'cart for transporting goods', thus 'driver of a cart'. Like Barber, an old occupational name.

Carvel From the Manx, 'song'.

Casey From the Celtic, 'brave in battle, aggressive'. **Variant:** Caswell. *See also* Casimir and Cassius.

Casimir From the Polish name, Kazimier, 'announcement of peace'. The patron saint of Poland (1458–84), son of King Casimir IV, rejected marriage in favour of celibacy and pursued his interests in theology and the arts of peace. This and another Polish name, Ladislas, from Vladimir, enjoyed a limited popularity in Britain in the 19th century. **Variants:** Casey, Cass, Cassie, Cassy, Kazimier.

Caspar From the German, 'imperial'. In medieval legend, Caspar was one of the three Magi who brought gifts to the baby Jesus (see Balthasar). **Variants:** Casper, Cass, Cassie, Cassy, Gaspar, Gaspard, Gaspare, Gasparo, Gasper, Jaspar, Jasper, Josper, Kaspar, Kasper.

Cassidy Possibly from the Welsh *castiwr*, 'ingenuous, trickster'. **Variants:** Cass, Cassie, Cassy.

Cassius In Roman history the name of many illustrious people, but made most famous – or infamous – by the general and politician,

Gaius Cassius Longinus (died 42 BC), who played a leading part in the conspiracy to assassinate Julius Caesar and later committed suicide at the battle of Philippi. Also a male form of Cassia. **Variants:** Case, Casey, Cash, Casius, Caskey, Cass, Cassie, Cassy, Cazzie, Cazzy, Cez, Chaz, Kaz.

Catalin In Irish legend, the magic name of a wizard.

Cecil From the Latin, *caecus*, 'blind'. The prominent family of ancient Rome with this name probably had a blind ancestor, although they often claimed their name derived from *caeculus*, 'hearthstone', a word with more homely associations and, in Roman mythology, the name of the son of Vulcan, god of fire and craftsmanship. The name was given to both boys and girls in the Middle Ages, then revived for boys only in the last century, leaving Cecilia for the girls. **Variants:** Caecilianus, Caecilius, Cece, Cecile, Cecilio, Cecilius, Ceese, Ces, Cis, Kilan, Seisyllt, Sissy, Sitsyllt.

Cedric From the Celtic, *cedrych*, 'pattern of bounty, model of generosity'; or possibly from the Old English name, Ceredig, 'amiable'. It was invented by Sir Walter Scott for his most successful novel, *Ivanhoe* (1819), a medieval tale in which Cedric is father of Wilfred and guardian to Rowena, who fall in love with each other. The chieftain Cerdic founded the kingdom of Wessex and is considered to be father of the British royal family. Literature further encouraged the name when Frances Hodgson Burnett gave it to the boy who unexpectedly became Earl of Dorincourt in her novel, *Little Lord Fauntleroy* (1886). **Variants:** Cad, Caddaric, Caradoc, Caradog, Ced, Cerdic, Ceredic, Rick, Rickie, Ricky.

Cedro Spanish, from the Greek, *kedros*, 'cedar,

juniper', a tree whose very fragrant wood produces an oil that is a protection against decay.

Celerino From the Latin, *celero*, 'quicken, haste, accelerate'.

Celo *See* Celosia *under girls.*

Chad From the Celtic, 'battle, warrior'. The British saint (died 672), also known as Ceadda, was noted for his humility and holiness. After studying with St Aidan, he became Bishop of York and Lichfield. The name was revived by the 19th-century Tractarian movement. **Variants:** Ceadda, Chaddie, Chaddy.

Chaim From the Hebrew, 'life'. **Variants:** Chayim, Chayyim, Chayym, Haim, Hayim, Haym, Hayyim, Hy, Hyman, Hymie, Mannie, Manny.

Chalmers In Scotland, an old occupational name for senior attendants at court. A name found mostly in Scotland. **Variant:** Chalmer.

Champion From the Latin, *campus*, 'flat open space', via the Middle English, *champion*, 'warrior'. In ancient Rome, sports and fighting contests were held on the campus. Thus the name implies someone who is a good defence or support. **Variant:** Champ.

Chancellor From the late Latin, *cancellarius*, 'secretary', keeper of records in a royal or noble household, later extended to mean a high-ranking official such as the chancellor of a university, government or bishop's diocese. **Variants:** Chaney, Cheney.

Chandler From the French, *chandelle*, 'candle', thus 'a maker or seller of candles, a dealer in provisions or special goods'. Like Barber, an old occupational name. **Variants:** Chan, Chaney, Cheney.

MAD, FAT AND SLOW

In the excitement of naming their babies, delighted parents may forget to check how Margaret Alexei Dunsford, Francis Allen Turner or Stephen Lewis Oliver Wapshott will read when only their initials are printed. The remedy is easy. Many people are known by their second name, so the names can always be switched around. They will probably still flow well, and the otherwise inevitable schooltime teasing will be neatly avoided.

Channing From the Latin, *canalis*, 'canal'. The broad and deep part of a river or passage between two seas. As a river is a common symbol for life, the name implies a straight and clear path through life. **Variants:** Chan, Chane.

Chanticleer From the Old French, *chanter*, 'to sing', and *cler*, 'clear', thus 'to sing out loud and bright'. The French medieval epic, *Reynard the Fox*, was hugely popular throughout northern Europe. All its characters are animals, headed by Nobel the lion; Chanticleer is the cock.

Chaplin From the Latin, *cappella*, 'chapel', thus 'the clergyman of a chapel', and also one of a large institution such as a hospital, ship or university. **Variants:** Capp, Chapin, Chopin.

Chapman From the Old English, *ceap*, 'trade', thus 'trader, shopkeeper, merchant'. **Variants:** Chap, Chappie, Chappy, Mannie, Manny.

Charles From the Old Norse, *karl*, via the Old English, *ceorl*, 'man, male, freeman', and the Old High German, *karal* and *carlo*. A name first used as Karl in Germany, Carolus in

France and Ceorl in Britain. As Charles, it was already one of the most popular names in medieval Europe, both for people and places, before being carried to Britain by the Normans in the 11th century. It gained favour under the Stuart kings, reaching a height of popularity in the 19th century. Despite its original meaning of an ordinary man, it has acquired pedigree royal associations through the centuries. The most important contributor to this was Charles the Great, known as Charlemagne (742–814), who founded the Holy Roman Empire, the first Western empire since the fall of Rome, and was crowned Emperor by Pope Leo III on Christmas Day, 800. At his enlightened court the revival of classical learning developed into the Carolingian Renaissance. Other monarchs bearing the name include Charles V (1500–58), King of Spain and Holy Roman Emperor; Charles I (1600–49), King of England, Scotland and Ireland who, after a troubled reign, was tried for treason and executed; and Charles II (1630–85), his successor after the monarchy was restored in 1660. In all, 10 French kings and 5 rulers of Sweden

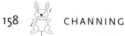

have been called Charles. Today, Queen Elizabeth's oldest son and heir to the British throne is called Charles Philip Arthur George (born 1948). The Italian saint, Charles Borromeo (1538–84), a cardinal at the age of 22 and Archbishop of Milan at 26, took a major and uncompromising part in the Roman Catholic Reformation. **Variants:** Alcuin, Carel, Carl, Carleton, Carlie, Carling, Carlisle, Carlo, Carlos, Carlson, Carlton, Carly, Carlyle, Carol, Carolle, Carolus, Carrol, Carroll, Cary, Caryl, Cathal, Cathaoir, Chad, Chaddie, Chaddy, Char, Charlet, Charley, Charlie, Charlot, Charls, Charlton, Charly, Charlys, Chas, Chay, Chic, Chick, Chicky, Chico, Chilla, Cholly, Chuck, Corliss, Curley, Curlie, Kalle, Karel, Karl, Karol, Karole, Karolus, Karoly, Siarl Tearlach, Turlogh.

Chauncey From the Latin, *cadere*, 'to fall, to happen', via the Old French, *cheaunce*, 'luck, chance'. **Variants:** Chance, Chancey, Chaune.

Chester From the Latin, *castrum*, 'fortress, castle, walled town'. The Romans built many fortress towns when they conquered Britain, including Chester itself, in Cheshire. Hence Chesley, 'camp by a meadow'. **Variants:** Caster, Castor, Chesleigh, Chesley, Chet.

Chevy From the Middle English ballad, *Chevy Chase*, recounting the story of the battle of Otterburn (1388) which had arisen from a hunt, or chase, around the Cheviot Hills that divide England and Scotland. **Variant:** Chase.

Chiel Scottish, from the Old English, *childe*, 'boy, lad'. The English gypsy form is Chal, the Russian, Chelovik. **Variants:** Chal, Chelovik.

Chik English gypsy name, meaning 'earth'.

Chip North American Indian, from *chippeu*, the name of a tribe of Algonquin-speaking Indians. **Variant:** Chipper.

Christian From the Greek, *Kristos*, 'anointed one'; in the Bible, the Greek translation of the Hebrew for 'Messiah'. Today, the word designates someone who professes belief that Jesus is Christ, the son of God, or who follows Christianity, the religion based on his teachings; also, a good, kind and generous person. A Christian name is one given to a child or adult at baptism (*see* Baptist). In the Christian world, the years are numbered from the year 1 AD, *anno Domini*, 'year of the Lord', the approximate year of Jesus' birth. In Denmark, Christian has been the name of 10 kings since the 15th century. In France, Chrétien of Troyes was the top romance writer of the 12th century. In England, Christian was the hero of John Bunyan's allegory, *The Pilgrim's Progress* (1678–84), but the name has always been less common than Christopher. **Variants:** Chretien, Chris, Chrissie, Chrissy, Christiaan, Christiano, Christie, Christien, Christy, Karston, Kerstan, Kit, Kito, Kreston, Kris, Krispin, Krista, Kristian, Kristo, Krystian, Zan.

Christobal Compound of Christ and *bal*, 'a dance, ball', thus 'dance of Christ'. **Variant:** Cristobol.

Christopher From the Greek, 'one who carries Christ'. Little is known of the 3rd-century martyr, St Christopher, but a later legend developed his cult and the name's popularity. It recounts that he was a huge man who sought the best of all masters; disappointed by a king and by Satan, he went to live beside a ford where travellers passed, hoping one might be Christ. One night, a child he was carrying across the ford grew increasingly heavy. The child was Jesus, who told him he was carrying the world on his back and had found the master for whom he was searching. It was a medieval belief that a

 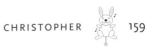

person who looked at an image of the saint would be safe all day – hence the quantity of pictures of him in churches. He is the patron saint of all travellers, including motorists. The Italian explorer, Cristoforo Columbo (1451–1506), known as Christopher Columbus in England and Cristobal Colon in Spain, discovered America whilst in the service of the Spaniards. Believing the world to be round, he had set off westwards hoping to find another route to the East, but arrived instead at the Bahamas, then Jamaica, Trinidad, Honduras, Costa Rica and Panama. The name survived the Reformation craze for biblical names, then rose to sustained heights of fashion in the last century. **Variants:** Chippy, Chris, Chrissie, Chrissy, Christal, Christie, Christoff, Christoffer, Christoforo, Christoph, Christophe, Christophorus, Christoval, Christovano, Christy, Chrystal, Cris, Cristoforo, Crystal, Gilchrist, Gillecriosd, Kester, Kit, Kristofel, Kristofer, Xit.

Chrysocomes From the Greek, 'with the golden locks'. One of many names given to the beautiful Apollo.

Chubb A river fish of the carp family which is short and thick, hence the implication of plumpness. **Variant:** Chubby.

Ciaran Two important Irish saints bear this name. Ciaran of Saighir lived in the 5th or 6th century, was probably one of the missionaries to Ireland before St Patrick, and is honoured as the first Bishop of Ossory. Ciaran of Clonmacnois (516–49), also called Kieran, trained under St Finnian before establishing a monastery at Clonmacnois, south of Athlone, which became one of the greatest in Ireland. **Variants:** Ciaren, Kiaran, Kiraren, Kyran.

Cicero From the Italian, *cicerone*, 'learned antiquarian, guide for sightseers'. A word derived from the great Roman orator and statesman, Marcus Tullius Cicero (106–43 BC), who was an exceptional scholar and a leading figure in the last years of the Roman Republic before Caesar became emperor. **Variants:** Cicerone, Ciceroni, Ciro, Cyrano.

Cid Spanish, from the Arabic, *sayyid*, 'master, lord'. In Spanish literature, the nickname given to Ruy Diaz, Count of Bivar, an 11th-century Christian hero who valiantly fought the Moors.

Clancy From the Gaelic, *clann*, 'offspring, family, tribe'.

Clarence Male form of Clare. St Clarus was a 7th-century French saint and martyr who lived as a hermit near Rouen in northern France; his name was taken by the villages nearby. The Norman family, de Clare, introduced the name to Britain and descendants gave their name to County Clare in Ireland. The title of the Duke of Clarence (1765–1837), later William IV, was taken from town of Clare in Suffolk when the dukedom was created in 1362. Sinclair is the anglicisation of St Clair. **Variants:** Clair, Claire, Clancy, Claral, Clare, Claron, Sinclair.

Clark From the Greek, *kleros*, 'inheritance', referring to the Levites' inheritance which was the Word of God and the Scriptures. The name then came to mean a person who could read and keep records – hence the 'clerical order' of the Church. **Variants:** Clarke, Claxton the name was brought more recently to the public's attention as Clark Kent, the name used by the cartoon superhero, Superman.

Claudius From the Latin, *claudus*, 'limping, lame, crippled, defective'. The Roman emperor and historian, Claudius I (10 BC–54 AD) was

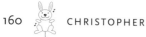

so-named because he was physically disabled and considered a simpleton. However, when Caligula was murdered in 41 AD, he became a sound and efficient emperor. A name found in Britain since the Roman occupation, it was then revived in the 16th century, when Lord Claude Hamilton (born 1543) was given the French form. **Variants:** Claud, Claude, Claudell, Claudian, Claudianus, Claudio, Claus, Glade.

Clay From the Old English, *claeq*, 'clay', a finegrained earth. In poetical language, a man's body as opposed to his spirit. **Variants:** Clayland, Clayton, Cle, Clea, Cletis, Cletus.

Cleanth Probably from the Old English, *claene*, 'clean, whole, pure, perfect'.

Clement From the Latin, *clemens*, 'kind, gentle, calm'. The British politician Clement Attlee (1883–1967) became leader of the Labour Party in 1935 and Prime Minister in 1945. Before him, other notable Clements include the first of 14 pope Clements, third successor to St Peter, who was a model of pastoral and paternal responsibility and who is seen as the first Apostolic Father. A name popular in the Middle Ages and the dedication for more than 40 English churches, it was revived by the Tractarians in the last century. **Variants:** Clem, Clemens, Clemente, Clementius, Clemmie, Clemmons, Clemmy, Clemon, Clim, Kal, Kalman, Kaloymous, Klemens, Klement, Kliment, Klimt.

Cleon *See* Clio *under girls.* **Variants:** Cleo, Cleophus, Clio, Kleon.

Clerebold Compound from the Latin, *clarus*, 'clear', and *bald*, 'bold'. Common from the 11th to the 14th centuries but rarely used since then. **Variants:** Clarembald, Clarenbald.

Clinton From the Middle English, *klint*, 'hill', and *tun*, 'town', thus 'hilltop town'. **Variant:** Clint.

Clive From the Old English, *clif*, 'steep, high and often overhanging rockface', hence Cleveland, 'place near the cliff', and Clifford, 'river crossing by the cliff'. The ambitious British soldier and statesman, Robert Clive (1725–74), known as Clive of India, was instrumental in establishing British power in Madras and Calcutta. He made the name popular with East India Company employees who gave it to their children as a first name in his honour. **Variants:** Cleavant, Cleavon, Cleve, Cleveland, Clevey, Clevie, Clif, Cliff, Cliffe, Clifford, Clifton.

Cloud The French prince and saint (520–60) was son of Clovis, King of the Franks, but resigned all claims to the Frankish throne by being tonsured a monk and devoting his life to good works and quietude.

Clovis *See* Clover *under girls.* Also a Latin form of Louis. Clovis (466–511), King of the Franks and greatest king of the early Merovingian dynasty, united Gaul and set up his capital at Paris. The Gallic form of his name is Louis, the name of 19 later French monarchs.

Cloyce From the Middle English, *acloien*, 'to obstruct, clog up, hamper'. **Variants:** Cloy, Cloyd.

Clure From the Latin, *cluere*, 'to be named in praise, earn good repute and fame'.

Clyde From the Welsh, 'heard from far away'. The Scottish river flows through Clydebank, the shipyard where the liners *Queen Mary* and *Queen Elizabeth* were built, and then Glasgow, before emptying into the

 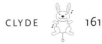

Firth of Clyde. The powerful Clydesdale breed of horse was developed in the Clyde valley. **Variants:** Cly, Clydell, Clywd.

Coburn From the Old English, *burn*, 'stream, fountain', thus 'where streams meet'. **Variant:** Coby.

Cody From the old English meaning 'helpful' and a 'pillow' or 'cushion'. Alternatives include Codey and Codie.

Colbert French, from the Latin, *collum*, 'neck' and the Old High German, *beraht*, 'bright, shining', thus 'a clear pass through a mountain'. **Variants:** Cole, Colvert, Culbert.

Colby From the old Norse meaning 'from the dark country'.

Cole From the Middle English, *col*, 'coal'. Thus Colby, 'coal town' and Coleman, 'coalminer'. **Variants:** Colby, Cole, Coleman, Colier, Colin, Colis, Collayer, Collie, Collier, Collis, Collyer, Colman, Colton, Colville, Colvin, Colyer.

Colin A French form of Nicholas; or the Gaelic form of Columba; or from the Welsh name, Colwyn; or from the Celtic, *cailean*, 'young hound, cub'. The name has grown in popularity since the 18th century. **Variants:** Cailean, Colan, Cole, Collie, Collin.

Columba From the Latin, *columba*, 'dove', the bird that symbolises peace (see Dove). The Irish saint (c. 521–597), also known as Colmicille, founded monasteries at Derry and Durrow before leaving Ireland with 12 companions for Iona, an island off the west coast of Scotland. Here he established another monastery which was the centre of his missionary work throughout Scotland. **Variants:** Colin, Colmicille, Colon, Colum, Columb, Columbus, Culva. *See also* Christopher.

Colwyn From the Welsh name, Collwyn, 'hazel grove', found in Wales since at least the 11th century.

Conal Irish, from the Celtic, 'high and mighty'.

Conan Irish, from the Celtic, *kuno*, 'high', or from the Middle English, *cunn* and *conn*, 'to know, learn, to be able to'. In Ireland, the name of a 7th-century chieftain, and in Britain, the name of several early bishops of London. More recently made famous by the Irish doctor and writer, Sir Arthur Conan Doyle (1859–1930), who created the character Sherlock Holmes. **Variants:** Con, Conant, Conn, Conney, Connie, Connor, Conny, Conor, Kinan, Kynan.

Conor Irish, from the Celtic, *conchubhar*, 'high desire'. The name of many figures in Irish legend and a common Irish name.

Conrad From the Old High German, *conja*, 'bold, wise', and *rad*, 'counsellor'. A name introduced to Britain from Germany during the Middle Ages. **Variants:** Con, Conn, Connie, Conny, Conrade, Conrado, Conroy, Cort, Koenraad, Konrad, Kort, Kurt.

Constantine From the Latin, *constare*, 'to stand together, remain steadfast, loyal and unchanging'. A name made immediately popular by the Roman emperor, Constantine the Great (285–337), who was converted to Christianity in 312, marking the end of Christian persecution. When he became sole emperor of both Western and Eastern empires in 324, he began to build a new eastern capital to rival Rome, which he named Constantinople (now called Istanbul). The name acquired further royal associations from Constantine MacFergus (died 820), King of the Picts, and from three early

Scottish kings. It was introduced into England by the Normans, and quickly spread. Unfashionable after the Reformation, it enjoyed a major revival in the last century. **Variants:** Con, Conney, Connie, Considine, Consta, Constans, Constant, Constantin, Constantinius, Constantino, Costa, Costain, Costane, Costin, Custance, Konstantin.

Consuel Male form of Consuela.

Cooper From the Latin, *cupa*, 'tub, vat, cask', thus 'a man who makes or repairs wooden tubs and barrels'. Like Barber, an old occupational name. **Variant:** Coop.

Corbet From the Latin, *corvinus*, 'raven'. **Variants:** Corb, Corbett, Corbey, Corbie, Corbin, Corby, Corwan, Corwin, Corwyn, Cory.

Cordell *See* Cordelia *under girls*. Also, from the Greek, *khorde*, 'string of a musical instrument'. **Variants:** Cord, Cordas.

Corin *See* Cora *under girls*. **Variants:** Caren, Carin.

Cormac From the Greek, *kormos*, 'tree trunk'. A name popular in Ireland. **Variants:** Cormack, Cormick.

Cornelius From the Latin, *corneus*, which can mean both 'cornell tree' and 'of horn, hardhearted, insensible'. In botany, the genus of trees that includes the cornell tree, or Cornelian cherry-tree. In ancient Rome, the Cornelius family were considered to include some of the most talented, distinguished and virtuous men and women. St Cornelius (died 253), known for his goodness and generosity, was pope amid troubled times in Rome and finally had to flee persecution in Rome. The name was introduced to Britain from Flanders where the pope's relics had been taken. **Variants:** Conney, Connie, Cornall,

Cornell, Corney, Cornie, Corny, Cory, Neil, Neilus, Nelly.

Cory From the Greek, *korys*, 'helmet'. In Greek pastoral poetry, the traditional name for a shepherd is Korudon, 'crested helmet'. **Variant:** Corey.

Cosmo *See* Cosima *under girls*. The martyred brother saints, Cosmas and Damian, were the patron saints of Milan, making the name popular in Italy. It was adopted as a family name by the powerful Medici family of Florence who were the dukes of Tuscany and great patrons of art. Probably introduced into Britain through Scotland where the father of the 3rd Duke of Gordon, a friend of Cosimo III of Tuscany, gave it to his son. **Variants:** Cosimo, Cosmas.

Count From the Old French, *conte*, 'companion, colleague'. **Variant:** Countee.

Covington From the Old English, *cofa*, 'cove', thus 'town in a cove'.

Cowan From the Middle English, *coule*, 'hooded robe' as worn by monks, implying a person who is a member of the clergy. **Variants:** Coe, Cowie.

Coy From the Latin, *quietus*, 'quiet', via the Old French, *coi*, 'shy, quiet, modest'. **Variant:** Coye.

Craig From the Celtic, *creag*, 'from the rocks'.

Cramer From the old English, *crammian*, 'to squeeze, fill up', whether the head with knowledge or the stomach with food. **Variants:** Cram, Kramer.

Crane From the Old English, *cran*, 'to stretch out, crane forward', showing eagerness and inquisitiveness. The name of birds belonging to the *Gruidae* family who have very long

THE MORE THE MERRIER

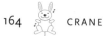

Parents usually give one, two or perhaps three names to their child. Some prefer to go for the short and clear. There is no harm in adding another John Smith to the estimated 10,000 already living, even if they do receive one another's mail occasionally. But some parents want something more dashing and memorable. For them, three names is just warming up. In the last century, the great-great-grandson of King Carlos III of Spain, Don Alfonso de Borbón y Borbón, was given 94 first names. In 1904, according to *The Guinness Book of Records*, a German boy with a ten-syllable surname was given 26 first names, one for each letter of the alphabet, beginning with Adolph and ending with Zeus. But he was usually known as plain Mr Wolfe + 585 (letters), Senior.

---

necks, legs and bills. **Variants:** Crandall, Crandell.

Crawford From the Old English, *crawan*, 'crow', and *ford*, 'a shallow river crossing', thus 'a ford where crows gather'. **Variants:** Craw, Crow.

Creole *See* Creola *under girls.*

Creon From the Greek, *kreon*, 'prince, ruler'. In Greek mythology, the name of several characters including the king of Thebes who offered the hand of his sister, Jocasta, to the person who could rid Thebes of the Sphinx.

Crichton From the Welsh, *crug*, 'hill', thus 'hilltop town'. **Variants:** Creighton, Creight, Crighton, Crite.

Crispin From the Latin, *crispus*, 'curled, crimped, wavy, curly-head'. SS Crispin and Crispian were brother shoemakers who were martyred in c. 285; they are the patron saints of shoemakers. Both names were popular during the Middle Ages, but less so since then. Crispus Attucks, a black man, is believed to have been the first American to die for Independence in the Boston Massacre. **Variants:** Crispian, Crispianus, Crispinian, Crispinianus, Crispus.

Croft From the Old English, *croft*, 'small field or pasture', or in Scotland, 'a small agricultural holding'.

Cromwell From the Welsh, *crwm*, 'bowed, arched', and *wella*, 'water', thus 'winding stream'. The British Puritan soldier and statesman, Oliver Cromwell (1599–1658), was Lord Protector of England from 1653 to 1658 and gave his name to the Cromwellian period of Puritan zeal and austerity.

Cronon From the Greek, *kronos*, 'companion'.

Crosby From the Middle English, *cros*, 'cross', probably referring to a market cross in a town centre.

Crowell From the Old English, *crawan*, 'to crow', implying to cry out with good news.

Cullen From the Celtic, 'cub, young animal', or from the Middle English, *cull*, 'to choose, pick out, gather'. **Variants:** Cull, Culley, Cullie, Cullin.

Curran From the Old English, *cyrin*, 'to churn, agitate'. **Variants:** Curr, Currey, Currie, Curry.

Curtis From the Latin, *curtis*, 'courtyard', via the Old French, *courtoner*, 'to be or reside at court, to flatter, entice, woo'. **Variants:** Cort, Cortie, Corty, Court, Courtenay, Courtland, Courtlandt, Courtney, Courts, Curcio, Curt, Curtell, Kurt.

Cuthbert From the Old English, *cuth*, 'famous', and *beohrt*, 'bright, shining, illustrious'. The English saint (c. 634–87), probably from Northumbria, was a young shepherd who had a vision of angels carrying the soul of St Aidan to heaven, which led him to become a monk under St Eata and to spread Christianity throughout northern Britain before becoming Bishop of Lindisfarne. He was known for his charm, preaching, and devotion to all mankind and to nature. A popular saint in medieval Britain, where 72 churches were named after him, his name fell out of use after the Reformation, to be revived by the 19th-century Tractarians.

Variants: Cudbert, Cudbright, Cuddie, Cuddy, Cumbert, Cuthbrid.

Cuyler From the Irish, *kyle*, 'chapel'.

Cyprian The martyr, St Cyprian (c. 200–58), was a barrister before he became Bishop of Carthage; he is regarded as one of the first great Christian Latin writers. The name was found in Britain in the 13th century and then became popular with the 19th-century Tractarians. Also the male form of Cypris.

Cyril From the Greek, *kyrios*, 'lord, like a lord'. The Macedonian missionary, St Cyril (827–69), and his brother, St Methodius, are known as 'the Apostles of the Slavs'. Cyril is thought to have invented both the Glagolitic and the Cyrillic alphabets in order to translate the Scriptures from Greek into the local language, thus laying the foundation of Slavonic literature. Introduced into Britain during the 17th century, the name was favoured by the 19th-century Tractarians but only became widespread in this century. **Variants:** Ciril, Cirill, Cirilo, Cirillo, Ciro, Cy, Cyriack, Cyrill, Cyrille, Cyrillo, Girioel, Kiril, Kyril, Syriack.

Cyrus From the Persian, *khuru*, 'throne'. The powerful king of Persia, Cyrus the Great (died 529), founded the Achaemenid empire and conquered the empire of the Medes, Babylon, Lydia and parts of Syria. Since his name is mentioned in the Old Testament, the name was fashionable with the Puritans. **Variants:** Ciro, Cy, Cyrie.

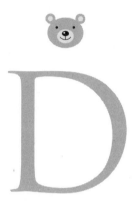

D

Dacey Irish, from the Gaelic, 'southerner'.

Daedalus In Greek mythology, the cunning Athenian sculptor who invented the axe and the saw. Jealous of his nephew's rival skills, he killed him and sought refuge with King Minos for whom be built the Labyrinth, a palace from which no-one could escape. But when he helped Theseus obtain a ball of thread so that he could escape from the Labyrinth, Minos punished him and his son, Icarus, by locking them up in it. They escaped by making an ingenious pair of wings out of wax, but Icarus flew too close to the sun, his wings melted and he fell into the Icarian Sea.

Dagan *See* Dagania *under girls.*

Dahi Welsh, from the Celtic, 'nimble'. The name became confused with, and finally absorbed by, David. **Variant:** Dathi.

Dai *See* David.

Dalbert From the Old High German, *tal*, 'valley, hollow', and *beraht*, 'bright, shining', thus 'bright valley'.

Dale From the Old Norse, *dahl*, 'broad valley, hollow', via the Old English, *dael*. Hence, Dalton, 'valley town' and Dallin, 'from the vale'. **Variants:** Dael, Dal, Dali, Dail, Dallan, Dallas, Dallin, Dalt, Dalton, Dalva, Delles, Dillon, Dolan.

Damon From the Greek, *daimon*, 'divine power, fate', via the Latin, *daemon*, 'spirit, evil spirit, demon', implying either a tormentor, devil or unclean spirit, or a genius, full of zeal, skill or energy; or from the Old English, *doeg*, 'day', hence Delbert, 'bright day'. In classical mythology, Damon and Pythias were such devoted friends that when Dionysius condemned Pythias to death, Damon took his place and offered to be executed if necessary while Pythias went home to arrange his affairs. Pythias returned in time, and the tyrant was so impressed by the friends'

 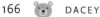

devotion that he freed them both. In Latin pastoral poetry, Damon is the type name for a rustic country youth. The popular American writer, Damon Runyon (1884–1946) wrote *Guys and Dolls* (1933), later a hit musical. A name found in Britain by the 13th century. **Variants:** Dag, Dagan, Dagget, Dailey, Daily, Daly, Dame, Damian, Damiano, Damien, Damlan, Damlano, Darmon, Day, Dayman, Daymon, Daymond, Dayton, Demian, Del, Delbert. *See also* Cosmo.

Dandie A nickname for Andrew, made popular by Sir Walter Scott who gave it to Dandy Dinmont, a sturdy Lowland farmer, in his novel, *Guy Mannering* (1815). **Variants:** Dandey, Dandy.

Dane From the Old Norse, *danh*, 'Dane', the inhabitants of Denmark. **Variants:** Dainard, Dane, Duane.

Daniel From the Hebrew, *dan*, 'judge', thus 'God is my judge'. In the Bible, the prophet whose faith protected him when he was condemned to die in a den of lions. St Daniel the Stylite (409–93), a disciple of St Simeon the Stylite, lived on top of two pillars outside Constantinople from where he gave shrewd and practical advice to those who came, including the emperors Leo I and Zeno. Crowds flocked to listen to his sermons which emphasised love for mankind and care for the poor. The name gained favour in the 12th century and was at its most popular during the Reformation vogue for Old Testament names. **Variants:** Dan, Dana, Dani, Danil, Danilo, Dannet, Dannie, Dannson, Danny, Deiniol, Denils, Dennel, Domhnall, Kamiela.

Dante From the Italian, *durare*, 'to endure, bear, be patient'. The Italian poet, Dante Alighieri (1265–1321) described his boyhood love for the unattainable Beatrice in *La Vita Nuova* (1292). His greatest work was *La Divina Commedia*, in which he described his journey through hell guided by Virgil, and through heaven with Beatrice again, now personifying perfect spiritual love. The name's romantic associations made it popular in the Middle Ages. During the medieval revival in the last century it was the first name of the Pre-Raphaelite painter, Dante Gabriel Rossetti (1828–82). *See also* Durand.

Dar From the Hebrew, 'pearl, mother-of-pearl'. *See* Pearl *under girls*.

Darcy From the French, *d'Areci*, the name of one of William the Conqueror's companions. **Variants:** D'arcy, D'Arcy, Dar, Darce.

Dardanos In Greek mythology, brother of Harmonia (see Harmony) and son of the all-powerful Zeus and Electra who founded Troy. The Dardans, or Daranians, were other names for the Trojans. **Variant:** Dard.

Darius Darius I (c. 558–486) seized the Persian throne after murdering the usurper. He divided the Persian empire into provinces and led an invasion into Greece which finally ended in defeat at the battle of Marathon in 490. **Variants:** Daare, Daren, Daria, Darian, Darien, Dario, Darin, Darrel, Darren, Daryl, Derry, Dorian. *See also* Darren.

Darrel Possibly from the Old English, *deor*, 'dear, beloved, special'. **Variants:** Dar, Dare, Darell, Darlin, Darling, Darol, Darold, Darrell, Darrill, Darrol, Darroll, Darry, Darryl, Daryl, Daryle, Derel, Derial, Derland, Derral, Derrel, Derrell, Derry, Dorrel.

Darren See Darius. **Variants:** Dar, Dare, Daren, Darin, Dario, Darn, Darnell, Daron, Darrin, Darring.

 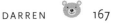

Darrow From the Old English, *daroth*, 'spear'. **Variant:** Daro.

Darton From the Old English, 'water', and *tun*, 'village, town', thus 'town near water'.

Darwin From the Old English, 'water', and *wyn*, 'friend', thus 'lover of the sea'. The British naturalist, Charles Robert Darwin (1809–82), put forward the revolutionary theory that evolution of nature and mankind was based on natural selection, the strongest, best and most adaptable surviving, the others not. His views were highly controversial, conflicting head on with the Christian idea that God was responsible for all creation. **Variants:** Derwin, Derwyn, Durwin.

Daven Scandinavian, meaning 'two rivers'.

David From the Hebrew name, Dodavehu, 'beloved by God', also used as a lullaby name. In the Bible, King David (died 962 BC) was born in Bethlehem. As a youth, he killed the giant Goliath. He later seized the throne, when Saul died, to become the second king of Judah. He later ruled Israel too, uniting the Israelites, and his son became King Solomon. A highly cultured man, he enjoyed music and possibly wrote the Psalms. The Star of David is the symbol of Judaism. A name first made popular in Wales and Scotland where its religious and royal associations grew. The patron saint of Wales is St David (520–600), also called Dewi. A teetotaller and vegetarian, he was primate of the Celtic church in South Wales, influenced monasticism in Ireland and founded a strict monastery at his headquarters, Mynyw (St David's). In Scotland, two kings bore the name: pious St David I (1084–1153), who invaded England but suffered defeat at the battle of the Standard (1138); and David II (1324–71), who tried again in 1346 but was defeated and taken prisoner. The name came to England only in the 12th century, possibly brought by the Normans, but its real popularity had to wait until this century. **Variants:** Dab, Dabbey, Dabby, Dabko, Dabney, Daffy, Dafyd, Dafydd, Dahi, Dai, Dakin, Dako, Dathi, Daud, Daue, Dav, Dave, Daveed, Davey, Davi, Davidde, Davide, Davidyne, Davie, Davin, Daviot, Davis, Davit, Davy, Davyd, Daw, Dawe, Dawes, Dawood, Dawoodji, Dawson, Dawud, Deakin, Deio, Devi, Devlin, Dewer, Dewey, Dewi, Dov, Dow, Dowe, Kavika, McTavish, Tab, Taffy.

Deacon From the Greek, *diakonos*, 'servant', implying a servant of God in the Christian church where a deacon ranks just below priest.

Dean From the Old English *dene*, 'valley' (the Forest of Dean in Gloucestershire, formerly a royal hunting preserve, became the first National Forest Park in Britain in 1938). Or from the Greek, *deka*, 'ten', via the Middle English, *deen*; the name implies 'one sat over ten', meaning a person of rank responsible for a collection of people. The American actor James Dean (1931–55) has probably popularised the name in this century; he starred in *East of Eden* (1954) and *Rebel Without a Cause* (1955) and his death at the age of 23 made him into a cult hero for the young. **Variants:** Deane, Dee, Dene, Dennit, Deno, Denton, Dino.

Decimus From the Latin, *decimus*, 'tenth'. A name often given to a tenth child.

Deiniol From the Welsh, 'charming, attractive'.

Dekel From the Arabic, 'palm tree, date palm', implying soaring height and straightness, and the capacity to produce nourishing fruit.

KNIGHTS AND LADIES

Heroes and heroines of favourite stories have always been a rich source of names. In the middle ages, one of many good legends focused on King Arthur and his Knights of the Round Table. It sparked the imaginations of parents dreaming of their sons' future chivalry and their daughters' beauty. Malory's epic *Le Morte Darthur*, printed on William Caxton's historic press, and Spenser's *The Faerie Queene*, kept the stories alive. Then came Tennyson's revival of the legend in the last century in the full gush of Victorian medieval mania. It was a huge popular success, selling 10,000 copies in the first week alone, and it revived names such as Arthur, Elaine, Enid, Gareth, Guinevere, Percival and Vivien.

Delano From the Irish Gaelic, 'healthy, dark man', suitable for a child of dark complexion. Or from the Old French, *de la nuit*, 'of the night', suitable for a child born during the night. **Variant:** Delaney.

Delmar From the Latin, *mare*, 'sea', thus 'from the sea'. **Variants:** Del, Delmer, Delmor, Delmore.

Delos From the Greek, *dhilos*, 'ring', a small Greek island in the Aegean Sea encircled by other islands. In Greek mythology, an island summoned from the depths of the ocean by Poseidon, god of the sea, then chained to the sea bed by the supreme god, Zeus; the gods Artemis and Apollo were born there. **Variants:** Deli, Delius. *See also* Delia.

Delvin From the Greek, *delphis*, 'dolphin'. **Variants:** Del, Delwin.

Demetrius From the Greek, 'earth mother'. In Greek mythology, the beautiful and fair-haired Demeter was goddess of fertile and cultivated soil and of its rich harvest, especially corn. She looked after agricultural labourers and was also the mother goddess of mankind who presided over marriages. St Demetrius of Rostov (1651–1709), a wealthy Cossack who became Bishop of Rostov, was an outspoken preacher and scholar who wrote drama and verse. **Variants:** Deems, Demetre, Demetri, Demmy, Dimitri, Dimitrios, Dimitry, Dmitri.

Dempsey From the Middle English, *demerite*, 'absence of merit, deserving of blame'. **Variant:** Demp.

Denby From the Old Norse, *denh*, 'Dane', thus 'Danish village, town'. **Variants:** Den, Denholm, Denney, Dennie, Denny.

Denis French form of Dionysius. The legend of St Dionysius of Paris (died c. 258), also known as Denis or Denys, recounts that he was a missionary sent from Rome to Gaul who after a few years was beheaded on Montmartre, 'martyr's hill', in Paris. The renowned abbey-church of St Denis, the French royal burial place, was dedicated to him and for many years he was regarded as the patron saint of France. The name was carried, with the cult, to Britain by the Normans and enjoyed popularity until the 17th century when it fell out of use, to be revived this century. **Variants:** Deenys, Den, Denison, Denit, Denman, Dennet, Dennis, Dennison, Dennit, Denny, Denote, Denys, Denzil, Denzel, Denzell, Diniz, Dion, Dionis, Diot, Donnet, Donoghm, Dwight, Enis, Ennis, Enzo, Tennis.

Denman Scottish, from the Middle English, *den*, 'small wooded dell', thus a man living in such a place.

Denver From the Middle English, *den*, 'small wooded valley', and the French, *vert*, 'green'.

Denzil Probably from the Celtic, *dinas*, 'stronghold', and the Old Cornish, *uhel*, 'high'. Alternatives include Denzel.

Deodatus From the Latin, *deodonatus*, 'gift of God'. An ecclesiastical name by the 7th century, and in general use from the 13th. **Variants:** Deodaonatus, Deodat, Dieudonne.

Derby From the Old English, *deor*, 'deer'; or from *dwr*, 'water', and *by*, 'habitation, village, town'; or a form of the Irish name, Dermot. The phrase 'Darby and Joan' means an elderly, placid, harmonious couple and originates from an 18th-century English ballad. **Variants:** Dar, Darb, Darby, Derland, Dero, Deron, Dorset, Dorsey, Dorsie, Dove, Dover, Dovey.

Derek From one of two Old High German names: Hrodrick, from *hrod*, 'famous', and *richi*, 'ruler, power, wealth', thus 'famous ruler'; or Thiudoricus, from *theuda*, 'people', thus 'the people's ruler' (see Theodoric). Found in Britain by the 15th century, to be revived this century. **Variants:** Darrick, Dederick, Dekker, Deric, Derick, Derrek, Derric, Derrick, Derrik, Derry, Deryck, Deryk, Diederick, Dirck, Dirk, Durk, Dyryke, Rick, Ricky, Theodoric, Thierry, Tedrick. *See also* Roderick.

Dermot From the Old Irish name, Diarmaid, from *di-fharmait*, 'free from envy'. In Irish legend, Diarmaid eloped with Grainne, Queen of Tara, only to die when her husband forced him to hunt a savage boar. A name most popular in Ireland. **Variants:** Darby, Der, Derby, Dermott, Diarmid, Diarmit, Diarmuit. *See also* Derby.

Deror From the Hebrew, 'freedom'. Also, the name given to the swallow, the fast-flying bird. **Variants:** Derori, Dror.

Derry Possibly from the Welsh, *deri*, 'oak trees'. **Variant:** Dare. *See also* Darrel.

Derwent From the Celtic, 'clear water'. The name of several rivers in Britain, the longest one flowing through Derbyshire into the River Trent.

Desiderio From the Latin, *desiderium*, 'ardent desire, deep longing, wish'. A name found in Britain since the Middle Ages. **Variants:** Desi, Desideratus, Desiderius, Diderot, Didi, Didier, Didon, Didot, Dizier.

Desmond From the Latin, *mundus*, 'the universe, the heavens, skies, earth, mankind', thus someone who is part of creation. In Ireland, it was originally a surname, from Deas Munter, 'man from South Munster', becoming a first name during the 18th century before crossing to England. **Variants:** Demon, Des, Desi, Dezi.

Devin From the Celtic, 'poet'.

Devir From the Hebrew, 'inner sanctum, inner room, holy place'.

Dexter *See* Dextra *under girls.* **Variants:** Decca, Deck, Dex.

Dhani From the Hindi, 'person of wealth and riches'.

Diamond *See* Diamanta *under girls.*

Didi *See* Desiderio and Dodo.

Diego *See* James. The Spanish Franciscan saint from Seville (c. 1400-63), was revered for his holiness and for his work with the poor in the Canary Islands.

Dietrich From the German, 'people of wealth, power and riches'. **Variants:** Dierk, Dieter, Dirk, Dtrik, Dytrych.

Digby From the Old French, *diguer,* 'to make a dyke or ditch', and, by inference, to unearth, investigate, discover, be curious. Used in Britain since the 19th century.

Diggory Probably from the French, *egare,* 'strayed, lost'. In Britain, Sir Degore was the hero of a medieval romance. Later, Oliver Goldsmith gave the name Diggory to a serving-man in his highly successful comedy, *She Stoops to Conquer* (1773). **Variant:** Digory.

Dinsmore From the Irish Gaelic, 'fortified hill'. **Variants:** Dinnie, Dinny, Dinsdale, Dinse.

Diogenes The Greek philosopher (412–322) was nicknamed *Kunus,* 'the dog', because he supposedly lived in a barrel–hence the name 'Cynics' for his followers. He rejected all forms of luxury and set up the Cynic school in Athens to promote self-denial, self-control, avoidance of physical pleasure, acceptance of suffering and a general return to nature.

Diomedes In Greek mythology, one of the chief heroes throughout the long Trojan war. He ran the Trojan camp with Odysseus, to whom he consistently gave wise and bold advice, and was helped by Athena to wound Aphrodite and Ares. **Variants:** Diomed, Diomede.

Dionysius From the Greek, 'god of the Nysa', a city in India or Afghanistan where he was born. In Greek mythology, god of wine, pleasure and frenzied revelry, later called Bacchus, whose cult celebrated the fertility of nature. The name therefore implies a person of terrific energy, spontaneity, passion and enjoyment of life. Several important saints have borne the name. The judge and martyr, St Dionysius the Areophagite, was converted by St Paul and became the first bishop of Athens. St Dionysius of Alexandria (died c. 265), was a brave bishop of Alexandria when there was much persecution. **Variants:** Dion, Dionisio, Dionysios, Dionysos, Dionysus. *See also* Denis.

Dixey *See* Dixie *under girls.* **Variants:** Dix, Dixie, Dixy.

Dixon Patronymic of Richard, 'son of Richard'. **Variant:** Diskin.

Dob Czech, from *dobro,* meaning 'to do good'; also a form of Robert. **Variants:** Dobb, Dobbs, Dobs.

Dobry Polish, meaning 'good'.

Dodo From the Hebrew *dodi,* 'beloved'. In the Bible, a member of one of the tribes of

 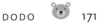

Israel. Or from the Portuguese, *duodo*, 'stupid, clumsy', the name given to the large, flightless bird found on the island of Mauritius in the Indian Ocean but extinct since the 17th century. **Variant:** Didi. *See also* Dudley.

Dominic From the Latin, *dominicus*, 'belonging to a lord or master'. In Christianity, 'belonging to God' and thus both 'servant of God' and 'God's day, Sunday'. The zealous but compassionate Spaniard, St Dominic (1170–1221), known as 'the burner and slayer of heretics', founded the Order of Preachers in 1216, a body of highly trained monastic priests devoted to teaching and preaching. They made an important contribution to intellectual life throughout medieval Europe. Later called Dominicans, or Blackfriars because of their black cloaks, they dominated the ruthless Spanish Inquisition. Although at first given only to children born on a Sunday, and then confined to Roman Catholics after the Reformation, the name is generally popular today. **Variants:** Dom, Domenic, Domenico, Domenyk, Domingo, Dominick, Dominik, Dominique, Dominy, Don, Nick, Nickie, Nicky.

Donald From the Celtic name, Domhnall, 'world ruler, proud ruler'. Especially popular in Scotland, helped by six early Scottish kings, of whom Donald I was their first Christian king. In Ireland, it is also a form of Daniel. **Variants:** Don, Donahue, Donal, Donalt, Donn, Donne, Donner, Donnie, Donny, Donahue, Donovan, MacDonald.

Donatus From the Latin, *donatus*, 'given, bestowed upon', implying a special present or even a sacrifice. According to tradition, St Donatus of Fiesole (died c. 876), was an Irishman who was miraculously instructed to become bishop of Fiesole, near Florence, when he was passing by on his return from Rome. A popular Saxon name, during the Middle Ages it was given to both boys and girls. **Variants:** Don, Donary, Donny.

Donnel From the Gaelic, *dun*, 'hill, hill-fort'. The Irish St Donnan (died 617) established a community of monks on the island of Eigg in the Inner Hebrides but a local gang of men martyred them all on Easter Eve. A name found in Scotland where several places and churches are also named after the saint. **Variants:** Donn, Donnell, Donnelly, Donny, Doon, Dun.

Dor From the French, *d'or*, 'made of gold'; also from the Hebrew, 'generation'.

Doran From the Greek, *doron*, 'gift'. **Variants:** Darren, Dore, Dorey, Dorian, Dorie, Doron, Dorran, Dory. *See also* Oscar.

Dorris See Doris under girls.

Dotan From the French, *dot*, 'dowry', a woman's marriage settlement; or from the Hebrew, *dat*, 'law'. **Variant:** Dothan.

Dotson Metronymic of Dorothy, 'son of Dot'. **Variant:** Doston.

Dougal From the Celtic name, Dugald, from *dubh*, 'dark colour', and *gall*, 'stranger'. The name given to Danes (compare Fingal). Even today, the name is used by an Irishman to mean an Englishman. Later, a nickname used by Lowland Scots for Highlanders. **Variants:** Doug, Dug, Dugald, Duggy.

Douglas From the Gaelic, *dubh*, 'dark colour', and *glas*, 'water', thus 'dark stream'. Douglas, capital of the Isle of Man, is at the junction of two streams, the Dhoo and the Glas. The ancient Scottish clan, whose legend goes back to the 8th century, acquired the earldoms of Douglas, Angus and Morton, and used the

TWO FOR TEA: NAMING TWINS

It is tempting to find two names to link twins perpetually, however different their personalities might be. Obvious pairs are Adam and Eve, Peter and Paul, Victoria and Albert, David and Jonathan, and Anthony and Cleopatra. Less obvious pairs abound in history, literature and legend: David and Bathsheba, Abelard and Heloise, Harlequin and Columbine, Romulus and Remus, Francis and Clare, Florus and Laurus, Apollo and Artemis, Dante and Beatrice, and Alexander and Philip. The same name for both twins has great style but might lead to amusing mix-ups: Henry and Henrietta, George and Georgina, Charles and Caroline, and Joseph and Josephine. Another trick would be to choose the same word but in different languages, such as Edan and Blaise, or Lipman and Philander. And then there are the more amusing pairs that perhaps none but the bravest parent would try: Mickey and Donald, Fortnum and Mason, Beau and Belle, Laurel and Hardy, Rose and Bush – or Charles and Diana.

---

name for boys and girls. The Douglas fir is named after the botanist, David Douglas (1798–1834), who in 1827 brought its seeds from North America to Scotland. **Variants:** Doug, Dougal, Dougie, Douglass, Dougy, Dugald, Duggie.

Dov From the Hebrew, 'bear'.

Dove From the Old English, *dufe*, 'dove', via *douve*. The many birds of the family *Columbinae*, especially pigeons. In the Bible, a dove brought back an olive leaf to Noah's ark, indicating peace after God's angry flood (Genesis 8). Thus all doves symbolise peace and messages of peace, and the turtle dove has the additional meaning of love – hence the affectionate term, 'my dove'. **Variants:** Dovey, Duff. *See also* Derby.

Dovey From the Hebrew, *davor*, 'to whisper', implying a quiet, reticent character.

Down From the Old English, *ofdune* and *dune*, 'from the hill'; the Old English, *dun*, 'rolling expanse of grassy hills', such as the North and South Downs in southern England; or from the Old Norse, *dunn*, 'down plumage', the very soft, fluffy feathers of a young bird. **Variant:** Doane.

Doyle From the Irish, *dail*, 'assembly, gathering'. A name boosted by the widespread popularity of Sir Arthur Conan Doyle's novels.

Drake From the Greek, *dracon*, 'serpent'. Vast serpent-dragons are an important part of the mythology of many countries – some have wings, like the red dragon of Wales, and most have claws and breathe fire. Dragons have different meanings in each tradition. In Japan, the ancestor of the royal family was the Dragon King of the Sea. In China and Scandinavia, dragons guard treasure and protect rulers. In Babylon and Egypt, they spell chaos. In Christianity, they were the devil incarnate – in England, St George was the Christian hero who slew the dragon.

Dre *See* Andrew. This diminutive version comes from the name Andre and means 'courageous'.

Drew *See* Andrew and Drogo.

Driscoll From the Celtic, *drystan*, 'sad, distressed'. *See also* Tristam.

Drogo From the Gothic German, *draga*, 'to carry'. Carried to England by the Normans as Drogo and in the French form, Dru. Used until the 17th century, to be revived in the 19th. **Variants:** Drew, Drewe, Drews, Dru, Druce, Drue, Drugo.

Dryden From the Middle English, *drye* and *denne*, 'dry secluded valley'.

Dude From the Irish, *duidin*, 'little pipe'; an English gypsy name, meaning 'moon'; or from German dialect, *dood*, 'fool'.

Dudley From the Old English, 'Dudo's meadow'. The 8th-century Saxon Prince Dodo supposedly built Dudley Castle. But it was Robert Dudley, Earl of Leicester and Queen Elizabeth I's favourite, who made the name popular. **Variant:** Dud.

Duff From the North English dialect, 'dough, uncooked pastry'. *See also* Dove.

Duke From the Latin, *dux*, 'leader, conductor, guide, commander'. A popular nickname for people who become leaders in their profes-

sion, especially in entertainment. **Variants:** Dukey, Dukie, Duky. *See also* Marquis.

Dukker English gypsy name, meaning 'to bewitch, tell fortunes'. **Variant:** Durriken.

Dumont From the French, *du mont*, 'from the mountain, hill'.

Duncan Scottish, from the Gaelic, *donn*, 'greyish-brown', and *chadh*, 'warrior', thus 'dark-skinned warrior'. Of several notable Scotsmen, the fame of King Duncan I (ruled 1034–40), supposedly slain by Macbeth at Pitvagenny, near Elgin, was revived and popularised in Shakespeare's tragedy, *Macbeth* (1606). The name's use, however, remains mostly confined to Scotland. **Variants:** Dun, Dunc, Dunkie, Dunn.

Dunstan From the Old English, *dunn*, 'greyish-brown'. The English saint (c. 909–88) was an exceptional man of his period, who stimulated the revival of monasticism in England with his work at Glastonbury monastery and then at Bath, Exeter, Westminster and elsewhere. He became Archbishop of Canterbury, principal adviser to the kings of Wessex, devised the coronation rite of English kings, and contributed to the *Regularis Concordia*, a more pastoral version of the Rule of St Benedict. He was also skilled in metal-work, calligraphy, played the harp and was an excellent and gentle teacher. **Variants:** Donestan, Dunn, Dunne, Dunst, Dustie, Dustin, Dusty.

Dupee From the French, *duper*, 'to deceive, trick'.

Dur From the Hebrew, 'to encircle, make a heap'. *See also* Derby.

Durand From the Latin, *durare*, 'to last, to endure'. Introduced to Britain by the

Normans. **Variants:** Dante, Durant, Durante, Duryea.

Duriel From the Hebrew, 'my house belongs to God', implying loyalty and faith.

Durril English gypsy name, meaning 'berry', most usually a gooseberry.

Durwald From the Middle English, *doer*, 'deer', and the German, *wald*, 'forest'. **Variants:** Durward, Durwood.

Dustin From old Norse. **Alternatives include** Dusty and Dustyn.

Dutton From the Celtic, 'fortified hill'.

Dwight From the Old English, *hwit*, 'white, fair', or from the French name, Diot, from Dionysius. A name especially popular in the USA where children of former students of Yale University were named after its president, Timothy Dwight (1795–1817). More recently, Dwight David Eisenhower (1890–1969), known as Ike, was Supreme Commander of the Allied Adventurous Forces during the Second World War and President of the United States from 1953 to 1961. **Variants:** Dewitt, DeWitt, Diot, Doyt, Wit, Wittie, Witty.

Dylan From the Welsh, 'the sea'. In Irish legend, the hero born of the sea-god who leapt back into the brine the moment he had been baptised. The name of the Welsh poet and writer from Swansea, Dylan Marlais Thomas (1914–53). More recently the singer American songwriter Bob Dylan has inspired many new parents. **Variants:** Dill, Dillie, Dillon, Dilly.

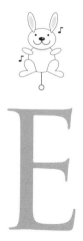

E

Eamon *See* Edmund and Edward.

Earl From the Old English, *eorl*, 'warrior, chief, nobleman'. In the British nobility, the rank between Marquis and viscount. **Variants:** Earland, Earle, Earlie, Early, Erl, Erle, Errol, Erroll, Rollo.

Eaton From the Old English, *ea*, 'river, running water', and *tun*, 'town, village', thus 'riverside town'.

Ebenezer From the Hebrew, 'stone of help'. In the Bible, the stone put up by Samuel to commemorate the defeat of the Philistines (1 Samuel 7). Popular with the Puritans, the name was brought into the limelight in the last century by Ebenezer Scrooge in Charles Dickens' story, *A Christmas Carol* (1843). Ebenezer is a mean man who is transformed by a visit from the ghost of Marley into a model of kindness and generosity. **Variants:** Benezer, Eb, Eban, Eben.

Edan From the Celtic, 'flame, fire'.

Eddy From the Old English, *ed*, 'again, back', referring to a whirlpool of water running against the tide. **Variant:** Edy. *See also* Edward.

Eden From the Hebrew, *eden*, 'delight'. In the Bible, God created the Garden of Eden, also called Paradise, for Adam (Genesis 2). *See also* Aidan.

Edgar From the Anglo-Saxon name, Eadgar, from the Old English, *eadig*, 'happy, fortunate, rich', and *gar*, 'spear' – 'ead' was the prefix of the Wessex royal family name. Alfred the Great's grandson, Edgar the Peaceful, King of Wessex, was the first publicly recognised King of England, uniting less powerful kings under him. The name lost favour after the Conquest but was revived by Shakespeare for his tragedy, *King Lear* (1606), in which Edgar is the virtuous legitimate son of Gloucester, and half-brother of Edmund who plots his disinheritance. Its second revival was when

Sir Walter Scott gave it to the Master of Ravenswood in his novel, *The Bride of Lammermoor* (1819), and it has been used frequently since. As Edga, it is also given to girls. **Variants:** Eadgar, Ed, Eddie, Eddy, Edgard, Neddie, Neddy, Teddie, Teddy.

Edlin *See* Adeline *under girls.*

Edmund From the Anglo-Saxon name, Eadmund, from the Old English, *eadig*, 'happy, fortunate, rich', and *mund*, 'guardian'. Three English kings have borne the name. First, the saint and King of East Anglia (840–70), a German adopted as heir by King Offa, who was defeated by the Danes and then supposedly martyred with arrows because he refused to share his Christian kingdom with heathens. Bury St Edmunds, in Suffolk, is named after him. Edmund I (921–46), King of England, forced the Danes out of Northumbria. Edmund Ironside (981–1016), King of England, resisted Knute's invasion in 1015 and then had to partition the country because his nobles supported Knute. The saint, teacher and preacher, Edmund of Abingdon (c. 1170–1240) was Archbishop of Canterbury. Despite a rather tumultuous political life, he wrote *Mirror of Holy Church*, which sets out the contemplative way to God in the English medieval mystic tradition. The name has been constantly in use down the centuries. **Variants:** Eadmond, Eamon, Ed, Edmon, Edmond. *See also* Edward.

Edom From the Hebrew, *adom*, 'red'. In the Bible, another name for Esau, Jacob's brother, whose descendants lived in Edom, an ancient country now forming parts of Jordan and Israel. Idumea is the Greek form. **Variant:** Idumea.

Edric From the Old English, *eadig*, 'happy, fortunate, rich', and *rice*, 'ruler'. Hence another Saxon name, Edred, 'fortunate and rich adviser'. **Variant:** Edred.

Edward From the Old English name, Eadward, from *eadig*, 'happy, fortunate, rich', and *weard*, which, like *mund*, means 'guardian, protector'. Edward the Elder (died 924), son of Alfred the Great, became King of Wessex and finally ruled all of England south of the Humber. Then came Edward the Confessor (1004–66), saint and King of England, who refounded the monastery and abbey at Westminster and was noted for his religious devotion, his generosity to the poor and sick and, later, his miracles. Whereas most Saxon names fell into disfavour after the Conquest, this – together with Edmund – did not, probably because of their Christian rather than their royal associations. Eight British kings bore the name after the Conquest. Edward I (1239–1307), King of England, set up the Model Parliament, considered to be the first English parliament. Edward VII (reigned 1901–10) gave his name to the lighthearted and elegant Edwardian period. The last was Edward VIII (1894–1972), King of Great Britain and Ireland, who forfeited the throne after 325 days to marry a divorced woman, Mrs Wallis Simpson. **Variants:** Duarte, Eamon, Ed, Edd, Eddard, Eddie, Eddy, Ede, Edik, Edison, Edouard, Edouardo, Edson, Eduard, Eduardo, Edvard, Edwardo, Edwardus, Emile, Ewart, Ned, Neddie, Neddy, Ted, Tedd, Teddie, Teddy.

Edwin From the Old English name, Eadwine, from *eadig*, 'fortunate, prosperous, happy', and *wine*, 'friend', thus 'happy friend'. St Edwin (died 633) was the first Christian King of Northumbria and the city,

 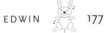

Edinburgh, is supposedly named after him. After falling into almost total disuse, except in Lancashire, the name was revived in the last century – *Edwin Drood* is the title of Dickens' last novel, unfinished when he died in 1870. **Variants:** Eaduin, Ed, Edred, Eduin, Eduino, Eduinus, Edwyn, Neddie, Teddie.

Egbert From the Old English, *ecq*, 'sword', and *beorht*, 'bright, shining', thus 'shining sword'. Another Saxon name to have been revived with the medievalism of the last century. **Variants:** Bert, Bertie, Berty.

Egmont From the Middle English, *egge*, 'corner, edge', and *mont*, 'mountain, hill', thus a person from the 'corner of the hill'. Hence Egerton, 'corner of the town'. The Flemish statesman and general, Lamoraal, Graaf van Egmont (1522–68), served under Philip II of Spain and is the subject of Goethe's tragedy, *Egmont* (1787). When the play was revived in 1810, Beethoven wrote incidental music for it which included overture, entr'actes, songs and the final 'Triumph Symphony'. **Variant:** Egerton.

Egon From the Old English, 'strong, formidable'. **Variants:** Egan, Egen, Keegan, MacEgan.

Ehud From the Hebrew, 'union'. In the Bible, the brave and left-handed Ehud belonged to the Benjamite tribe. He freed the children of Israel from servitude under the fat King Eglon of Moab by stabbing him in the belly with a double-sided dagger (Judges 3).

Elan *See* Elana *under girls*. **Variants:** Ela, Elah, Elai, Elon.

Elazar From the Hebrew, 'God helped'. In the Bible, the son of Aaron who was chief priest of Israel. **Variants:** El, Elazaro, Eleazar, Elie, Eliezer, Ely, Lazar, Lazarus.

Eldon *See* Aldous. **Variants:** Edlen, Edlon, Elder, Eldor, Elton.

Eldwin From the Old English, *eald*, 'old, respected', and *wine*, 'friend', thus 'old and valued friend'.

Elford From the Old English, *aethel*, 'noble', and *ford*, 'river crossing'. The same prefix is used for other landmark names: Elbridge, 'noble bridge'; Elton, 'noble town', and Elwood, 'noble wood'. *See also* Aldous. **Variants:** Aldridge, Elbridge, Eldridge, Elton, Elwood.

Elgar From the Old English, *aethel*, 'noble', and *gar*, 'spear', thus 'noble spear', implying protection and defence. The British composer, Edward Elgar (1857–1934), wrote five marches called *Pomp and Circumstance* (1901–30), of which the first is a setting for the song *Land of Hope and Glory*. **Variants:** Algar, Alger, Elger.

Elgin From the Old English, *aethel*, 'noble', and the Celtic, *gwen*, 'white, pure'. It was the 7th Earl of Elgin who paid £35,000 in 1816 on behalf of the British Museum for the Greek sculptures from the Acropolis in Athens, now known as the Elgin Marbles.

Eli From the Hebrew, *al*, 'height'. In the Bible, the last of the Old Testament high priest Judges, who brought up Samuel. A popular 17th-century name.

Eligius The French saint (c. 588–660) was an engraver and silversmith at the royal court who made enough money to found a monastery at Soulignac and a convent at Paris. He later became a bishop and was known for his wisdom and generosity. He is patron saint of metal-workers, smiths and farriers. **Variant:** Eloi.

Elijah From the Hebrew, 'the Lord is my God'. In the Bible, one of the early Hebrew prophets, later referred to as Elias in the New Testament. Eliot, the common English form, was very popular during the Middle Ages, but the original Hebrew name was taken up again in the 17th century by the Puritans. **Variants:** El, Eli, Elia, Elias, Elie, Eligio, Elihu, Elio, Eliot, Eliott, Elis, Elisio, Elison, Eliyahu, Elliot, Elliott, Ellis, Ellison, Elly, Elsen, Elson, Ely, Elyas, Elye, Elyot, Elys, Ilie, Ilija, Ilya.

Elisha From the Hebrew, 'God is my help, is generous'. In the Bible, the early Hebrew prophet who succeeded Elijah. Although the Hebrew form is found in 17th-century Britain, Ellis is the more common English form. It was a pupil of Rugby School, William Webb Ellis (1807–72), who in 1823 picked up the ball and ran with it while playing football, thereby inventing Rugby football. Several other names have the same 'El' prefix: Elihu, 'he is my God'; Elizur, 'my God is my rock'; Elkana, 'God has acquired', and Elrad, 'God is ruler'. **Variants:** Elias, Eliot, Elis, Elisee, Eliseo, Elison, Elizur, Elkan, Elkanah, Ellas, Elliot, Elliott, Ellis, Ellison, Elly, Elrad, Elrod, Elsden, Elsen, Elson, Elston, Ely, Hrod.

Ellard From the Old High German, *elira*, 'alder tree', and *hart*, 'strong'. Several other names have the same prefix: Elden, 'valley of alders'; Ellsworth, 'homestead near alder trees', and Elwood, 'alder wood'. **Variants:** Alden, Aldon, Elden, Ellary, Ellerey, Ellery, Ellsworth, Ellwood, Elsden, Elsdon, Elston, Elton, Elwill, Elwood.

Ellis *See* Elisha.

Elmer From the Old English name, Aethelmaer, from *aethel*, 'noble', and *maere*, 'famous'. **Variants:** Ailemar, Aylmar, Aylmer, Aymer, Edmar, Edmer, Eilemar, Elma, Elman, Elmo, Elmore.

Elmo *See* Elmer and Erasmus.

Elrad From the Old English, *aethel*, 'noble', and *rad*, 'counsel, advice'. **Variant:** Elrod.

Elroy From the Spanish, 'the king'. Leroy, from *le roi*, is the French form.

Elston From the Old English, *aethel*, 'noble', and *tun*, 'town, village', thus 'the noble's town'; or from English forms of Elijah and Elisha, thus 'Eliot's town', 'Ellis' town', and so on. **Variants:** Elsden, Elsdon, Elton.

Elton *See* Elford, Elston.

Elvin From the Old English name, Aelfwine, from the Old High German *aelf*, 'elf-like, spritely, clever, quick-witted', and *wine*, 'friend'. The American rock-and-roll star, Elvis Aaron Presley (1935–77), who made more than 30 films and sold more than 150 million records, certainly made the name a popular choice during the 1950s and 1960s. **Variants:** Al, Alvis, El, Elva, Elvert, Elvis, Elwin, Elwyn.

Elvis *See* Elvin.

Emanuel From the Hebrew, 'God is with us'. In the Bible, God tells Ahaz that a virgin will bear a son, called Immanuel, meaning Christ (Isaiah 7). The name was found in Cornwall during the 15th and 16th centuries, then became more widespread. It was always more popular with Jews than Christians. The real name of the actor, Edward G. Robinson (1893–1973), was Emanuel Goldenberg. **Variants:** Emanuela, Emanuele, Emmanuel, Imanuel, Immanuel, Mani, Manny, Mannye, Mano, Manoel, Manuel, Manuela.

Embert From the Old English, *him* and *heom*, 'to them', and *beraht*, 'bright', thus someone who will bring brightness and happiness to other people.

Emerald *See under girls.*

Emery From the Old German name, Emmerich, from the Old High German, *richi*, 'ruler, power, wealth'. Also a male form of Emily, from Amelia. The Normans carried it to Britain where it was used for both girls and boys until the end of the last century. **Variants:** Almericus, Almery, Amalrich, Amerigo, Amory, Emerick, Emericus, Emerson, Emil, Emile, Emilio, Emlin, Emlyn, Emmerich, Emmerlich, Emmory, Emory, Imray, Imre.

Emmet From the Hebrew, *emet*, 'truth'. **Variants:** Emmett, Emmit, Emmitt.

Endelon *See* Gwendolen *under girls.*

Endymion From the Greek, *endumion*, 'diver', as when the sun dives down as it sets. In Greek mythology, a handsome youth, possibly a sun god, who is the subject of several conflicting stories. In the nicest, he is a prince who, while out hunting, lies down to rest beside a cool grotto and falls asleep. Selene, goddess of the moon, espies him, falls in love, and steals a kiss from her sleeping beauty. He wakes and asks Zeus for immortality and perpetual youth, a wish granted on condition that he also sleeps for eternity. However, Selene continues to come every night, silently, to contemplate her sleeping lover – which is why the rays of the loving moon caress sleeping mortals. The name was found in the 16th and 17th centuries, but rarely since then.

Engelbert From the Old German, *engel*, 'angel', and *beraht*, 'bright', thus 'bright as an angel'. The German composer, Engelbert Humperdinck (1854–1921), wrote the opera *Hansel and Gretel* and was both friend and assistant to his fellow composer, Richard Wagner. **Variants:** Bert, Bertie, Berty, Englebert, Ingelbert, Inglebert.

Enoch From the Hebrew, 'educated, dedicated'. In the Bible, the son of Cain, born after Cain had killed Abel, and father of Methuselah. A name favoured by the 17th-century Puritans and today found mostly in northern England and the Midlands.

Enos From the Hebrew, *enosh*, 'man'. In the Bible, a son of Seth (Genesis 4). **Variant:** Enosh.

Ensign From the Latin, *insigne*, 'badge of decoration, class, office or honour', and also 'an honour, a standard, national flag, a uniform'.

Ephraim From the Hebrew, 'fruitful'. In the Bible, Joseph has two sons by Asenath: Manasseh, 'restful', and then Ephraim. St Ephraim (c. 306–73) was a poet and theologian whose didactic homilies and hymns, rich in imagery, are still used in the Syrian church. A name first found in Britain during the 17th century. **Variants:** Efim, Efraim, Efrat, Efrem, Efren, Efron.

Er From the Hebrew, 'aware'. **Variant:** Eri.

Erasmus From the Greek, *erasmios*, 'loved, desired'. The Dutch scholar and humanist, Desiderius Erasmus (1466–1536), reacted against the materialism and ostentation of the medieval church by reviving classical texts and emphasising a simple Christian faith based on studying the Scriptures. Little is known about St Erasmus or Elmo (died c. 303), but his cult in the 6th century developed a legend recounting that his intestines

 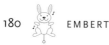

had been wound out on a windlass. Hence he is patron saint of sailors, and the occasional electrical discharge at the masthead of a ship is called 'St Elmo's fire', signifying his protection. **Variants:** Elmo, Erasme, Erasmo, Eraste, Erastus, Ras, Rastus.

Erhard From the Old German, 'resolution'. **Variant:** Erhart.

Eric From the Old Norse name, Eirkir, from the Old High German, *ehre*, 'honour', and *richi*, 'power, ruler', thus 'honourable ruler'. Alternatively, the name may mean 'island ruler'. Eric the Red was a Norse chieftain who sailed to the west and discovered Greenland where, in 986, he established a colony of about 500 people. The name was consistently popular with the Danes and Swedes, but only used widely in Britain since the last century, possibly helped by the Victorian vogue for medievalism and by Rider Haggard's Norse romance set in Iceland, *Eric Brighteyes* (1891). **Variants:** Air, Ehren, Erich, Erie, Erik, Eryk, Eryle, Euric, Richie, Rick.

Erland From the Old High German, *ehre*, 'honour', thus 'honourable country'. Hence, Ermal, 'honourable meeting place' and Erling, 'my honourable son'. **Variants:** Erling, Ermal.

Ermin *See* Emma *under girls*. **Variant:** Erme.

Ernest From the Old High German, *ernust*, 'keenness in battle, intense desire, seriously determined'. A favourite name among the German aristocracy, carried to Britain in the 18th century by the Hanoverian kings. In Oscar Wilde's last play, a comedy, *The Importance of Being Earnest* (1895), the hero finally has to admit before Lady Bracknell that, when a baby, he was left on Victoria Station 'in a hand-bag'. **Variants:** Earnest, Ern, Erneis, Erneste, Ernesto, Ernestus, Ernie, Ernis, Erno, Ernst, Erny.

Eros From the Greek, *eros*, 'love, desire, sexual love'. In Greek mythology, son and companion of the goddess of love, Aphrodite, and the god who brings harmony to chaos and permits life to develop. As the youngest and naughtiest of the gods, the winged Eros played pranks by shooting his arrows into men and gods to strike instant, fiery passion into their hearts. The aluminium figure of Eros in Piccadilly Circus, London, was designed by Sir Alfred Gilbert in 1893 as a monument to the philanthropist, the 7th Earl of Shaftesbury (died 1885).

Errol Possibly a German form of Earl, or from a Scottish place name. Popularised this century by the Australian actor, Errol Flynn (1909–59), noted for his swashbuckling roles in such films as *Captain Blood* (1935). **Variants:** Erroll, Rollo, Rolly.

Erskine From the Gaelic, 'from the height of the cliff'. **Variants:** Kin, Kinny.

Esau From the Hebrew, *esau*, 'hairy'. In the Bible, the son of Isaac and Rebecca. A good hunter and farmer, he sold his birthright to his twin brother Jacob (Genesis 25).

Esmund From the Old English, *mund*, 'guardian, protector', thus 'very good or gracious protector', or from the Norse name, Asmundr, 'divine protection'. The hero of Thackeray's novel, *The History of Henry Esmond* (1852), brought the name back into vogue in the last century. **Variant:** Esmond.

Esteban From the Spanish meaning a 'crown' or 'garland'.

Estel Male form of Estelle.

Estes Spanish, from the Latin, *aestas*, 'summer, summer heat, midsummer'; or from *aestus*, 'the waves of passion, heat, desire or the sea; or the waves and changes of emotions'. **Variant:** Eston.

Ethan From the Hebrew, 'permanent, assured', a word used to describe streams that flow the year round without drying up during the summer. **Variants:** Etan, Ethe.

Ethelbert From the Old English name, Aethelbryht, from *aethel*, 'noble', and *beorht*, 'bright'. St Ethelbert of Kent (c. 560–616), King of Kent and the most influential ruler in southern England, welcomed St Augustine, was converted and gave him land at Canterbury. He built the cathedrals of St Andrew's in Rochester and, in the territory of the East Saxons, the first St Paul's of London. It was to another St Ethelbert (died 794), a king of the East Angles who was murdered at Sutton Walls in Herefordshire, that Hereford cathedral was dedicated. Like other Saxon names, it underwent a 19th-century revival. See also Adelbert and Albert. **Variants:** Elbert, Elbie.

Ethelred From the Old English name, Aethelthryth, from *aethel*, 'noble', and *thryth*, 'strength'. Ethelred the Unready (c. 968–1016), King of the English, spent most of his reign fighting off Danish invasions without much success. Another medieval name to be revived in the last century. **Variants:** Aethelraed, Ailred, Alret, Edred, Ethelred.

Eubule From the Greek, *euboulos*, 'good and beneficial adviser'. In Greek mythology, a name given to Zeus. A name found in Britain after the Reformation. **Variants:** Euball, Eubie, Ewball.

Eucal From the Greek, *eus*, 'good', and *kaluptos*, 'covered', thus 'well covered'. In botany, the blooms of the eucalyptus plant are covered before they open; the plant is valued for the aromatic oil pressed from its leaves which is used in medicine, perfume and as a flavouring.

Euclid See Euclea under girls. The major contribution of the Greek mathematician Euclid (3rd–4th century BC) was the use of deductive principles of logic in geometry.

Eudo From the Greek, *eu*, 'good, pleasant', and *daimon*, 'spirit', thus 'lucky spirit, happiness, well-being'. Introduced by the Normans, the name has only rarely been used since the 16th century. **Variants:** Eudes, Eudon, Udo, Udona.

Eugene See Eugenia under girls. The name of four popes, which influenced its use until the Tudor period. Napoleon III's consort Eugenie brought the name back into popularity in England, both for boys and girls, although the boy's form is now often shortened to Gene. **Variants:** Eugen, Eugenio, Eugenius, Gene, Genie, Owen, Yevgeny.

Eulis *See* Eulalia *under girls.*

Eusibius From the Greek, *eusibes*, 'pious'. A popular name in ancient Greece, where Eusibius of Caesarea (264–349) was a noted historian.

Eustace From the Greek, *eustachios*, 'plentiful corn, fruitful'. The popular medieval legend of the martyr, St Eustace, recounts that he was a 2nd-century Roman general who, while out hunting, had a vision of a cross hovering between the antlers of a stag. This brought instant conversion to Christianity, loss of his job, poverty and misfortune, until he was

HOMELAND NAMES

To meet a Hilda from Kent would be unusual – she should come from northern England. And a Meraud in Cumbria would be far from his native Cornwall. For, although Britain is a small island, several names have remained manily regional. Ferdinand is still confined to the Midlands. Enoch is found there and further north, but Aldous is an East Anglian name, Beck is up north with Hilda, and across the border are Alistair, Angus, Fergus, Hamish, Janet, and many more. Like the Scottish Alison and Andrew, the Welsh David has spread throughout the island, but Aneurin and Bronwen are still found mostly in their homeland.

---

reinstated and led his troops to victory. However, when he refused to participate in the victorious thanksgiving to the Roman gods, he and his family were roasted to death. **Variants:** Eustache, Eustasius, Eustathius, Eustatius, Eustazio, Eustis, Stacey, Stacie, Stacy.

Evald From the name, Everildis, from the Old English, *eofor*, 'boar', and *hild*, 'battle'. **Variants:** Evaldo, Everildis, Ewald, Ewaldo, Ival, Ivol.

Evelyn Given to both boys and girls; its use as a Christian name for boys dates from the 17th century. The novels of Evelyn Waugh (1903–66) include the satire, *Decline and Fall* (1928) and the later work, *Brideshead Revisited* (1945). **Variants:** Evel, Evelio, Evelle.

Everard From the Old High German name, Eburhart, from *ebur*, 'wild boar', and *hard*, 'strong', implying 'strong warrior'. Introduced to Britain by the Normans, it has been used ever since. **Variants:** Averitt, Devereux, Eberhard, Eberhart, Eberle, Ebert, Everart, Everet, Everett, Everette, Everhard, Everley, Evert, Eward, Ewart.

Ewart From the Old French, *eviere*, 'ewer, large pitcher or jug'. **Variants:** Euel, Ewell.

Ewen Welsh form of John. **Variants:** Eaven, Ev, Evan, Evander, Evans, Evin, Evo, Evon, Ewan, Owen.

Ezekiel From the Hebrew, *Y'hezkel*, 'may God strengthen'. In the Bible, a major Hebrew prophet who lived in the 6th century BC and wrote the Book of Ezekiel in the Old Testament. **Variants:** Ezechial, Ezell, Eziechiele, Haskel, Haskell, Hehezkel, Yehezekel, Zeke.

Ezra From the Hebrew, 'help'. In the Bible, a Hebrew high priest of the 5th century BC. The name was taken up in 17th-century Britain. **Variants:** Esdras, Esra, Ezar, Ezer, Ezri, Ezzard, Ezzret. *See also* Wyndham.

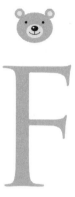

Fabius Possibly from the Latin, *faba*, 'bean'. In ancient Rome, the name of a noble family whose several distinguished members included Quintus Fabius Maximus (died 203 BC), known as Cunctator, 'Delayer', the Roman General who managed to defeat Hannibal without direct fighting. It is from him that the Fabian Society, founded in 1883, takes its name – it is dedicated to the gradual spread of democratic socialism and its members advocate caution, strategy and progress without conflict. Respect for St Fabianus, who was pope from 236 to 251, kept the name alive and it is found intermittently in Britain from the 12th century on. **Variants:** Fabe, Faber, Fabian, Fabiano, Fabien, Fabio.

Fadeyka Russian, meaning 'stout-hearted, courageous'. **Variants:** Fadey, Fadeyushka.

Fahey From the Old English, *foegen*, 'joyful, glad, happy'.

Falkner From the Greek, *phalkone*, 'falcon'. The highly prized birds of the family *Falconidai* have especially powerful wings and beady eyes, and falconers have trained them for hunting since the Middle Ages. **Variants:** Falcon, Falkner, Faulkner, Fowler.

Faramond From the Old German name, Faramund, from *fara*, 'journey, travel, distance', and *mund*, 'guardian', thus 'protected traveller'. Hence Farland, 'distant land'. Faramond was the name of the legendary first king of France. **Variants:** Fara, Farman, Farmannus, Farr, Farrimond, Phareman.

Farley From the Old French, *feire*, 'fair', a special place and day for a market or celebration, kept by custom or law; or from the Old Norse, *faqr*, 'beautiful, pleasing', or from the Old English, *faer*, 'wayside'. The second part of the name comes from the Middle English, *leye*, 'meadow'. **Variants:** Fair, Fairbanks, Fairleigh, Fairley, Far, Farl, Farlie, Farly.

Farquhar From the Gaelic name, Fearchar, from *fer*, 'man', and *car*, 'friendly'. The name of an early Scottish king, which accounts for its continued use in the Scottish highlands.

Farrar From the Latin, *ferrarius*, 'blacksmith' and *ferrum*, 'iron'. **Variants:** Farrel, Farrell, Farris, Ferris, Ferrol.

Farrel From the Celtic, 'valiant man'. See also Farrar. **Variants:** Farr, Farrell, Ferrel, Ferrell.

Fate From the Latin, *fata*, 'the Fates'. In classical mythology, the three Fates controlled human destiny (see Moira). From the same root comes the English word fairy, meaning a supernatural being who can help – or hinder – a person's future. **Variants:** Fait, Faye, Fayette.

Faunus In Roman mythology, one of the earliest rural rustic gods, presiding over nature and, above all, fertility. He invented the rustic pipe, had powers of prophecy and was worshipped by farmers and shepherds. His festival on February 15 was one of the most important in the Roman calendar, especially for women who wished to become pregnant. The equivalent Greek god is Pan.

Faustus From the Latin, *faustus*, 'fortunate'. The 16th-century German astrologer and magician, Johann Faust, was the inspiration for Goethe's play, *Faust* (1808), whose hero is a magician and alchemist who sells his soul to the devil to gain power and knowledge.

Felix See Felicia under girls. The early popularity of this name is reflected by four popes, and 67 saints listed in the Roman Martyrology. Felix of Dunwich (died 648) was a Burgundian missionary in East Anglia who gave his name to the town Felixstowe. Popular during the Middle Ages, the name is still used today but is less common than the girl's form. Felix is also the animal type-name for a cat (compare Bruno the bear). **Variants:** Fee, Felice, Felicio, Felike, Feliks, Felis, Felizio, Phelim.

Felton From the Old Norse, *fjall*, 'hill', and the Old English, *tun*, 'town, village', thus 'town on or near a hill'. **Variants:** Fell, Felt, Feltie, Felty.

Fenton From the Old English, *fenn*, 'marshy, swampy land', and *tun*, 'town, village', thus 'town near marshland'. **Variants:** Fen, Fennie, Fenny.

Ferd From the German, *pferd*, 'horse'. **Variants:** Ferde, Ferdie, Ferdy. *See also* Ferdinand.

Ferdinand From the Latin, *ferox*, 'wild, bold, courageous, warlike, gallant, headstrong, insolent'. A name kept popular by European royal families. Significant bearers of it include the saint, King Ferdinand III of Castile (1199–1252), who pushed the Moors out of southern Spain to make it a Christian state; and King Ferdinand V of Castile, Aragon and Naples (1452–1516), who ruled with his wife, Isabella. The name was at its most popular from the Middle Ages until the 17th century, especially in the Midlands. **Variants:** Fardie, Fardy, Fearn, Ferd, Ferde, Ferdie, Ferdinando, Ferdy, Fern, Fernand, Fernandas, Fernando, Fernandus, Ferrand, Ferrando, Ferrant, Ferrante, Ferren, Ferrentus, Hernan, Hernando.

Fergus From the Gaelic, *ver qusti*, 'manly choice, best choice'. According to legend, Feargus was one of three brothers who led the Scots from Ireland to the country later called Scotland (see Angus). Ten Celtic saints were called Fergus and the name is still popular in Ireland and Scotland. **Variants:** Fearghas, Feargus, Ferguson.

Fermin From the Latin, *firmus*, 'firm, strong'. St Firmius, Bishop of Metz during the 5th century, is the reason for the name's use in Britain from the 12th to 16th centuries. **Variants:** Feridon, Firmin, Furman.

Festus From the Latin, *festus*, 'festive, joyful, merry'.

Fidel See Faith under girls. In Beethoven's only opera, *Fidelio* (1805), the heroine, Leonora, assumes the male name to rescue her husband from prison. **Variants:** Fidele, Fidelio.

Fielding From the Old English, *feld*, 'field', a broad open expanse of land often used for agriculture or for sport. **Variants:** Fee, Fie, Field, Fielder.

Fingal From the Gaelic, *fionn gall*, 'fair stranger'. A term used by Celts to describe the fair-complexioned Norwegians (compare Dougal).

Finlay From the Gaelic, 'fair-haired soldier'. **Variants:** Fin, Findlay, Findley, Finley, Finn.

Finn *See* Fiona *under girls*. In Irish Celtic mythology, the hero Finn and his band of young warriors were mortals with supernatural powers, and ideals of the real Celtic warrior. They gave help where needed, often to the gods, and were regarded as defenders of Ireland. Several Irish saints have borne the name, including St Finnian of Clonard (died c. 549), the initiator of monasticism in Ireland and the most important saint after St Patrick; St Finbarr (died c. 633), who founded the monastery and see of Cork; and St Finan (died 661), missionary to Northumbria. **Variants:** Eifion, Finan, Finbar, Finbarr, Finian, Finnegan, Finnian, Fion.

Fisk From the German, *fisch*, 'fish'. **Variants:** Fish, Fiske.

Fitz From the Old English, 'son'. The many compounds include **Fitzgerald, Fitzpatrick** and **Fitzroy**.

Flan From the Old French, *flaon*, 'flat metal', via the Old English, 'arrow'. **Variants:** Flan, Flann, Flannery.

Flavian *See* Flavia *under girls*. **Variants:** Flavio, Flavius.

Florian *See* Florence *under girls*. The saint twins, Florus and Laurus, were Greek stone-masons who were working on a heathen temple when they were converted. They threw out the idols and were then martyred by being drowned in a well. A name found in Britain during the Middle Ages. **Variants:** Ferenc, Fiorello, Florence, Florentino, Florents, Florentz, Florenz, Flory.

Flyn From the Gaelic, 'son of the red-haired man'. **Variants:** Flin, Flinn, Flynn. *See also* Errol.

Fonda *See under girls*. **Variant:** Fon.

Forbes From the Greek, *phorbe*, 'fodder', any plant besides grass that grows in a field or meadow. A name especially popular in Scotland.

Ford From the Old English, 'shallow river-crossing'. The British writer and editor, Ford Madox Ford (1873–1939), founded the *English Review* in 1908, but the name is more popular in the USA where Henry Ford (1863–1947), founded the Ford Motor Company in 1903 and produced the first of the model Ts in 1908.

Fordel English gypsy name, meaning 'forgive'.

Fordon From the Old High German, *fartuon*, 'to destroy'.

Fortney From the Latin, *fortis*, 'strong', a bastion, fortified place, fort. **Variants:** Fort, Fortnum.

Fortune *See* Fortuna *under girls*. **Variants:** Fortunato, Fortune, Fortunio.

Foster From the late Latin expression, *forestis silva*, 'outside forest', the royal forest and game preserve of Emperor Charlemagne (see Charles). From this came the English word, forest, which as Forester became an occupation name, like Barber. **Variants:** Forest, Forester, Forrest, Forrester, Forster, Foss.

Fountain From the Latin, *fons*, 'spring, fountain, source of a well'.

Foy From the Middle Dutch, *foye*, 'journey, parting feast', adapted in Scotland to mean a farewell entertainment, feast or present given before a wedding, at harvest-time or before parting.

Francis *See* Frances *under girls*; also a nickname meaning 'with the airs and graces of a Frenchman'. A name carrying both religious and royal connotations. St Francis of Assisi (c. 1181–1226), born Giovanni Bernardone, was nicknamed Francesco. The son of a wealthy draper, he was a carefree youth, then a soldier, before devoting his life to God. In 1210, he founded the order of the Friars Minor, later called Franciscans or Greyfriars from the colour of their habits. At first, they consisted of just twelve travelling preachers who emphasised simplicity, poverty and humility–a sharp contrast to other monks who lived cloistered, comfortable lives. Their headquarters were at Assisi but their ideas spread like wildfire and soon there were centres throughout Europe. A man of spiritual power and insight, St Francis' *Canticle to the Sun* expresses his love of nature. In 1980, he was made patron saint of ecology. St Francis Xavier (1506–52) was the co-founder of the Jesuit order with Ignatius Loyola, and missionary to India, Sri Lanka and Japan. Among the royals, Francis I (1494–1547) was the first of several French rulers of the name. In Britain, the name was taken up and made popular under the Tudors, and borne by three exceptional men: the admiral and navigator, Sir Francis Drake; the statesman, Sir Francis Walsingham (1536–90); and the philosopher and politician, Francis Bacon (1561–1626). After that, it fell out of favour, to be revived early in the last century. The form Frank, found in Britain since the Conquest, seems to have the direct meaning, 'a Frank'. **Variants:** Chico, Fenenc, Fran, Franca, Francesco, Franchot, Francie, Francisco, Franciscus, Franciskus, Franck, Francklin, Francklyn, Franco, Francois, Frank, Frankie, Franklin, Franklyn, Franky, Frannie, Frans, Frants, Franz, Frenz, Firsco, Pancho.

Fraser Possibly from the Old French, *fraisil*, 'charcoal cinders', thus 'charcoal maker'. Like Barber, an old occupational name. **Variants:** Frasier, Fraze, Frazer, Frazier.

Frederick From the Old High German, *frithu*, 'peace' and *rik*, 'king, ruler', thus 'peaceful ruler'. Several King Fredericks – there have been 10 Danish ones–have failed to live up to the meaning of their name, including Frederick Barbarossa ('redbeard') (c. 1123–90), Emperor of the Holy Roman Empire, who went into Italy but was defeated by papal armies, and Frederick the Great (1712–86), King of Prussia and enlightened despot, who was a brilliant soldier and laid the foundations of the powerful Prussian military state. In Britain, the Anglo-Saxon form, Freodhoric, did not survive the Conquest. The name was reintroduced by the Hanoverian kings in the 18th century (it was given to George II's son) and became a favourite in the 19th. **Variants:** Eric, Erich, Erick, Erik, Federico, Fred, Freddie, Freddy, Fredek, Frederic, Frederich, Frederico, Frederigo, Frederik, Fredric, Fredrick, Freed, Freeman, Fridrich, Friedrich, Frits, Fritz, Fritzi, Rich, Rick, Rickie, Ricky.

Frey From the Old Norse, 'noble man'. In Norse mythology, the god Frey, also known as Ing, is husband of Freya and presides over peace and fertility. *See* Ingram.

Fry From the Old Norse, *frjo*, 'seed, offspring'. **Variant:** Frye.

Fulbert From the Old German name, Filibert, from *filu*, 'very, much', and *beraht*, 'bright'. Introduced into Britain by the Normans.

Variants: Bert, Berty, Filbert, Filberte, Filibert, Fulbright, Phil, Philbert, Philibert.

Fulk From the Old English, *folc*, 'people, relatives, a nation or a tribe'. A Burgundian favourite, the name was carried to Britain by the Normans. **Variants:** Fulco, Fulke.

Fuller From the Latin, *fullo*, 'cloth-fuller', a person who shrinks and thickens cloth. Like Barber, an old occupational name.

Fursey The Irish saint (died 648) was a monastic missionary. With his brothers, the saints Foillan and Ultan, he came to England and established a monastery at Yarmouth, then a second at Lagny, near Paris. The chronicler Bede describes him as 'renowned for his words and works, outstanding in goodness'.

Fuzzy From the Low German, *fussiq*, 'spongy', meaning both indistinct and very tightly curled, frizzy hair.

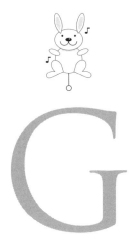

G

Gabbo From the Old Norse, *gabba*, 'to mock'.

Gabriel Name of the archangel who told the Virgin Mary she would be the mother of Jesus; see Gabriela under girls. Among the notable people bearing the name are Gabriel Daniel Fahrenheit (1686–1736), the German physicist who invented the temperature scale, and Gabriel Fauré (1845–1924), the French composer and organist. A name found mostly in Ireland. **Variants:** Gab, Gabbie, Gabby, Gabe, Gabel, Gabell, Gabi, Gabie, Gabrielle, Gabriello, Gabryel, Gavrila. *See also* Dante.

Gad From the Hebrew, 'fortunate', and 'warrior', hence Gadiel, 'God is my fortune'. In the Bible, Gad is one of the 12 sons of Joseph, and thus the ancestor of one of the tribes of Israel. **Variant:** Gadi.

Gael Probably from the Old Welsh, *gwydd*, 'wild', via *Gwyddel*, 'Irishman'. The collective name for the Gaelic-speaking people of Ireland, Scotland and the Isle of Man. Also, a name for a Scottish Highlander.

Gage From the Old French, *gage*, 'pledge', especially as a formal challenge for a fight, duel or battle.

Gaines From the Old French, *gaigner*, 'to obtain', implying someone who increases in ability, prestige and honour as well as in wealth.

Gal From the Hebrew, 'wave, mound'; hence Gali, 'my wave'. Also given to girls. **Variant:** Gali.

Galahad From the Gaelic, 'hawk in battle'. In Arthurian legend, Sir Galahad was the son of Lancelot and the epitome of virtue, chivalry and courage; he was the only knight of Arthur's Round Table who reached the Holy Grail. Thus the name implies chivalry, nobility and purity. *See also* Arthur.

Gale From the Old French, *galant*, 'gallant, brave, noble, ostentatious, dashing, courteous to women, amorous'. Also a male form of Abigail. **Variants:** Gael, Gail, Gaile, Gallard, Gay, Gayelord, Gayle, Gayler, Gaylor, Gaylord.

Galen From the Greek, *galerios*, 'still, tranquil'. The Greek physician Galen (c. 130–200) compiled the treatises of Greek medical knowledge, including the theory of the four humours, that formed the basis of European medicine until the Renaissance. **Variants:** Gaelan, Gale.

Gall The Irish saint (died c. 640) accompanied St Columba on his mission to Europe, finally settling at Bregenz, near Lake Constance. His cult brought forth a quantity of legends, notably the claim that he founded the nearby monastery of St Gallen, but it was actually founded a century later.

Gallagher From the Celtic, 'eager helper'. Related to Gale.

Galvin From the Gaelic, 'sparrow'. **Variants:** Gal, Galvan, Galven.

Gamal From the Arabic, *jamal*, 'beauty'. **Variants:** Gamali, Gamli, Gamul, Gil, Gilad, Gilead, Jammal.

Gamliel From the Hebrew, 'my reward is God'. Since it is found in the Bible and has a suitable meaning, the name was taken up by the 17th-century Puritans.

Gammel From the Old Norse, *gamal*, 'old'. Gamel was a common name in the north of England during the Middle Ages but is now confined to Scotland in the form of Gemmel. **Variants:** Gamel, Gemmel.

Gardiner Probably from the Latin, *hortus gardinus*, 'enclosed garden', via the Middle English, *gardyn*. Traditionally, a garden is a symbol for a man's path through life: well-tended, it flourishes; ignored or abused, it goes to ruin. **Variants:** Gar, Gard, Garden, Gardener, Gardie, Gardnard, Gardner, Gardy.

Gareth From the Welsh name, Gwaredd, 'gentle'. An old name revived in the last century by the medieval vogue and Tennyson's poem, *Gareth and Lynette* (1872). Today, it is found mostly in Wales. **Variant:** Garth.

Garfield From the Old English, *gara*, 'promontory'. **Variants:** Gar, Field.

Garland From the Old French, *garlande*, 'an ornament of gold threads', but later meaning a wreath of flowers and leaves worn as a prize or hung up for a festival. Also given to girls. The name became fashionable this century when Judy Garland (1922–69), born Frances Gumm, starred in the film, *The Wizard of Oz* (1939), for which she received an Academy Award. **Variants:** Garlen, Garlon.

Garnet *See under girls.* **Variants:** Garner, Garnett, Gram.

Garret From the French, *garir*, 'to observe'. **Variants:** Gar, Garreth, Garrett, Garrott, Garry, Gary.

Garridan English gypsy name, meaning 'you hid'.

Garson From the Old French, *quarir*, 'to protect', especially when soldiers occupy a military post. **Variant:** Garrison.

Garth From the Old Norse, *gyrthr*, 'enclosure of land', meaning a field or a garden. **Variants:** Garret, Garton, Garvey, Garvie, Garvin, Garry, Gary.

Garvin From the Old English, *gar*, 'spear', and *wine*, 'friend', thus 'friend in battle, ally'.

Variants: Gar, Garwin, Vin, Vinnie, Vinny, Win, Winnie, Winny.

Gascon From the French, 'from Gascony'. The people of the ancient province of south-west France were originally Vascones, or Basques, and earned a reputation for garrulity, boastfulness and swaggering – hence a 'gascon', meaning a boastful person. **Variant:** Gaston.

Gavin From the Welsh name, Gwalchmai, 'hawk of the plain'. In Arthurian legend, Gawain was King Arthur's nephew and a knight of the Round Table. The name has been consistently popular in Scotland. **Variants:** Gauen, Gauvin, Gav, Gavan, Gaven, Gavvy, Gawain, Gawaine, Gawen, Gawin, Walwain, Walwyn. *See also* Arthur.

Gaylord *See* Gale.

Gaynor From the Irish, 'son of the fair man', thus a name suitable for a son whose father has fair hair or complexion. **Variants:** Gainer, Gainor, Gay, Gayner.

Gedalia From the Hebrew, 'God is great'. **Variants:** Gedaliah, Gedaliahu, Gedelio.

Geddes From the Old Norse, *gaddr*, 'spear, goad, bar of metal', and also 'rod, wand, fishing rod'.

Gefania From the Hebrew, 'vineyard of the Lord'. **Variants:** Gefaniah, Gephania, Gephaniah.

Genesius From the Greek, *genesis*, 'creation, generation, horoscope'. The first book of the Bible, describing the creation of the world. Two Roman martyr saints helped spread the name: Genesius the Actor, who was converted while doing a stunt mocking the baptism ceremony, and Genesius of Arles, a clerk who admitted his faith when instructed to write down an imperial edict against Christians. **Variant:** Genesis.

Geoffrey A name formed from several other names, so that its meaning is now unclear. The Old German name was Gaufrid, from *gavja*, 'district', but it was confused with Godafrid, from *guda* and *frithu*, 'peace of God'. Other names that contributed to the tangle include Walafrid, 'peaceful traveller', and Gisfrid, 'vow of peace'. The English poet, Geoffrey Chaucer (1342–1400), a diplomat and customs official by trade, wrote *The Canterbury Tales*, in which a party of pilgrims recount stories on their way from London to Canterbury. For this and his other works he is regarded as the father of English poetry. An earlier writer, Geoffrey of Monmouth (1100–54), wrote a *History of the Kings of Britain* in which he managed, with much imagination, to trace a direct line from the Trojans to King Arthur; he was an important influence on later medieval romance writers. The name fell out of favour with the Tudors, to be revived in the last century. Godfrey is the modern form of Godafrid. **Variants:** Geoff, Giotto, Gisfrid, Godfrey, Godofredo, Gottfried, Gotz, Govert, Jef, Jeff, Jefferies, Jefferson, Jeffery, Jeffie, Jeffrey, Jeffries, Jeffry, Jeffy. *See also* jeffrey.

George From the Greek, *georgos*, 'farm labourer'. Almost nothing factual is known about the patron saint of England, soldiers and boy scouts and one of the most renowned of the early martyrs who lived in the 3rd or 4th century. This soldier-saint was probably martyred in Lydda in Palestine, from where crusaders soon spread his cult across Europe. He acquired several ripe legends: in England, he was thought to be a knight from Cappadocia who rescued Una from a dragon while in Libya, worked quantities of miracles and was finally tortured and beheaded at Nicodemia – all recounted in the *Golden Legend,* a medieval collection of the lives of the saints by Jacobus de Voragine (1230–98). In 1415 his saint's day entered the highest rank in the English church calendar, with a public holiday. The popularity of the name and its solid royal associations began in 1714 when the Elector of Hanover (1660–1727) became George I, King of Great Britain and Ireland. The Protestant Hanoverian line produced five more kings of the same name; George V (1865–1936) changed the family name to Windsor during World War I and in 1932 began the tradition of the monarch's annual Christmas broadcast. In the USA the statesman and general, George Washington (1732–99) fought in the War of Independence and in 1789 became the first President of the United States. **Variants:** Egor, Geo, Geordie, Georg, Georges, Georgie, Georgio, Georgius, Georgy, Goran, Igor, Jarge, Jerzy, Jiri, Jorge, Jorgen, Jurg, McGeorge, Seiorse, Sior, Yorick, York, Yuri.

Geraint Welsh, from the Old English name, Gerontius, from the Greek, *geron,* 'old'. A medieval name revived in the last century (*see* Arthur).

Gerard From the Old German, *gairu,* 'spear', and *hardu,* 'hard', implying a warrior; hence the French and German names Gerald, 'spear rule'; Gerbert, 'bright spear'; Gerbold, 'bold spear', and Gervaise, 'servant of the spear'. A name introduced by the Normans, although the form Gerald seems to have come from Ireland and Wales. All forms enjoyed popularity in the Middle Ages, then underwent a revival in the last century. The British poet, Gerard Manley Hopkins (1844–89), was con-

verted to Roman Catholicism and became a Jesuit priest. **Variants:** Erhard, Garabed, Garcia, Gardell, Garey, Garo, Garrard, Garrick, Garry, Garvey, Garvie, Gary, Gearard, Gerald, Geraldo, Gerardo, Geraud, Gerbert, Gerbold, Gerhard, Gerhardt, Gerold, Gerret, Gerrie, Gerrit, Gerry, Gervais, Gervase, Gervis, Gerwald, Gherardo, Giraldo, Giralt, Girard, Giraud, Girault, Giraut, Goran, Graham, Jarett, Jarrett, Jerald, Jerrald, Jerrall, Jerrard, Jerre, Jerrel, Jerrell, Jerrie, Jerrold, Jerry.

Germain *See* Gemma *under girls.*

Gibor From the Hebrew, 'strong'. **Variant:** Gibson.

Gideon From the Hebrew, 'maimed' or 'mighty warrior'. In the Bible, a judge and hero of Israel who conquered the Midianites (Judges 6). **Variant:** Gidi.

Gifford Either from the Old High German name, Gebahard, 'to give openly and boldly', or from the Middle English, *gille,* 'ravine', and *ford,* 'river-crossing', thus 'crossing near a ravine'. Old English variants: Gebahad, Giff, Giffard, Gifferd, Giffie, Giffy, Gilford, Gilmore, Gilroy.

Gil From the Hebrew, 'joy'. **Variants:** Gili, Gill, Gilli. *See also* Gilbert.

Gilbert From the Old German name, Gisilbert, 'bright pledge'; or from another old German name, Willibehrt, from *wellen,* 'desire, will', and *beraht,* 'bright, illustrious', thus 'the desire to be illustrious'; or from the Celtic, *gillie,* 'lad, servant', perhaps from servant of St Gilbert. A name introduced by the Normans to become a firm favourite throughout the Middle Ages. St Gilbert of Sempringham, Lincolnshire (c. 1085–1189) founded the Gilbertian Order, the only specifically English religious order. He started several communities with men's and women's houses side by side, as well as leper hospitals and orphanages, all of which were closed by Henry VIII. In the Robin Hood stories, Gilbert of the White Hand was one of the band of men who robbed the rich to give to the poor. **Variants:** Bert, Bertie, Berty, Burt, Burtie, Burty, Gib, Gibb, Gibbie, Gibbon, Gibby, Gibson, Gil, Gilberto, Gilburt, Gill, Gilli, Gillie, Giselbert, Guilbert, Wilbert, Wilbur, Wilburt, Will.

Gilchrist From the Gaelic, *gillie*, 'lad, servant', thus 'servant of Christ'.

Gilder *See* Gilda *under girls*. Like Barber, an old occupational name. The hermit who lived on an island in the Bristol Channel, St Gildas the Wise (c. 500–570), wrote *Concerning the Ruin and Conquest of Britain* as a warning lesson for kings and clergy to start behaving themselves.

Giles From the Latin name, Aegidius, from the Greek, *aigis*, 'kid goat, goat skin' and, by extension, children and descendants. In Greek mythology, the aegis was the shield of the supreme god, Zeus, which he shook to create storms and thunder, making it a symbol of divine protection. It was made of the skin of Amalthea who had suckled the god and was also worn as a cloak by his daughter, Athena. The cult of the hermit, St Giles (possibly 9th century), was very strong in the later Middle Ages – about 150 British churches are dedicated to him including the High Kirk, Edinburgh. His wondrous legend (almost pure fiction) tells of the Visigothic king, Wamba, shooting an arrow at the saint's pet deer which instead wounded the saint himself; he is patron saint of cripples and the poor. Gilles was a renowned 18th-century French clown. **Variants:** Egide, Egidio, Egidius, Gide, Gidie, Gil, Gile, Gilean, Gileon, Gill, Gilles, Gillette, Gillian, Gyles.

Gillie English gypsy name, meaning 'song'. *See also* Gilroy.

Gilmore From the Old Norse, *gil*, 'deep glen', and the Old English, *more*, 'tree stump, root'. **Variants:** Gill, Gillie, Gillmore, Gilmour.

Gilroy From the Gaelic, *gillie*, 'servant', and the French, *roi*, 'king'. **Variants:** Gill, Gilly, Roy.

Giora From the Aramaic, 'convert'.

Glade From the Old English, *glaed*, 'being happy and giving happiness'. **Variants:** Gladdie, Gladdy, Gladstone, Gladwin, Gladwyn, Glat, Win, Winny, Wyn. *See also* Claudius.

Glen From the Gaelic, *gleann*, 'narrow mountain valley', usually one with a stream at the bottom. The highly popular Scottish romances and histories by Sir Walter Scott (1731–1832) popularised the word as a name. **Variants:** Glenard, Glenn, Glennard, Glennon, Glyn, Glynn.

Goddard From the Old English, *god*, 'good', thus 'good advice'. A common name in the Middle Ages, but hardly used since the 17th century. **Variants:** Godard, Godart, Gothart.

Godfrey *See* Geoffrey.

Godric From the Old English, from *god*, 'good', and *rice*, 'ruler, power, wealth'. A nickname for Henry I (1068–1135). St Godric (1065–1170) was a prosperous merchant and trader who turned hermit to make amends for his dishonest business practices. He acquired powers of prophecy, tamed animals and was also a considerable lyric poet and composer of hymns. **Variants:** Godrich, Goodrich.

Godwin From the Old English, *god*, 'good', and *wine*, 'friend' or 'friend of God', meaning a Christian. One of the most popular

 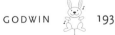

medieval names, and one that survived the Conquest. **Variants:** Godewyn, Goodwin, Win, Winny, Wyn.

Gold *See* Golda *under girls.* Hence Goldwin, 'one who loves gold', a popular form in the Middle Ages. **Variants:** Golden, Goldman, Goldsmith, Goldwin, Goldwyn.

Goliath From the Hebrew name, Golyat, 'stranger, exile'. In the Bible, the Philistine giant slain by David (1 Samuel 17), giving the name its second meaning of 'giant'.

Gomer From the Hebrew, 'to complete', thus suitable for the last child of a family. Also given to girls.

Gordius In Greek mythology, a peasant who was elected king of Phrygia. He tied an extremely complicated knot in his chariot; when Alexander learnt that the man who could untie the Gordian knot would rule over all Asia, he sliced it with his sword. Thus the name implies the ability to resolve a complex problem with one decisive action. **Variants:** Gordion, Gordon.

Gordon From the Old English, *gor*, 'marsh', and *denn*, whose Scottish meaning is 'small wooded dell'. The ancient Scottish clan is named after the Gordon lands in Berwickshire, and their titles include Duke of Gordon and Earl of Aberdeen – the Gordon setter hunting dog was named after the 4th Duke. Used as a first name outside the clan only since 1885, the year the hero General Gordon (1833–85) was killed defending Khartoum against the Mahdists. **Variants:** Goran, Gordan, Gorden, Gordie, Gordy, Gore, Gorham, Gorrell, Gorton.

Gowan From the Old Norse, *gullin*, 'golden'. The Scotish name for small yellow or white flowers, especially the daisy. **Variants:** Gowall, Gower.

Gozal *See* Gozala *under girls.*

Grady From the Latin, *gradus*, 'step, position, degree, grade'.

Graham From Grantham, from the Middle English, *grant*, 'agree, promise, bestow', and the Old English, *ham*, 'town, village, manor, home'; or from the Greek, *grais*, 'old'; or from the Latin, *granum*, 'grain'; or, finally, a form of Gerard. The original members of the ancient Scottish clan were Anglo-Normans who moved north in the 12th century. **Variants:** Graeme, Graemer, Graenem, Graenum, Gram.

Graily From the Latin, *gradalis*, 'dish'. In medieval legend, the chalice used by Christ at the Last Supper and the quest of many a chivalrous medieval knight, finally reached by Sir Galahad. *See* Arthur.

Granger From the Latin, *granum*, 'grain', which came to mean farmhouse or the granary where corn paid as tithes was stored, hence a person who works on a farm. Like Barber, an old occupational name.

Grant From the Old French, *granter*, 'to agree, promise, bestow'. A name especially popular in the USA, where General Ulysses Grant (1822–85) was President from 1868 to 1876. **Variants:** Grantland, Grantley. *See also* Graham.

Granville From the French, *grand*, 'large, full-grown', and *ville*, 'town', a place in Normandy. The English playwright, actor, producer and critic, Harley Granville-Barker (1877–1946), was co-manager of the Royal Court theatre and produced a string of Shakespeare plays at the Savoy Theatre. **Variant:** Grenville.

Gray From the Old English, *graeg*, 'grey'. Greyfriars was the English nickname of the Cistercian and Franciscan monks, whose habits were that colour. **Variants:** Graydon, Greg, Grey, Greyson.

Greeley From the Old English, *grene*, 'green', and *leah*, 'meadow, grassland'. **Variant:** Greely.

Gregory From the Greek, *gregorios*, 'watchman'. The diminutive Greg was popularised by the doctor, pope and saint, Gregory I (540–604), known as Gregory the Great and the first of 16 popes of the name. Born into wealth, he founded a monastery in Rome and a few more in Sicily before becoming a monk aged 35 and then the first monk to be elected pope. During his epoch-making 14-year reign he reformed the papal administration, sent missionaries to England (*see* Augustine), outlined the clergy's duties in *Pastoral Care* and presided over the development of the Gregorian chant, or plainsong. In all, his life and ideals were a model for the medieval clergy. Under Pope Gregory XIII the Gregorian Calendar was introduced in 1582, a corrected version of the Julian Calendar (*see* Caesar). After the Conquest, the name spread outside the monasteries, but then fell out of favour during the Reformation, when it was considered too popish. **Variants:** Gero, Greg, Gregg, Gregoire, Gregor, Gregorio, Gregorius, Gregour, Gregos, Gregus, Greis, Grischa.

Griffith From the Welsh name, Gruffydd, from the Welsh, *udd*, 'lord'. In Greek mythology, a griffin is an animal with a lion's body and an eagle's head and wings – a combination of strength, swiftness and intelligence. **Variants:** Griffin, Gruffydd, Gryphon.

Grimbald From the Old High German, *grimm*, 'fierce', and the Old English, *beald*, 'bold'. **Variants:** Grimbel, Grimbold, Grimm.

Griswald From the Old German, *grisja*, 'grey', and *wald*, 'wood, forest'. **Variants:** Gris, Gritz, Griz.

Grove From the Old English, *graf*, 'small thicket of trees'. Hence Grover, 'someone who grows trees'. **Variant:** Grover.

Guillermo From the Spanish meaning a 'strong and resolute protector'. Alternatives include Guglielmo (Italian), Guillaume (French), Gwilym (Welsh), Uilleam (Scottish Gaelic).

Gundulf From the Old Norse, *gunnarr*, 'war'. In the Norse legend, the Burgundian King Gundulf (also called Gunner) is finally slain because he refuses to reveal where he has hidden the Nibelung's treasure. The legend was possibly based on the historical hero, Gundaharius, who was defeated by the Huns in 436. It was revived last century in Wagner's epic opera, *The Ring of the Nibelung* (1876). **Variants:** Gonzales, Gonzalo, Gunn, Gunner, Guntar, Gunther, Guntur.

Gurion From the Hebrew, *gur*, 'lion', implying strength. Hence Gurial, 'God is my strength and protection'. **Variants:** Gur, Guri, Guriel. *See also* Ben-Gurion.

Gurney From the Latin, *grunnire*, 'to grunt'. A gurnet is a marine fish that grunts when it is caught. **Variants:** Gornus, Gourney.

Gustave From the German, 'staff of the Goths'. A popular name in Germany and Sweden, promoted by the royal families. The king and general, Gustavus II of Sweden (1594–1632), popularised the name throughout Europe. **Variants:** Gus, Gustaf, Gustav, Gustavo, Gustavus.

 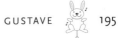

TOP OF THE POPS

Like hem-lines and hair-styles, names go in and out of fashion. But there are always some classics that weather all the changes. John and William have been two consistent favourites since the 12th century, and Alexander has sustained its popularity in Scotland. For girls, Anne and Mary have been steady favourites. Around them others have risen and fallen in fashion, and sometimes risen again. Guy was quite popular until Guy Fawkes tried to blow up the Houses of Parliament on November 5, 1603 (thus 'Bonfire Day'). The hero of Bloomfield's poem *The Farmer's Boy* (1800) threw Giles out of fashion. Both names have since recovered their popularity. But Boniface, good enough for popes to adopt, was permanently reduced to being a type name for inn-keepers just because of George Farquhar's play, *The Beaux' Stratagem* (1707). Betty, a hot Tudor favourite, became so common that it lost its prestige value and was often given to chambermaids in the 18th century. Abigail and Jane suffered the same fate, while Gillian became a synonym for a flirt.

Guthrie From the Celtic, 'war hero'.

Guy A name introduced to Britain by the Normans as Guido and Wido, which possibly derived from 'wide', 'wood' or 'guide'. It became associated with the Latin, *vitus*, 'lively' and thus acceptable to clergy and Christians. Guy Fawkes was the member of the plot to blow up Parliament in 1605 who was discovered in the cellars just in time; the failure of the Gunpowder Plot is celebrated each November 5 with effigies of Guy Fawkes burnt on bonfires and with fireworks. The name is thus also given to a person who is the object of ridicule, but before the plot Guy had been a popular name. It then fell right out of favour, to be revived in the last century, possibly helped by Sir Walter Scott's novel, *Guy Mannering* (1815). St Guy is patron saint of comedians and dancers. **Variants:** Guido, Guyon, Vitus, Viti, Wido.

Gwyn *See* Gwyneth *under girls*. **Variant:** Gwynne.

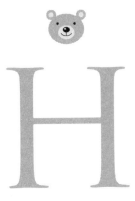

H

Habakkuk A name that appears only in the Bible, and later taken up by Methodists in Wales. Habakkuk was a prophet who lived in the late 7th century BC; his prophecies are in the book of his name. **Variant:** Hubacue.

Hadar From the Hebrew, 'glory'.

Haddon From the Scottish, *hadder*, 'heather', thus 'heathland'. Hence Hadley, 'meadow of heather, moorland'. **Variants:** Had, Hadden, Hadlai, Hadleigh, Hadley, Hatchen, Heath, Lee, Leigh.

Hadrian The Roman emperor (76–138) was an enlightened scholar, poet and musician. He came to Britain in about 122 and had Hadrian's Wall built from Wallsend to Bowness, marking the northern boundary of his vast empire (see also Adrian under both boys and girls).

Hakeem From the Arabic, 'wise'. One of the 99 names and qualities of Allah listed in the Qur'an. **Variant:** Hakim.

Hakon From the Old Norse, *hag*, 'useful'. Haakon VII (1872–1957), King of Norway, maintains the royal character of the name. The name was introduced to Britain by the Danes but fell out of favour in the 13th century, except in Shetland. **Variants:** Haakon, Hacon, Hak.

Hale From the Old English, *hal*, 'safe, sound, healthy and whole'. **Variants:** Hal, Haley, Halford, Halley, Hallie, Halsey, Halsy, Hollis, Holly.

Halil From the Hebrew, 'flute'. **Variant:** Hallil.

Hall From the Old English, *heall*, 'to cover', meaning a large, covered and usually public place. Hence Hallberg, 'snow-capped mountain'. **Variant:** Hallberg.

Ham From the Old English, *ham*, 'home, home town'; also from the Hebrew, 'warm, swarthy'. In the Bible, Shem, Ham and Japheth were the sons of Noah, born when Noah was 500 years old. Ham is considered by some to be the father of the Egyptians (Genesis 5).

Hamal From the Arabic, 'lamb'.

Hamish From the Irish, Shamus, from James.

Hamlet From the Old High German, *heim*, 'home', via the Old English *ham*, thus 'small village', hence Hamlin, 'home near a brook', and Hampden, 'home in the valley'. A name introduced by the Normans and well-used until the 18th century. The hero of Shakespeare's tragedy, *Hamlet* (1602), is based on the Danish prince, Amleth, and gave the name another meaning, 'indecisiveness'. Shakespeare's own son was called Hamnet, after his godfather. **Variants:** Amleth, Amlothi, Haimes, Ham, Hamelin, Hames, Hamil, Hamilton, Hamlin, Hammond, Hamnet, Hamo, Hamon, Hamond, Hampden, Hampton, Haymund, Haymo, Tony.

Hannibal The soldier and statesman from Carthage (247–183 bc) who in 218 BC crossed the Alps with some 35,000 men and 37 elephants to rout the Roman armies. But instead of continuing to Rome, he had to return to defend Carthage. The name thus implies feats of travel and organisation. It has been used in Cornwall since the 16th century. **Variants:** Annibal, Annibale, Hanniball, Honeyball.

Hans From the German, Johannes, from John. **Variants:** Hanan, Handley, Hanes, Hanley, Hanns, Hansel, Hansen, Hanson, Haynes, Heinz, Henlee, Honus.

Harcourt From the Old German, *heri*, 'army', thus 'military quadrangle'. A name popular during the Restoration. **Variants:** Harry, Court.

Hardwin From the Old German, *hardu*, 'hard, strong', and *wine*, 'friend', thus 'strong and

loyal friend'. Introduced by the Normans, the name became widespread as Harding. **Variants:** Harding, Hardwyn.

Hardy From the Old French, *hardir*, 'to grow bold', thus 'courageous, robust'. **Variants:** Harden, Hardin, Harding.

Harel From the Hebrew, 'mountain of God'. **Variant:** Harrell.

Harlequin From the Old English mythical figure, King Herla, another name for Woden, who led a troop of demon horsemen through the night. The name was taken by the Old French as *harlequin*, 'a brightly dressed, masked buffoon', a character in the *commedia dell'arte* which became the English pantomime. With his quick wit, honest love, agility, faithfulness and fearlessness, he was one of the best-loved characters. *See also* Columbine *under girls*.

Harley From the Middle Low German, *harle*, 'hemp, flax', thus 'hemp field'. The library of the two bibliophiles, Sir Robert Harley, Earl of Oxford (1661–1724) and his son, Edward, was bought by the British Museum in 1753 and includes some of its most valuable manuscripts. Harley Granville-Barker was a playwright, actor and producer. **Variants:** Harl, Harlan.

Harmon *See* Harmonia *under girls*.

Harold From the Old German name, Heriwald, 'army power', thus 'leader or commander of an army'. A name probably carried to Britain by the Danes, with its royal associations. King Harold I (died 1040), known as 'Harefoot', was the illegitimate son of the Danish King Knute and died just as Knute's legitimate son, Hardecanute, King of Denmark, was preparing to claim the English throne. Harold II (c. 1022–66), succeeded to the throne in 1066 but the same year William of Normandy invaded and Harold was killed at the Battle of Hastings. The name then fell into disuse, to be revived in the last century, perhaps helped by the poem that made Byron famous, *Childe Harold's Progress* (1812–18). **Variants:** Araldo, Arold, Eral, Hal, Haldon, Halford, Harald, Harivlad, Hariwald, Harlow, Hardoldus, Harolt, Harry, Heral, Hereweald, Hiraldo, Parry, Rigo.

Harper From the Old English, *hearpe*, 'harp', the musical instrument played especially in Ireland; or from the Latin, *harpa*, 'sickle'.

Harrison From the Old English meaning 'son of Harry' or 'ruler of the army'. Alternatives include Arailt (Scottish Gaelic), Haral, Harald (Scandinavian), Harrold, Herold, Harris, Harisen, Harrissen, Harrysen, Harysen and Harry.

Harte From the Germanic, *hirsch*, via the Old English, *heort*, 'mature male deer, stag', especially one more than five years old. A hart royal was a stag chased during a royal hunt. **Variants:** Hart, Hartley, Hartman, Hartwell, Hartwig, Heartley, Hersch, Herschel, Hersh, Hershel, Hertz, Hertzl, Herzl, Heschel, Heshel, Hirsch, Hirsh.

Harvey From the Breton name, Haerveu, 'worthy of battle', implying a mature, strong and well-trained man. St Harvey (6th century), known as Harve or Huwan, was a blind monk and wandering minstrel whose cult was very popular in Brittany, making the name popular in Britain after the Conquest. **Variants:** Erve, Harv, Harve, Harveson, Harvie, Hervey, Hervi.

Hasad Turkish, meaning 'harvest, reaping'.

Haskell *See* Ash and Ezekiel. **Variants:** Haskel, Hassel.

Haslett From the Old English, *haesel*, 'hazle', a tree bearing edible nuts which have given their name to the yellowish-brown colour.

Hassan From the Arabic, 'pleasant, good'. **Variants:** Asan, Hasan.

Hasting From the Old Norse, *husa*, 'house'; or from the Latin, *hasta*, 'spear'. At Hastings, the coastal town in East Sussex, William of Normandy defeated Harold II in 1066. **Variants:** Hastie, Hastings, Hasty.

Haven From the Old English, *haefen*, 'harbour, refuge, sanctuary'. **Variants:** Hagan, Hagen, Hazen, Hogan.

Hayden From the Old English, *hieg*, 'hay, dried grass', thus 'grassy dell, pastureland'. The phrase 'to make hay while the sun shines' means to take advantage of a good thing. **Variants:** Haydn, Hayes, Hays, Hayward, Haywood, Heywood.

Hector From the Greek, *hektor*, 'holding fast, anchor'. In Greek mythology, the strong Trojan prince, son of Priam, who led the army in the long Trojan war but who was slain after 10 years by a single blow from Achilles who dragged his body triumphantly round the walls of Troy three times. Later, the name acquired the meaning 'blusterer, swagger, bully'. The real name of the British writer, Saki (1870–1916), was Hector Hugh Munro. The name has most popularity in Scotland, where it is also a translation of the Gaelic name, Eachdonn. **Variants:** Ector, Ettore.

Hedley From the Old English dialect word, *heder*, 'male sheep', especially one aged between eight months and the time of its first shearing; thus, 'meadow for sheep'.

  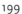

Helaku North American Indian, meaning 'sunny day'.

Helgi In Norse mythology, the warrior Helgi was deeply in love with one of the Valkyries, Kara, who accompanied him to war in the form of a swan. When she sang sweetly above the battlefield, the enemy lost their drive to win. But one day Helgi raised his sword to slay an adversary and fatally wounded Kara by accident, ending their happiness.

Heli From the Greek, *helios*, 'sun'. In Greek mythology, Helios is god of the sun, all-seeing and all-knowing. Daily he emerged from a swamp in Ethiopia to ride across the vault of the heavens in his golden chariot drawn by nine dazzling white horses. By evening, he reached the land of the Hesperides and sailed the ocean all night, to arrive back in time for his next day's journey. **Variant:** Heller. *See also* Selene and Sol.

Helmut From the Old French, *helme*, 'strong defensive cover for the head'. A name implying a warrior. **Variants:** Hellmut, Helm.

Heman From the Hebrew, 'faithful'.

Henry From the Old High German names, Haimirich and Heimerich, from *haimi*, 'house', and *richi*, 'ruler, wealth, power'. A name with solid European royal associations that have maintained its popularity. In Britain, the first of eight kings of England, all nicknamed Harry, was Henry I (1133–89), youngest son of William the Conqueror. Of the others, Henry IV (1367–1413) regained the throne from Richard II and founded the Lancastrian dynasty; Henry V (1387–1422) won the Battle of Agincourt in 1415; Henry VII (1457–1509) united the enemy families of Lancaster and York and founded the Tudor line; and Henry VIII (1491–1547) put the royal stamp of approval on divorce when Catherine of Aragon, the first of his six wives, failed to produce an heir. His Act of Supremacy in 1536 marked the break with Rome and the beginning of the dissolution of the monasteries. A name confined to the aristocracy until the popularity of Henry V, the merry Prince Hal of Shakespeare's *Henry IV* (c. 1597). In Norse mythology, Heimadall guards Asgard, the heavenly abode of the gods. The patronymics include Barry and Darris. **Variants:** Arrigo, Enrico, Enrique, Enzio, Erizio, Erizo, Ezio, Guccio, Haimirich, Hal, Halkin, Hank, Harris, Harrison, Harry, Hawkin, Hedric, Hedrick, Heimadall, Heiman, Heindrick, Heine, Heinemann, Heinie, Heinrich, Heinrick, Heinrik, Heinz, Hendri, Hendric, Hendrick, Hendrik, Heneli, Henke, Henning, Henny, Henri, Henric, Henricus, Henrik, Henriot, Henryk, Henty, Heriot, Herriot, Herry, Rico, Rik, Rogberto. *See also* Thomas.

Herbert From the Old German, *heri*, 'army', and *beraht*, 'bright, illustrious', thus 'outstanding military man'. St Herbert of Cologne (c. 970–1021) was an exceptional bishop of his time and an adviser to Emperor Otto III. He was known for his generosity, discipline and pacificism. A name carried to Britain by the Normans to enjoy favour until the 14th century, it was revived in the last century, possibly because, like Howard, it carried overtones of nobility. **Variants:** Bert, Bertie, Berty, Eberto, Harbert, Heber, Hebert, Herb, Herbertus, Herbie, Herby, Heriberto.

Hercules In Greek mythology, the extraordinarily strong son of the supreme god, Zeus, and Alceme, who won immortality by performing 12 arduous labours which included capturing a golden horned stag and the mad Cretan bull; killing the Nemean lion, the

HARRY AND THE ROYAL HENRYS

When the Prince and Princess of Wales announced that their second son would be known as Harry, they were following a long British royal tradition. All eight King Henrys have been nicknamed Harry. Although the future Henry V was known as Prince Hal in Shakespeare's play, the battle cry when he became king was 'God for Harry! England and Saint George'. The latest Prince Harry was born on September 15, 1984. His full name is Henry Charles Albert David and the birth certificate carefully notes his father's occupation as 'Prince of the United Kingdom'.

---

serpent with nine heads, a wild bull and flesh-eating birds and cows; and stealing the golden apples of the Hesperides. Thus, a herculean feat means success against all the odds, and a herculean person is very strong and courageous. A name found in England in the 16th and 17th centuries, rarely since. **Variants:** Herc, Hercule.

Herman From the Old High German, *heri*, 'army', thus 'soldier'. **Variants:** Armand, Armando, Armant, Armin, Armina, Ermanno, Ermin, Harman, Harmen, Harmon, Herenan, Hermann, Hermanze, Hermie, Herminio, Hermon, Hermy. *See also* Armand and Herman.

Hermes *See* Hermione *under girls.* **Variant:** Hermus.

Hern From the Middle English, *heroun* and *herne*, 'heron'. The birds of the *Ardeidae* family wait for their prey standing motionless on one foot, then dive down for fish, frog or rodent. As herons were believed to be shy of their fellows, stone herons used to be stood

beside fishponds to frighten off real herons and safeguard the fish. **Variants:** Herndon, Herne, Heron, Hornsby.

Herod From the Greek, 'to protect, guard'. The Greek historian, Heroditus (484–425 BC), laid the foundations of secular narrative history and is regarded as the father of history. In ancient Rome, there are two less appealing Herods: Herod the Great (73–74 BC), who is supposed to have been jealous of Christ's birth and ordered the slaying of all children under two years old in Bethlehem; and Herod Antipas (died c. 40) who married his niece Herodias who then schemed to kill the disapproving John the Baptist (*see* Salome).

Hershell From the traditional Jewish meaning 'deer'. Alternatives include Herschel, Herschyl and Hersyl.

Hesketh From the Hebrew name, Hezekiah, 'my strength comes from God'. A name taken up by the 17th-century Puritans. **Variants:** Hezeki, Hezekiah.

Hilal From the Arabic, 'new moon'. **Variant:** Hilel.

Hilary *See also under girls.* Of several saints, St Hilary of Arles (c. 400–449) was an energetic and almost too zealous bishop who was twice rebuked by Pope Leo I. **Variants:** Hilaire, Hilar, Hilarid, Hilario, Hilarius, Hill, Hillard, Hillary, Hillery, Hilliard, Hillie, Hilly, Ilario, Laris.

Hildebrand From the Old German, *hildi*, 'battle', and *brant*, 'fire, torch, sword-blade', implying a warrior whose sword flashes with action during battle. A popular name in medieval romances, boosted by St Hildebrand, another name for Pope Gregory VII (1000–85). After a period of disfavour, it enjoyed a small revival in the last century. **Variants:** Hildebrand, Hildreth.

Hillel From the Hebrew, 'renowned, acclaimed'.

Hilmer From the Old English, *hyll*, 'hill, remote high area', thus 'hill near the sea or water'. **Variants:** High, Hill, Hyland, Hyman.

Hippolytus From the Greek, *ippolutos*, 'freeing the horses'. In Greek mythology, son of Hippolyta, Queen of the Amazons, and Theseus. **Variants:** Ippolitus, Ypolit, Ypolitus.

Hiram From the Hebrew, 'noble brother, born to nobility'. **Variant:** Ahiram.

Hiroshi Japanese, meaning 'generous'.

Hisoka Japanese, meaning 'secretive, shy'.

Ho Chinese, meaning 'good'.

Hod From the Hebrew, 'vigour, splendour'. Hence Hodiah, 'my splendour is from God'. Also given to girls. **Variant:** Hodiya.

Hodges *See* Roger.

Hoffman From the German *hof*, 'courtier, man of influence and flattery'. The German romantic novelist, Ernst Theodor Amadeus Hoffmann (1776–1822) was also a composer who changed one of his names, Wilhelm, to Amadeus in honour of Mozart. He is the hero of Offenbach's opera, *The Tales of Hoffman* (1881).

Holden From the Old English, *hol*, 'valley', and *denn*, 'sheltered place', hence Holbrook, 'valley with a stream'. Or from the Old English, *halden*, 'one who keeps watch', especially over pastures and sheep. **Variant:** Holbrook.

Holleb Polish, meaning 'like a dove', therefore a symbol of peace (see Dove). **Variants:** Hollub, Holub.

Holm From the Old Norse, *holmr*, 'meadow, small island', meaning low land beside water, or a river island. **Variants:** Holmes, Hume.

Holt From the Old English, *holt*, 'wooded hill, a copse'.

Homer From the Greek, 'being hostage or led', and, by inference, 'blind person'. The Greek poet (8th century BC), wrote the two epic poems, *The Iliad* and *The Odyssey*, a rich mixture of the fact, fantasy, legend and myths of the oral tradition which recount the history of the Trojan War and Odysseus's journey afterwards. Thus the term Homeric implies work on an enormous scale, while Homeric laughter refers to the loud and unrestrained laughter of the Greek gods. A name found in Britain in the last century but made more popular recently in the USA by the creation of cartoon character Homer Simpson. **Variants:** Homero, Omero.

Honester From the Old English, *han*, 'stone', meaning a whetstone for sharpening tools, thus 'tool sharpener'.

Honi From the Hebrew, 'gracious'.

Honor *See under girls.*

Horace Possibly from the Latin, *hora*, 'time, hour'. A popular name in ancient Rome. In the great Roman Horatius family, there was a story that three brothers fought to the death three relatives from a nearby city, the ultimate display of their loyalty to their city and father. The legendary Roman hero, Horatius Cocles, supposedly held back the Etruscan army until the wooden bridge over the Tiber was demolished, then swam across to safety. And Horace (65–8 BC), or Horatius, was the Roman poet whose gentle and humane philosophy is expressed in his Satires and Carmina (Odes). Renaissance Italy revived the name which then spread to England–Horatio is friend to Hamlet in Shakespeare's play, and Horace Walpole (1717–79) was the writer and wit whose novel, *Castle of Otranto* (1765), began the gothic literary fashion. **Variants:** Horacio, Horatio, Horatius, Orazio. *See also* Neil.

Horst From the German, *horst*, 'leap'.

Horton From the Latin, *hortus*, 'garden'. *See* Gardiner.

Horus In Egyptian mythology, god of the sky whose eyes were the sun and moon. As ruler of the united Egypt, Horus was the ancestor of the pharaohs who considered themselves to be his representatives on earth.

Hosea From the Hebrew, 'salvation'. In the Bible, the first of the minor prophets. He lived in the 8th century BC and foretold the rise of the Kingdom of Israel. **Variants:** Hoshal, Osia, Osias.

Hototo North American Indian, meaning 'the whistler'.

Howard From the Old English, *hogg*, 'wild boar, domestic swine', and *weardian*, 'warden', thus 'hog-warden', the medieval official who kept a check on the district's pigs. The American multi-millionaire and magnate, Howard Robard Hughes (1905–76), founded the Hughes Aircraft Corporation, broke the airspeed record in 1935 and the round-the-world record in 1938, but lived as a recluse from 1951 until his death. Although long popular in the USA, Howard has been a first name in Britain only since the nineteenth century, and was possibly taken up for its associations with the noble family of Howards. **Variants:** Hogg, Howey, Howie, Ward.

Howell From the Old English, *hog*, 'wild boar, domestic swine', and *hyll*, 'high, hill', thus 'hill where boars or swine roam'. Or from the Welsh, *hywel*, 'eminent'. **Variants:** Hoel, Hough, Houghton, Howe, Howel, Howey, Howland, Hulett, Hywel, Powell.

Howi North American Indian, meaning 'dove'.

Hoyle From the Middle Dutch, *hoei*, 'heavy barge'. Sir Edmund Hoyle (1672–1769) wrote *A Short Treatise on the Game of White* (1742), the standard work on card-games for over a century. **Variant:** Hoyt.

Hudson Patronymic of Hudd, from Richard.

Hugh From the Old High German name, Huguberht, from *hugu*, 'spirit, mind', and *beraht*, 'shining, illustrious', thus 'intelligent and noble-spirited'; or from the Celtic names, Hu and Hew, 'fire, inspiration'. The name of several saints, including Hugh of Liège (8th century), a noble who enjoyed hunting as much as holiness and was therefore popular with the aristocracy–his festival on November 3 marked the opening of the stag-hunting

NAMING THE PLAYERS

The Tudor plays of William Shakespeare, Ben Jonson, and the duo, Beaumont and Fletcher, were by no means intended for the élite. They were enjoyed by large crowds and were a popular source of public entertainment. Shakespeare's romantic Juliet was his own translation of the Italian name, Giulietta. He also made up Perdita for the rags-to-riches princess in *A Winter's Tale*. Films have the same impact today, making fashionable the names of both the stars and the parts they play. *The Wizard of Oz* brought the names Judy and Garland into the limelight as much as that of her fairytale character, Dorothy. And *Gone With the Wind* surely encouraged the names of both the romantic leads, Scarlett and Rhett, as well as the real names of their players, Vivien and Clark.

---

season. St Hugh of Cluny (1024–1120) was a more remarkable man, who became Abbot of Cluny monastery and thus of all Benedictine houses at the age of 25, a post he retained for 60 years. He was a reformist, diplomat and adviser to popes, and took Cluny to its peak of influence and power. More recently, the British politician, Hugh Todd Naylor Gaitskell (1906–63), was leader of the Labour Party from 1955 to 1963. The name enjoyed its greatest popularity during the Middle Ages, to be revived at the beginning of the last century. **Variants:** Bert, Bertie, Berty, Hew, Hobard, Hobart, Hub, Hubbard, Hubbell, Hube, Huberd, Hubert, Huberto, Hubie, Huet, Huey, Hughie, Hugi, Hugibert, Hugo, Hutchin, Huw, Uberto, Ugo.

Humbert From the Old High German, *heim*, 'home', and *beraht*, 'shining, bright'. **Variants:** Hum, Humberto, Umberto.

Humphrey From the Old German, *hun*, 'strength', and *frythu*, 'peace'. A name implying a quiet but solid strength of character. It was used by the aristocracy in the Middle Ages, when Henry IV's son was called Humphrey, Duke of Gloucester. He was starved to death by political opponents, hence the phrase, 'to dine with Duke Humphrey', meaning to go without supper. Humpty Dumpty is the nursery rhyme character, so those nicknames imply a short, tubby boy. The name may have been popularised in this century by the screen actor Humphrey Bogart (1899–1957). **Variants:** Dumpty, Hum, Humfrey, Humfrid, Humfried, Hump, Humph, Humphry, Humpty, Hundredo, Hunfrey, Onfre, Onfroi, Onofredo, Umphrey.

Hunter From the Old English, *huntian*, 'to search diligently, pursue, track down', especially chasing animals to kill them for food or sport. **Variants:** Huntington, Huntley, Lee, Leigh.

Hussein From the Arabic, *husn*, 'good'. **Variants:** Hosein, Hossein, Husain, Hussain.

Huxley From the Old English, *aesc*, 'ash tree', and *leah*, 'meadow, grassland', thus 'field of ash trees'. *See also* Ash. **Variants:** Haskel, Haskell, Hux, Lee, Leigh.

Hyde From the Old English, *hid*, 'measure of land'. This was the amount needed by one man to keep a family. Hyde Park in central London covers 146 hectares and was one of Henry VIII's royal deer parks until Charles I opened it to the public in 1635. **Variant:** Hyder. *See also* Jekyll.

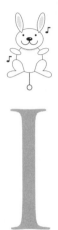

Ian Scottish form of John. **Variant:** Iain.

Ib English form of Abba.

Ignatius From the Greek, *ignis*, 'fire'. Several saints have borne the name but it is the Spaniard, Ignatius of Loyola (1491–1556), known as Inigo, who influenced the name's later use. Born into nobility, he was a soldier before giving his life to Christ. After a pilgrimage to Jerusalem and four-years' study, he became the inspiration of seven students in Paris, who included Frances Xavier. In 1540 this movement became official as The Society of Jesus, known as the Jesuits. It spread throughout the world from Rome, emphasising learning and prayer with the help of Ignatius' book, *Spiritual Exercises*. The British architect Inigo Jones (1573–1652) introduced the Palladian style from Italy to Britain and designed the Queen's House, Greenwich. **Variants:** Eneco, Iggie, Iggy, Ignace, Ignacio, Ignatz, Ignaz, Ignazio, Inigo, Inigue.

Igor *See* George. **Variants:** Inge, Ingmar.

Ike *See* Dwight and Isaac.

Ilan From the Hebrew, 'tree'.

Ilbert From the Old German, *hildi*, 'battle', and *beraht*, 'bright', thus 'distinguished warrior'. Introduced by the Normans, the name did not catch on and is rare after the 13th century.

Imbert From the Old German name, Isenbard, 'iron bard'. Like Ilbert, an unsuccessful import by the Normans.

Imri From the Hebrew, 'tall'. **Variants:** Imric, Imrie.

Ingram From the Old Norse, 'Ing's raven'. In Norse mythology, Ing is a name for Frey, god of peace and fertility, whose strong cult in Sweden produced splendid temples and elaborate festivals with music, dancing and games. Among Ing's possessions were a sword that flashed through the air of its own accord, a horse that crossed mountains faster than the wind, and a ship large enough to take all his companions but small enough to fold into his pocket. He fell desperately in love with the giant, Gerda and, after a long period of agonised wooing, won her as his wife. As the Angles saw Ing as their ancestor, the name was popular throughout the Middle Ages, and then went out of fashion with the Reformation. **Variants:** Ingamar, Ingemar, Inglis, Ingmar, Ingo, Ingra, Ingrim. *See also* Inge under girls.

Innes From the Gaelic, 'island'. **Variants:** Innes, Innis.

Intrepid From the Latin, *intrepidus*, 'not alarmed', meaning resolute, brave and courageous.

Iolo Welsh, probably from Iorwerth, 'worthy lord'. *See also* Julian.

Ira From the Aramaic, 'stallion'.

Irvin From the Gaelic, 'handsome, fair'. **Variants:** Earvin, Erv, Erve, Ervin, Erwin, Irv, Irvine, Irving, Irwin, Irwyn. *See also* Washington.

Isaac From the Hebrew, *yishaq*, 'he laughs'. In the Bible, the son of Abraham and Sarah, born when Abraham was 100 years old, much to Sarah's surprise. Isaac was in turn father of Jacob and Esau (Genesis 21). Popular with early Christians in Eastern Europe, the name only gained favour in Britain after the Reformation. Izaac Walton (1593–1683) wrote the classic fishing manual, *The Compleat Angler* (1653). Sir Isaac Newton (1642–1727), mathematician and physicist, devised calculus and wrote a treatise on the theory of gravitation. **Variants:** Eisig, Ike, Ikey, Isaacus, Isaak, Isac, Isacco, Isak, Itzik, Izaak, Izak, Yirtzhak, Yithak, Yitzchak, Zak.

Isaiah From the Hebrew, *Yeshayah*, 'salvation of the Lord'. In the Bible, one of the foremost prophets, living in Judah in the 8th century BC. Isaiah, Jeremiah (see Jeremy) and Ezekiel were the three major prophets. **Variants:** Esaias, Ikaia, Is, Isa, Isaias, Issa, Yeshaya, Yeshayahu.

Ishmael From the Hebrew, *Yismael*, 'God hears'. In the Bible, Abraham's son by the maid of his wife, Sarah (Genesis 16). At the time, Sarah believed she could not have children, but she later gave birth to Isaac, after which Ishmael and his brother Hagar were thrown out of the house – hence Ishmael also means 'outcast'. **Variant:** Ismail.

Isidore *See* Isadora *under girls*. St Isidore of Seville (c. 560–636), influential scholar and Bishop of Seville, strengthened the Spanish church and his writings included *Origins*, an encyclopaedia of medieval knowledge. **Variants:** Dore, Dory, Isador, Isidor, Isidoro, Isidro, Izzy.

Israel From the Hebrew, *Yisrael*, 'he who struggles with God' or 'may God prevail'. In the Bible, the name given to Jacob by the angel with whom he fought (Genesis 32). The Israelites are the descendants of Jacob, the whole Hebrew people, regarded as heirs of the covenant of Jacob. The State of Israel, created in 1947, declared independence the following year, and is the only state in the world where Judaism is the official religion. **Variant:** Srully. *See also* Jacob.

Itamar From the Hebrew, 'palm grove'. **Variants:** Ithamar, Ittamar.

Itiel From the Hebrew, 'God is with me'.

Ivan Russian form of John. **Variants:** Evo, Evon, Ivo, Yvan, Yvon.

Ivar From the Old Norse, 'archer'. **Variants:** Ive, Iver, Ivor, Yvon, Yvor.

Ivor From the Latin, *ebur*, 'ivory'; also from the Welsh name, Ifor, 'lord'. **Variants:** Ivair, Ivar, Ive, Iver.

J

Jabez A Hebrew name, possibly meaning 'I bore him in sorrow', which would account for its use by the Puritans and, later, the Dissenters.

Jacinto Male form of Hyacinth, from the Spanish.

Jackson *See* Jacob.

Jack *See* Jacob.

Jacob From the Hebrew, 'supplanter, follower'. In the Bible, son of Isaac and Rebecca and twin brother of Esau. Jacob was born after Esau and came out of the womb holding his brother's heel (Genesis 25). Later, he took Esau's inheritance and then tricked their father into giving him the first blessing. The third of the Patriachs, with Abraham and Isaac before him, Jacob had 12 sons who were the fathers of the 12 tribes of Israel–Israel being another name for Jacob. Jacob's Ladder is a ladder that Jacob saw in a dream, with angels going up and down it and God at the top who told Jacob he would be the father of a blessed people who would live in God's chosen land (Genesis 28). Highly popular with Jews in the post-biblical period, the name was introduced to Britain among the clergy and then spread out after the Conquest, to become a popular Old Testament name during the Reformation. The British sculptor, Sir Jacob Epstein (1880–1959) created many bronzes for public buildings, including *St Michael and the Devil* for Coventry Cathedral. **Variants:** Akevy, Akiba, Akiva, Akkoobjee, Akkub, Cob, Cobb, Cobbie, Cobby, Como, Coppo, Diego, Gemmes, Giacobbe, Giacobo, Giacomo, Giacopo, Hamish, Iago, Jaap, Jacinto, Jack, Jacke, Jackie, Jackman, Jackson, Jacky, Jaco, Jacobo, Jacobos, Jacobs, Jacobson, Jacobus, Jacoby, Jacopo, Jacque, Jacques, Jago, Jake, Jakie, Jakob, Jakon, Jakov, James, Jamie, Jaques, Jaquot, Jascha, Jaschenka, Jasha, Jayme, Jeb, Jemmy, Jock, Jocko, Joco, Kivi, Kub, Kubaa, Lapo, Santiago, Seumuis, Yaacov, Yaagov, Yaakov, Yago, Yuki. *See also* James.

Jaden Meaning 'God has heard'.

James English form of Jacob. A thoroughly Christian and royal form of the name. In the Bible, James is a brother of Jesus, sometimes confused with St James the Less (died c. 62), and he was one of the Apostles. St James the Greater (died 44), also an Apostle, was brother of St John and the first Apostle to be martyred. Both brothers and St Peter witnessed the transfiguration and had slight precedence over the other Apostles. In Spain, it was claimed that he came to preach there and that after his death his body was carried to Santiago de Compostela, still a great pilgrimage centre. The British royal influence on the name's popularity began in Scotland, where the name first took hold. James IV (1473–1513) led his people to their greatest defeat by the English at Flodden (1513). James VI of Scotland (1566–1625) became James I of England in 1603. He was a devout Roman Catholic who founded the Stuart dynasty and believed in the divine right of kings. James II (1633–1701), an even more zealous Roman Catholic, was the victim of the Duke of Monmouth's rebellion and eventually had to flee to safety in France. Its fashion with the middle classes in this century is reflected in the announcements on the Court page of *The Times* newspaper: for the last 21 years James has been the most popular boy's name. The form Hamish is used in the Scottish Highlands; Seamus and its variants in Ireland. **Variants:** Dago, Diego, Hamish, Iago, Jaime, Jaimie, Jam, Jamesy, Jamey, Jamie, Jan, Janny, Jay, Jayme, Jas, Jem, Jim, Jimbo, Jimmie, Jimmy, Seamus, Seumas, Seumus, Shamus, Zebedee. *See also* Jacob.

Jamil From the Asian-Indian name meaning 'handsome'. Alternatives include Jamal.

Janus From the Latin, *janus*, 'passage, arcade, gateway'. In Roman mythology, the god of gateways who looked both in and out. He was therefore god of endings and beginnings and gave his name to the month of January. In art, he was portrayed with two heads, back to back. St Januarius (died c. 305) has an exceptional relic, kept in Naples Cathedral: for the last 500 years, a glass phial containing some of his dried blood is displayed 18 times a year, and after each showing it liquefies. So far, there is no scientific explanation. **Variant:** Januarius.

Japheth From the Hebrew, 'beautiful', implying youth. In the Bible, the youngest of Noah's three sons, Shem, Ham and Japheth. A name used by the 17th-century Puritans. **Variants:** Japhet, Yafet, Yaphet.

Jardine From the French, *jardin*, 'garden'. *See* Gardiner.

Jareb From the Hebrew, 'he will maintain'. **Variant:** Jarib.

Jared From the Hebrew meaning 'descendent'.

Jaron From the Hebrew, 'to cry aloud, sing out'. **Variant:** Yartron.

Jaroslav Czech, meaning 'glory of spring'. One of the most popular names in Czechoslovakia.

Jarvis *See* Gerard. **Variants:** Gary, Gervais, Gervase, Gervise, Jary, Jerve, Jervis.

Jason Greek form of Joshua. In Greek mythology, Jason led the Argonauts, a collection of Greek heroes, in the quest for the Golden Fleece. The fleece had belonged to a fabulous ram which had been sacrificed and was now in the hands of Aeetes. Jason fell in love with Medea, Aeetes' daughter, who helped him obtain the fleece and escape to safety. In the Bible, one Jason wrote the book of Ecclesiasticus; another was a relative of St Paul. A name found in Britain since the 17th century. **Variants:** Jaeson, Jay.

Jaspar From the Arabic, *yashb*. A semi-precious stone of red or reddish-brown opaque quartz. **Variants:** Caspar, Gaspar, Gaspard, Gaspare, Jasper, Kaspar. *See also* Caspar.

Jay From the Latin, *gaius*, 'jay'. The bird's harsh chirping has given the name a second meaning, 'cheeky chatterer', and its bright colours a third, 'absurdly and flashily dressed person'. Gaius was the first name of Julius Caesar. **Variant:** Gaius. *See also* Jason.

Jed From the Arabic, *yed*, 'hand'.

Jedaiah From the Hebrew, 'God knows'. Hence, Jedidiah, 'beloved of God', a name for Solomon, and Jehiel, 'may God live'. **Variants:** Didi, Jed, Jeddy, Yehiel.

Jefferey *See* Geoffrey. The form Jefferson became popular in the USA when Thomas Jefferson (1743–1826) drafted the American Declaration of Independence in 1776; he was third president of the United States from 1801 to 1809.

Jephthah From the Hebrew, 'he will open', referring to a first-born child of a family. The Puritans used the name sometimes. **Variants:** Jephtah, Yiftach, Yiftah.

Jeremy From the Hebrew name, Yirmayahu, or Jeremiah, 'God is uplifted'. In the Bible, a major prophet (7th–6th centuries BC), whose book contains his prophecies and who also wrote the Lamentations. Found in Britain by the Middle Ages, the name was popular with the Puritans, to be revived this century. The political theorist and philosopher, Jeremy Bentham (1748–1832), laid the foundations of utilitarianism, the theory that human endeavour should strive for the greatest happiness for the greatest number of people. **Variants:** Gerome, Gerrie, Gerry, Hieremas, Hieronymus, Jere, Jereme, Jeremiah, Jeremias, Jerre, Jerrie, Jerrome, Jerry, Yirmeeyahu. *See also* Jerome.

Jerome From the Greek name, Gerome, 'holy and sacred name'. St Jerome (c. 342–420), whose real name was Eusebius Hieronymus, is among the greatest of all biblical scholars and doctors of the church. He became secretary to Pope Damascus (c. 304–384), for whom he began revising the Latin translation of the New Testament. This project was enlarged to produce in 404 the Vulgate, a new version of the complete Latin Bible. A name found in Britain since the 12th century. The English writer Jerome K. Jerome (1859–1927) wrote the best-selling humorous novel, *Three Men in a Boat* (1889). **Variants:** Gerome, Geronima, Gerry, Jeromo, Jeronim, Jerram, Jerrie, Jerry. *See also* Jeremy and John.

Jesse See Jessie under girls. Another popular post-Reformation name. Jesse James (1847–82) was a famous American outlaw in the days of the wild west. **Variants:** Jess, Jessamine, Jessie.

Jesus From the Hebrew name, Yehoshua, or Joshua. In the Bible, the son of Mary, and the Messiah who was the Son of God. *See also* Christian.

Jethro From the Hebrew, 'wealth, abundance'. In the Bible, the father-in-law of Moses. Like so many Old Testament names, popular after the Reformation. Jethro Tull (1674–1741) was an English agriculturalist who invented a new kind of drill for sowing seeds. **Variants:** Jeth, Jett.

Jibben English gypsy name, meaning 'life'. **Variant:** Jivvil.

Jivanta From the East Indies, meaning 'long-lived'. **Variant:** Jivin.

Joab From the Hebrew, 'God is father'. In the Bible, nephew of King David. **Variant:** Yoav.

Joachim From the Hebrew, 'God will establish'. In the Bible, a King of Judah. In early apocryphal writing, the saints Joachim and Ann are the parents of the Virgin Mary. **Variants:** Akim, Giachimo, Jehoiachin, Jehoiakim, Joa, Jochim, Joaquin, Yehoiakim.

Job From the Hebrew name, Iyyobh, from *ayabh*, 'to be hostile', thus 'hated, persecuted, oppressed'. In the Bible, Job's faith in God saw him through a series of calamities, making him the model of patience – hence the term 'patience of Job' to describe almost superhuman qualities of tolerance and endurance. An Old Testament name that enjoyed post-Reformation popularity.

Jocelin *See under girls.*

Joel *See under girls.* **Variant:** Yoel.

John From the Hebrew name, Jochanan, 'God is kind and merciful'. One of the most consistently popular English names since the first crusaders carried it back to Britain, and the most popular name of all since the 17th century. Its peak was between 1650 and 1699, when about a quarter of all male baptismal names were John. It has been ratified down the centuries by 82 saints, 23 popes, and countless notable and literary figures. Of the saints, John the Baptist (died c. 29) was the herald of Christ (see Baptist). John the Divine (died c. 100), or Theologian, was the fisherman who, with his brother St James and St Peter, became one of the preferred Apostles. Tradition then made him the favourite whom Jesus asked to take care of his mother Mary after his death. He possibly wrote the Fourth Gospel, three epistles and the Book of Revelations. When too old to preach, Jerome records that John simply said: 'Love one another. That is the Lord's command: and if you keep it, that by itself is enough.' The two saints between them have the dedications of almost 700 British churches. The only English king called John (1167–1216) was forced by his barons to sign the Magna Carta in 1215, the foundation of British civil liberty. In literature, John Bull is without doubt the foremost John character: honest, straightforward and trusting, he personifies England and the English. He was created by John Arbuthnot for his political satire, *The History of John Bull* (1712), advocating peace and an end to the war with France. The ballad *John Gilpin* (1782) was written by William Cowper. John O'Groats is named after the Dutchman, John de Groat, who built an octagonal house there in the 16th century. Because it is at the north-eastern tip of Scotland, the phrase 'from Land's End to John O'Groats' means the length of Britain. The name Jack seems to have arrived in Britain through wool-trading with the Low Countries, where Jankin was the nickname for Jan, the female form of John. Quickly popularised, it became a favourite children's hero name, as in Jack the Giant-killer, Jack and Jill and Jack Sprat. Ian is the Scottish form; Sean the Irish. See also Ewen, Hans, Ivan, Jacob, James, Jonathan and Yank. The compounds include **Gian-Carlo** and **John-Paul**. **Variants:** Evan, Ewan, Gehan, Gennaro, Geno, Gian, Giovanni, Haines, Hanan, Hans, Iain, Ian, Ion, Ivan, Jack, Jackie, Jackman, Jakon, Jan, Janes, Janne, Janos, Jean, Jeanno,

Jehan, Jenkin, Jenner, Jennings, Jens, Joannes, Jochanan, Jock, Jocko, Johan, Johanan, Johann, Johannes, Johnnie, Johnny, Jon, Jone, Jovan, Juan, Owen, St John, Sean, Shaughn, Shaun, Shawn, Yan, Yana, Yancy, Yank, Yankee, Yanni, Yochanan, Yohanan, Yves, Zan, Zane, Zebedee.

Jonah From the Hebrew, *yonah*, 'moaning, dove', see Dove. In the Bible, the prophet who disobeyed God during a storm at sea was thrown overboard, swallowed by a whale and regurgitated three days later unharmed. Hence the name can imply bad luck. A popular Reformation name, but rare today. **Variants:** Jonas, Yona, Yonah. *See also* Peter.

Jonathan From the Hebrew, *nathan*, 'God's gift'. In the Bible, the eldest son of King Saul. His deep friendship with his brother-in-law, King David, gave rise to the comparison of a loyal and brotherly friendship being 'like David and Jonathan' (1 Samuel 20). With the vogue for Old Testament names, Jonathan became popular after the Reformation. The Irish-born writer Jonathan Swift (1667–1745) wrote *Gulliver's Travels* (1726), a powerful satire attacking contemporary politics, science and philosophy. **Variants:** Jon, Jonathan, Jonny, Yonatan. *See also* John and Nathaniel.

Jordon *See* Jardena *under girls.* **Variants:** Ira, Giordano, Jared, Jarrod, Jerad, Jordain, Jori, Jory, Judd, Yarden.

Joseph From the Hebrew name, Yosayf, 'God will multiply'. In the Bible, the 12th and favourite son of Jacob and Rachel who was sold by his brothers into slavery (Genesis 37). Also, the carpenter and upright husband of the Virgin Mary (Matthew 1), who as a saint still has a strong cult in Europe and acquired a good quantity of apocryphal stories. The French Franciscan friar and diplomat, Joseph Frère (1577–1638) was adviser to Cardinal Richelieu and gained the nickname 'Eminence Grise' from his grey habit. Like other Old Testament names, it became really popular in Britain only after the Reformation. The British painter, Joseph William Mallard Turner (1775–1851), is noted for his ability to capture atmosphere through light, colour and space. **Variants:** Beppe, Beppo, Che, Giuseppe, Iosep, Iosif, Jaska, Jo, Joce, Jody, Joe, Joey, Joie, Josce, Jose, Josephus, Joses, Josko, Jozef, Osip, Pepe, Pepito, Peppo, Yosayf, Yosef, Yosel, Yoseph, Yosi, Yossel, Yossele, Yussuf.

Joshua From the Hebrew name, Yehoshua, 'God is my salvation'. In the Bible, the successor to Moses who led the Israelites to the Promised Land. A very popular name in the post-biblical period, when Jesus and the Greek form, Jason, were also used. In Britain, it was favoured as an Old Testament name after the Reformation. The painter Joshua Reynolds (1723–92) was the first President of the Royal Academy. **Variants:** Hosea, Hoshayah, Jason, Jesous, Jesus, Josh, Josua, Josue, Mosha, Yehoshua. *See also* Jason.

Josiah From the Hebrew, 'May the Lord heal and protect', in the sense of restoring a mother after she has given birth. In the Bible, the King of Judah (638–608) who succeeded to the throne aged eight. Used in Britain by the 17th-century Puritans. **Variants:** Josh, Josias.

Jotham From the Hebrew, 'God is perfect'.

Jotun *See* Utgard.

Joubert From the Old English name, Godbeorht, from *beorht*, 'bright, shining, illustrious', thus 'God's radiance'. **Variant:** Jovett.

Joyce *See* Joyce and Jocelin *under girls*.

Jubal *See* Yovela *under girls*. In the Bible, a descendant of Cain who invented the lyre, harp, organ and other musical instruments (Genesis 4). **Variant:** Yovel.

Jude *See* Judith *under girls*. The apostle and martyr, St Jude (1st century), is the intercessor for people with problems and the patron saint of lost causes. The name was encouraged by Thomas Hardy's novel, *Jude the Obscure* (1895). **Variants:** Jud, Judah, Judas, Judd, Jude, Judson, Yehuda, Yehudah.

Julian Probably from the Greek, 'soft-haired, fair-complexioned'. Gaius Julius Caesar was the first emperor of the Roman Empire. Several saints include Julian the Hospitaller, after whom countless hospitals and churches are named. He was the popular hero of a medieval romance recounting how he expiated the mistaken murder of his parents by helping travellers and the poor, and finally earned God's blessing. The name arrived in Britain in the 13th century but its great popularity is recent. The form Jolyon was possibly helped by the character Jolyon Forsyte in John Galsworthy's novel, *The Forsyte Saga* (1906–28). **Variants:** Giuliano, Giulio, Guliano, Iola, Iolo, Jellon, Jolin, Jollan, Jollanus, Jolyon,

Jule, Jules, Julianus, Julien, Julio, Julius, Julot, Julyan.

Jumbo From the African, *jumba*, 'elephant'. One of London Zoo's first and most popular elephants was named Jumbo, which then became the animal's traditional name. **Variants:** Jamba, Jum, Jumba.

Jun Chinese, meaning 'truth', and Japanese, meaning 'obedience'.

Junior *See* June *under girls*. In the USA a familiar term for 'boy' or 'son'. **Variant:** Junius.

Jupiter *See* Zeus.

Justin From the Latin, *justus*, 'upright, righteous, true, lawful'. The philosopher and travelling preacher, St Justin (c. 100–165), was the most important Christian apologist of the 2nd century, martyred in Rome when he refused to sacrifice to the gods, saying 'No right-minded man forsakes truth for falsehood.' His name was soon widespread. The great Byzantine emperor, Justinian I (483–565), expanded his empire, achieved temporary unity of the Christian church, began to build the church of St Sophia and revised Roman law into the Justinian Code. **Variants:** Giustino, Giusto, Justinian, Justino, Justis, Justus, Jut, Jute.

Juventino From the Latin, *juvenalis*, 'youthful'.

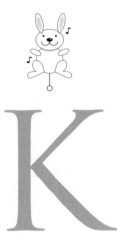

K

Kadmiel From the Hebrew, 'God is ancient'.

Kahil From the Arabic, 'friend, lover'. **Variant:** Kalil.

Kaikane Hawaiian, from *kai*, 'ocean', thus 'man of the ocean'. **Variant:** Kai.

Kalani Hawaiian, meaning 'the heavens'.

Kalil From the Greek, *kalos*, 'beautiful'; also the male form of Kelila. **Variants:** Kahil, Kahlil, Kailil, Kal, Kallie, Kalton.

Kalle Scandinavian, meaning 'strong and manly'.

Kalman *See* Clement.

Kaloosh Armenian, meaning 'blessed arrival'.

Kamil From the Arabic, 'perfect'. One of the 99 qualities of God listed in the Qur'an.

Kane From the Gaelic, 'tribute'. **Variants:** Kain, Kaine, Kayne.

Kaniel From the Arabic, 'spear'. **Variant:** Kani.

Karif From the Arabic, *kharif*, 'autumn'.

Karim From the Arabic, *karam*, 'generous, noble'. In the Qur'an, one of the 99 names for God. **Variants:** Kareem, Kario.

Karl *See* Charles.

Karma From the Tibetan meaning a 'star'.

Karmel *See* Carmel.

Kasimir From the Slavonic, 'commands peace'.

Katriel From the Hebrew, 'God is my crown'. **Variant:** Kati.

Kaufman From the German, 'merchant'. **Variant:** Kaufmann.

Kay *See under girls*. The Welsh form is Kai, in Arthurian legend the name of one of the knights of the Round Table (*see* Arthur).

Keane From the Old English, *cene*, 'wise, clever, brave, strong'. **Variants:** Kane, Kani, Kayne, Kean, Keenan, Keene, Kene, Kienan.

Kedem *See* Kedma *under girls.*

Keefe Irish, from the Arabic, *kayf*, 'euphoria, enjoyment', implying a self-conscious state of pleasant idleness or intoxication. **Variants:** Keever, Kief, Kif.

Keith From the Gaelic, 'forest, wood'. A name that gained favour in Scotland before spreading recently to the rest of Britain.

Kelly *See under girls.*

Kelsey From the Middle English, *kele*, 'keel', the backbone of a ship's structure. The name thus implies strength and reliability. **Variants:** Kelcey, Kelley, Kellog, Kellow, Kelo, Kelson, Kelton.

Kelvin From the Middle English, *kele*, 'keel of a ship', and *wine*, 'friend', thus 'fond of ships'. **Variant:** Kelwin.

Kendal From the Old English, *cyn*, 'ruler, royal', and *dell*, 'wooded valley', thus 'royal valley'. Kendal green is a coarse, woollen cloth originally woven in Kendal, Westmorland. **Variants:** Ken, Kendall, Kendell, Kenn, Kennie, Kenny.

Kendrick From the Old English name Cynric, from *cyne*, 'royal, ruler', and *rice*, 'ruler, power, wealth', implying a strong combination of power and influence. A name found often during the Middle Ages, falling into disfavour after the 17th century. **Variants:** Ken, Kendig, Kenn, Kennie, Kenny, Kenric, Kenrick, Kenward, Rick, Rickie, Ricky.

Kenelm From the Old English name, Cenhelm, from *cene*, 'brave', and *helm*, 'helmet', thus 'courageous warrior'. St Kenelm (died 819), King of Mercia, made the name popular in the Midlands before the Normans arrived.

Kennedy From the Old English, *cyne*, 'royal, ruler'. A name made popular in this century by the American Kennedy family: the Democratic politician, John Fitzgerald Kennedy (1917–63), known as Jack, became the youngest, and the first Roman Catholic, President of the United States in 1961, and was assassinated in 1963. **Variants:** Kemp, Ken, Kenman, Kenn, Kennard, Kennie, Kenny, Kent, Kenton, Kenyon.

Kenneth From the Gaelic name, Caioneach, or Cynnedd, both meaning 'handsome, fair'. It was the Irish St Caioneach (5th century) who gave his name to Kilkenny. Kenneth McAlpine (died c. 860) spread the name when he became the first to rule both Picts and Scots, and it is still a Scottish favourite. In Sir Walter Scott's novel, *The Talisman* (1825), Sir Kenneth is the hero, a Christian crusader known as Knight of the Leopard. **Variants:** Canice, Cennydd, Cenydd, Ken, Kene, Kenn, Kennie, Kenny, Kent, Kenton, Kenward. *See also* Canice.

Kent From the Old Celtic, *kanto*, 'white', and later referring to the people or dialect of Kent.

Kentigern From the Gaelic name, Ceanntigher, 'chief lord'. The Scottish saint (died c. 612), whose nickname was Mungo, 'most dear', supposedly founded the church at Glasgow and a monastery at Llanelwy, and also performed a collection of miracles. He is patron saint of Glasgow. A medieval name, rarely found later.

Kenward From the Old English name, Cenweard, from *cene* 'brave', and *weard*, 'guard'. The Normans modified the name, but it then fell out of use.

Kerey English gypsy name, meaning 'homeward bound'.

Kermit From the Dutch, *kermis*, 'church', but in England its meaning has changed to a noisy and merry carnival or fair. **Variants:** Ker, Kermie, Kermy, Kerr.

Kern From the Old Irish, *ceitern*, 'band of infantry', usually referring to light-armed, rustic Irish soldiers. **Variants:** Kearney, Kearny.

Kerry *See under girls.*

Kevin Irish, from the name Caomhghin, from the Old Irish name, Coemgen, 'handsome birth'. A name first made popular by St Kevin (died 618), or Coemgen, who founded the monastery at Glendalough, near Dublin, which was renowned for its scholarship and the beauty of its setting. **Variants:** Caomhghin, Coemgen, Kev, Kevan, Keven.

Key From the Old English, *caeg*, 'key', symbolising the key to the world's riches. **Variant:** Keyes.

Kid From the Middle English, *kide*, 'young goat'. A slang term for a child, but sometimes used as a first name, particularly in the USA. **Variant:** Kidd.

Kiefer From the old English meaning a 'cooper' or one who makes barrels. The name has been popularised after actor, Kiefer Sutherland. Alternatives include Keefer and Keifer.

Kieran *See Ciaran.*

Kilian From the Gaelic, 'small and warlike'. **Variants:** Killian, Killie, Killy, Kilmer.

Kim *See Kimball and Kipling.*

Kimball Possibly from the Greek, *kymbalon*, 'hollow vessel'. Or from the old English ruler, Cymbeline or Cunobelinus (died 42), 'high and mighty', chief of the Catuvellauni tribe,

who ruled the area covered today by Hertfordshire. The form Kim was popularised by the clever, all-knowing hero of Rudyard Kipling's novel set in India, *Kim* (1901). **Variants:** Kim, Kimmie, Kimmy.

Kin Japanese, meaning 'golden'. **Variant:** Kane.

Kinchen From the Old Norse, *kyn*, 'family, clan, relatives'.

Kingsley From the Old English, *cyning*, 'king', thus 'king's meadow'. The British novelist, Charles Kingsley (1819–75), wrote *Westward Ho!*, *The Heroes* and *The Water Babies*, all firm favourites with children. **Variants:** King, Kingsleigh, Kingston, Kinnaird, Kinsey.

Kinta North American Indian, meaning 'beaver'. *See Beverley under girls.*

Kipling Possibly from the Old English, *cypra*, 'smoked herring' or 'male salmon during the spawning season'. The journalist, poet and novelist, Joseph Rudyard Kipling (1865–1936), wrote for adults and children, including the *Jungle Books*, *Kim* and *Just So Stories*, all set in India where he spent the first part of his life. **Variant:** Kip.

Kipp From the Old English, 'pointed hill, peak'. H. G. Wells' novel, *Kipps: the Story of a Simple Soul* (1905), perhaps encouraged the name's use early in this century. **Variants:** Kippie, Kippy.

Kiral Turkish, meaning 'king'.

Kirk Scottish, from the Old English, *cerice*, 'church' (see Kirsty). Hence Kirkland and Kirtland, 'place near the church', and Kirby, 'village with a church'. **Variants:** Kerby, Kirby, Kirkland, Kirtland, Kirtly.

ONE, TWO, THREE ...

When one family named the last of several children Exit, all their friends knew just what it meant. A name can reveal exactly where someone sits on the family tree. In the days of large families, Septimus, Octavius and Nonus – Latin for seven, eight and nine – would indicate the place in an ever-increasing family. Perhaps Primo or Prima up to Quentin and Quinta – one to five – would do for most modern families. Primo Carnera (1906–67) was 6ft 5in tall and World Heavyweight Boxing Champion in 1933–34 – Number One! If Octavia, or Octavius, is a favourite but eight children are out of the question, there are other tricks to keep the child prominently in the family charts: a birth during the eighth month, on the eighth day of the month, in the eighth year of the marriage – or even at house number eight in a street.

Kistur English gypsy name, meaning 'rider'.

Kitron From the Hebrew, 'crown'.

Kiyoshi Japanese, meaning 'quiet'.

Kline From the German, 'small'.

Knoll From the Old English, *cnoll*, 'hillock, mound'. **Variant:** Koll.

Knute Possibly from the Old Danish name, Knud, from *kint*, 'race, type, kind'. The mighty Danish king, Knute II (c. 994–1035), also called Canute, ruled England, Denmark and Norway, fighting off Viking attacks to the south and Scots to the north. St Knute IV (died 1086), raided Yorkshire (1075) and planned a serious invasion but his opponents killed him in St Alban's Church at Odense, an act seen by his supporters as martyrdom. As Nute and Note, the name was used until the end of the Middle Ages. **Variants:** Canute, Canutus, Knud, Knut, Note, Nute, Nutkin, Nutt.

Korah From the Hebrew, 'bald'. **Variant:** Korach.

Kramer *See* Cramer.

Kurt *See* Conrad.

Kyle From the Gaelic, 'narrow strait, channel between islands'. Also given to girls. **Variants:** Kile, Ky.

Kyloe From the Old English, *cy*, 'cow', and *leah*, 'meadow', thus 'cow pasture'.

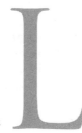

Laban *See* Lewanna *under girls.* In the Bible, father of the beautiful Rachel.

Lachlan Possibly from the Gaelic, *laochail*, 'warlike'. *See also* Loch and Locke.

Laddie From the Middle English, *ladde*, 'boy, young man, servant'. Also, a friendly general term for any boy or man. Laddie is found mostly in Scotland, Lad in England. **Variants:** Lad, Ladd, Laddy.

Laertes In Greek mythology, the hero respected for his wisdom who was also the father of Odysseus. The name became known in Britain when Shakespeare gave it to Ophelia's brother in his tragedy, *Hamlet* (1602). He avenges his sister's death by killing Hamlet – and, in the process, himself.

Laffit From the Old French, *la fei*, 'the faith'. The Marquis de La Fayette (1757–1834), whose formidable string of first names was Marie Joseph Paul Yves Roch Gilbert, was a French soldier and politician who worked for Washington during the American War of Independence; he also designed the French flag. Thus the name is associated with fighting for freedom but it is found more in the USA than in Britain. **Variants:** Lafayette, Lafitte.

Laird Scottish form of Lord.

Lake From the Latin, *lacus*, 'basin, pond, lake'.

Lal Indian name, meaning 'beloved'.

Lale From the Latin, *lallare*, 'to sing to sleep, to sing a lullaby'. **Variant:** Lalo.

Lambert From the Old High German, *landa*, 'land', and *beraht*, 'bright, shining', meaning someone as bright as the beautiful landscape. The zealous missionary, St Lambert of Maastricht (c. 635–705) was greatly revered in the Middle Ages and spread the name's use, but it fell out of favour in the 16th century, to be revived recently. **Variants:** Bert, Bertie, Berty, Lamberto, Lammie, Landbert.

 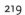

Lamont From the Old French, *la mont*, 'the mountain', implying greatness. **Variants:** Lammond, Lamond, LaMont, Lemont, Monty.

Lancelot From the Latin, *lancea*, 'lance', a sharp spear on a very long handle, used by cavalry to charge at full speed against the enemy; thus the name implies a brave warrior. Or, from the German, *ansi*, 'god'; see Ancel. In Arthurian legend, the dashing Sir Lancelot, a knight of the Round Table, had an affair with Queen Guinevere which led to war with King Arthur. This romantic figure made the name popular in the Middle Ages and again in the last century, during the medieval vogue, when it was especially used in northern England. **Variants:** Lance, Lancing, Lansing, Launcelot.

Landan From the Old High German, *lant*, 'land, open space, territory', especially agricultural land. **Variants:** Lander, Landers, Landis, Landman, Landon, Landor, Landry, Langtry, Lunds, Lunt.

Lane From the Old Frisian, *lana*, 'to move', thus a path to move through, symbolising the straight and narrow path of life. **Variants:** Lanie, Leney.

Lang From the Old English, *lang*, 'long'. Hence Langdon, 'long town'; Langford 'wide river crossing', and Langley, 'long meadow'. **Variants:** Laing, Langdon, Langer, Langford, Langhorne, Langley, Langsdon, Langston, Langtry, Lanny, Largo, Longfellow.

Langundo North American Indian, meaning 'peaceful'.

Larron From the Old French, *laron*, 'robber'. **Variants:** Latheron, Lathron.

Larvall From the Old Italian, *lavare*, 'to wash', thus a well or place for washing, a low-lying wet area of land. **Variant:** Larvell.

Latham From the Old English, *laeth*, 'land that is owned, district'. Hence Latimer, 'district by the sea'. **Variants:** Lathe, Lather, Lathrop, Latimer, Lattie, Latty, Lay.

Laval From the Old English, *hlaford*, 'lord' (*see* Lord). Or from the Italian, *lava*, 'sudden stream', meaning either water after a storm or molten rock from an erupting volcano. **Variants:** Lave, Lavrans.

Lavern From the Latin, *vernum*, 'springtime', via the French, where it picked up the prefix, *la*, 'the'. **Variants:** Laverne, LaVerne, Lavrans, Luvern. *See also* Vernon.

Lawrence *See also* Laurel under girls. A name promoted by the example of several saints. They include the Roman martyr, Lawrence (died 258), Deacon of Rome, one of the most venerated of all Rome's martyrs; Lawrence of Canterbury (died 619), who came with St Augustine in the first mission to southern England; and the austere but righteous Irish saint, Lawrence O'Toole (c. 1128–1226). Despite these early saints, the name only took off after the Normans arrived, becoming popular by the Tudor period, when Shakespeare gave it to the kindly friar who marries the young lovers in *Romeo and Juliet* (1595). This century, the name has been popularised by the novelist, David Herbert Lawrence (1885–1930), whose controversial sex scenes in *Lady Chatterley's Lover* (1928) caused the book to be banned in Britain until 1961. The romantic hero figure, Thomas Edward Lawrence (1888–1935), was the British soldier and writer known as Lawrence of Arabia. The real name of the American comedian, Stan Laurel, was Arthur Stanley Jefferson (1890–1965). **Variants:** Lanty, Larikin, Larkin, Larns, Larry, Lars, Larson, Laurel, Lauren, Laurence, Laurens, Laurent, Laurie,

Lauriston, Lauritz, Lauro, Lawrey, Lawry, Lenci, Lon, Lonnie, Lonny, Lorant, Loren, Lorence, Lorens, Lorentz, Lorenz, Lorenzo, Lorin, Loring, Lorn, Lorne, Lorrie, Lorry, Lowrence, Rance.

Lawton From the Old English, *hlaew*, 'hill, mound', and *tun*, 'village, homestead', thus 'village or houses on a hill'. **Variant:** Lawford.

Lazarus Greek form of Elazar, which came to mean 'leper, beggar'. In the Bible, the brother of Mary and Martha whom Jesus raised from the dead (John 11); also the beggar in the parable of the rich man and the beggar (Luke 16). The name has connotations both of recovery to health and the heavenly rewards of living a life of poverty, and was therefore taken up by the Puritans. **Variants:** Lazar, Lazare, Lazaro, Lazer, Lazlo, Lesser.

Leander From the Greek, *leon*, 'lion', and *andros*, 'man', thus 'man of lion's strength'. In the tragic Greek tale, the handsome and strong Leander fell in love with beautiful Hero, a priestess of Venus. Every night he swam across the Hellespont to see her. One night he was drowned and in her misery she threw herself into the sea to join him. **Variants:** Ander, Lea, Leandre, Leandro, Leanther, Lee, Leo, Maclean. *See also* Andrew.

Leben From the Yiddish, 'life'.

Ledell *See* Leda *under girls.*

Lee *See under girls. See also* Leo, Leroy and Lesley. **Variants:** Lea, Leigh.

Leek From the Old English, *leac*, 'garden of herbs, kitchen garden', hence *laecward*, 'gardener'; *see* Gardiner.

Leeland From the Old English, *hleo*, 'shelter, cover', thus 'sheltered land'. **Variants:** Layland, Layton, Leighland, Leighton, Leland.

Legrand From the Old French, *le grand*, 'the big, grand or great one'. **Variant:** Legrant.

Lel English gypsy name, meaning 'he takes'.

Lemuel From the Hebrew, 'devoted to God'. Like Jedaiah, another name for Solomon. Used in Britain by the Puritans, and by Jonathan Swift for the hero of *Gulliver's Travels.* **Variants:** Lem, Lemmie, Lemmy.

Len From the Old English, *len* and *leen*, 'tenant house', usually on a farm or homestead. Hence Lenvil, 'tenant house near a village'. **Variants:** Lendal, Lendall, Lendon, Lennon, Lennox, Lenvil, Lenwood. *See also* Leonard.

Lenis From the Latin, *lenis*, 'gentle, moderate, calm, soft'.

Lennon *See* Len. Also now popular after John Lennon, singer and songwriter with English band The Beatles.

Lennor English gypsy name, meaning 'spring, summer'.

Lennox See Len. A name with growing popularity after British heavyweight boxer Lennox Lewis.

Lensar English gypsy name, meaning 'with his parents'. The similar Lendar means 'from his parents'.

Leo From the Greek, *leon*, 'lion', implying strength of character, will and physique, thus a popular name given to two constellations of stars, the fifth sign of the zodiac, six Byzantine emperors and 13 popes of whom five are saints. The most influential was Pope Leo I (c. 400–461), known as Leo the Great, who was valued for his ability, energy and noble character. By negotiating first with Attila and then Gaiseric and Vandal, he twice saved Rome from attack. Leo IX (1002–54)

reformed and invigorated the papacy after a lax patch in its history. And, in 1890, Pope Leo XIII was the first authority to set out the duties and rights of employees and employers. Like Bruno the bear, Leo is the children's typename for a lion. Loeb is the German form; Leon, the Greek and Spanish form, doubles for Levi, and is often given to Jews. **Variants:** Label, Lee, Leib, Leibel, Len, Leni, Lenn, Lennie, Leodis, Leon, Leondaus, Leone, Leonid, Leonidas, Leonis, Lev, Lion, Lionel, Lionello, Llewellyn, Llywellyn, Loeb, Loew, Loewy, Lon, Lonnie, Lowe, Lyons, Lyonel, Lyron.

Leofric From the Old English, *leof*, 'dear', and *rice*, 'ruler, wealth', thus 'beloved ruler'. It survived the Conquest, but died out soon afterwards.

Leofwin From the Old English, *leof*, 'dear', and *wine*, 'friend'. Unlike Leofric, this survived into the 13th century before falling into disuse.

Leonard From the Old High German name, Lewenhart, from *levon*, 'lion', and *hart*, 'strong', thus 'strong as a lion', a good manly quality. The nickname of Richard I (1157–99) was *Coeur de Lion*, 'Lionheart'. It was he who made the treaty that allowed Christians into Jerusalem on the Third Crusade (1190). During the later Middle Ages, there was in France and England a strong cult of St Leonard, a hermit about whom nothing is known but who attracted a string of miracles and powers which eventually made him patron saint of prisoners. The name has been popular since then. The extraordinary Italian artist and scientist, Leonardo da Vinci (1452–1519), who painted the *Mona Lisa* and designed a forerunner of the tank, was one of the great geniuses of the Renaissance. **Variants:** Len, Lenard, Lenn,

Lennard, Lennart, Lennie, Lenny, Leo, Leon, Leonala, Leonardo, Leonerd, Leonhard, Lionardo, Lon, Lonnard, Lonnie, Lonny. *See also* Leo.

Leopold From the Old High German, *leudi*, 'people', and *balda*, 'bold', with the inference of lion-like boldness and strength. Many Austrian rulers, of whom the first was also a saint, bore the name. But it was only introduced into Britain in the last century, when Queen Victoria named her third son after her uncle, Leopold of Belgium. **Variants:** Leo, Leopoldo, Leupold, Poldi, Poldo.

Leor *See* Leora *under girls*. **Variant:** Lior.

Leron From the Old French, *la ronde*, 'the circle', traditionally symbolising perfection and the circle of life. *See also* Ring. **Variants:** Lerond, Lerone, Lerin, Lerrin.

Leroy From the French, *le roi*, 'the king'. **Variants:** Elroy, Lee, Lee Roy, Lerol, Roy.

Leshem From the Hebrew, 'precious stone'.

Leslie *See* Lesley *under girls*. **Variants:** Lee, Les, Lesley.

Lester Contraction of Leicester, from Chester. **Variants:** Leicester, Les, Letcher, Leycester.

Lev From the Hebrew, *lev*, 'heart'. *See also* Leo and Levi.

Levant From the Latin, *levare*, 'to rise up, to raise', especially the rising sun that marks each new day and is the essential nourishment for crops. **Variants:** Lebert, Lev, Levander, Lever, Leverett, Levert, Livingstone.

Levi *See* Levia *under girls*. **Variants:** Lavey, Lavi, Lavy, Leavitt, Lev, Levic, Lever, Lewi.

Lewis English form of Louis. The remarkable Lewis Carroll (1832–98), whose real name was Charles Lutwidge Dodgson, not only wrote *Alice's Adventures in Wonderland* (1865) and *Through the Looking Glass and What Alice Found There* (1872), but was a leading mathematician, a pioneering portrait photographer and an ordained deacon. The 'Alice' books were written for Alice Liddell, daughter of the Dean of Christ Church, Oxford.

Lex From the Greek, *lexis*, 'word', hence lexicon, 'dictionary', a valuable source of knowledge. **Variants:** Laxton, Lexton.

Lian Irish, from the French, *lier*, 'to bind, protect'. **Variants:** Liam, Lyam.

Liang Chinese, meaning 'good, excellent'.

Liddon From the Old English, *hlidan*, 'to shelter, hide'.

Lief Meaning beloved from the Old Norse, *leifr*, via the Old English, *lufian*, 'to praise, regard highly, hold dear, love'. **Variants:** Leif, Lie, Lif.

Lind *See* Linden *under girls.* Hence Lindley, 'meadow with linden trees', and Lindbert, 'hill of linden trees'. **Variants:** Linc, Lincoln, Lindall, Lindbergh, Lindbert, Linde, Lindel, Lindell, Linden, Lindley, Lindo, Lindon, Linton, Lynd, Lynde, Lyndall, Lynden, Lyndon.

Lindsey *See under girls.* **Variants:** Lind, Lindsay, Lindsy, Lindy, Linsey, Linzy.

Linfred From the German, 'gentle peace'.

Lingrel From the Old English, *hlinc*, 'hill, rising ground, bank', especially the undulating sandy ground near the seashore. **Variants:** Linc, Link.

Linus *See* Linnett *under girls.*

Lipman From the German name, Liebman, from *lieb*, 'love', thus 'lover of mankind'.

Variants: Lever, Lieber.

Liron *See under girls.* **Variants:** Leron, Liron, Lyron.

Lisle From the French town, Lille, famous for the fine cotton threads made there, thus 'strong, top quality, fine thread'. A name implying a fine character. **Variants:** Lille, Lyall, Lyell, Lyle.

Litton From the Old English, *lytel*, 'little', and *tun*, 'town, village'. **Variants:** Lyle, Lytel, Lytton.

Llewellyn Welsh, from *llew*, 'lion', or *llyw*, 'leader', and *eilun*, 'likeness'. There are two great Welsh princes by this name. Llywelyn ap Iorwerth (1173–1240), known as Llywelyn the Great, paid homage to King John of England before giving his position to his son and becoming a monk. Llywelyn ap Gruffudd (died 1282), known as Llywelyn the Last, died in battle with Edward I of England, marking the loss of Welsh independence. The English form is Leoline; *see also* Leo. **Variants:** Fluellen, Leoline, Lewlin, Lleelo, Llew, Llywellyn, Llywelyn.

Lloyd From the Welsh, *llwyd*, 'brown, grey', implying a dark complexion. A name especially popularised outside Wales at the beginning of this century when the Cockney music-hall artiste Marie Lloyd (1870–1922) was singing *Oh, I Do Like to be Beside the Seaside*. At the same time, the American actor Harold Lloyd (1893–1971) was star of the silent screen. The Welshman, David Lloyd George (1863–1945), Prime Minister of Britain from 1916 to 1922, created a reputation with married ladies that led to the song 'Lloyd George knew my father, father knew Lloyd George'. But one of the most famous Lloyds is an institution, the association of insurance underwriters founded in Lloyd's Coffee House, London, in 1688. **Variants:** Floyd, Loy.

Locadio From the Latin, *locus*, 'place'.

Loch From the Gaelic, *loch*, 'lake or arm of the sea'. **Variants:** Lachlan, Lough.

Locke From the Old Norse, *lok*, 'lid, end, conclusion', and now meaning a fastening or enclosure, thus a suitable name for the last child. A lovelock is a tress of hair exchanged by lovers as a vow of constancy. **Variant:** Lachlan.

Lodge From the Old French, *loge*, 'cottage, hut', referring especially to cottages on a large estate.

Logan From the Middle English, *logge*, 'record or journal of performance, experience or an expedition', implying someone who will lead a life worth recording. The American horticulturist, James H. Logan (1841–1928), crossed a blackberry and a raspberry to produce a loganberry.

Lombard From the Old High German, *lang*, 'long', and *bart*, 'beard', thus 'long-bearded', implying the wisdom and respect of old age. The Lombards, a Germanic tribe, settled in the Po Valley, Italy, and became known as bankers and moneychangers. **Variants:** Lombardo, Bard, Bardo.

Lon *See* Alphonse, Lawrence and Leo.

Loral From the Old High German, *lera*, 'to teach or instruct doctrines', or a male form of Lorelei.

Lord From the Old English name, Hlaford, from *hlaf*, 'bread', and *weard*, 'guardian', meaning the head of the household, lord of the manor, who provides the keep for his dependants, thus the name implies power and authority.

Loredo From Loreto, a north Italian town. In the apocryphal stories of the Virgin's life, her house was miraculously moved to Loreto from Nazareth in 1295, and the name was used from that time. **Variant:** Lorado.

Lorimer *See* Lorice *under girls*. **Variants:** Lorrie, Lorry.

Lot From the Hebrew, 'covering'. In the Bible, Lot's wife is turned into a pillar of salt when she defies instructions and looks back as they both flee from Sodom (Genesis 19). **Variant:** Lotan.

Louis From the Old French name, Loeis, and the Old High German name, Hluodowig. They become Clovis and Ludovicus in Latin. Hluodowig, from *hluda*, 'famous, glory', and *wiga*, 'war', means 'renowned warrior'. A name with the royal stamp of the kings of France from the 8th to 19th centuries. St Louis of France (1214–70) was also King Louis IX and married the sister-in-law of Henry III of England, fostering close relations between the countries. He was deeply religious, believed in individual rights, led two crusades and was the epitome of the medieval Christian king. But the greatest Louis was Louis XIV (1638–1715), known as the Sun King, who at his brilliant court at Versailles ushered in an age of magnificence that permeated Europe during his long reign from 1643 to 1715. The name reached Britain as Lowes in the Middle Ages, and has been reasonably popular ever since. The boxer Joe Louis Barrow (1914–81), known as the Brown Bomber, held the world heavyweight title from 1937 to 1949. Louis Armstrong (1900–71), known as 'Satchmo', was one of the best-known jazz musicians, both as a trumpeter and a singer. *See also* Lewis. **Variants:** Aloys, Aloysius, Clovis, Elois, Lew, Lewellen, Lewes, Lewi, Lewie, Lewis, Liewelyn, Llywellyn, Loeis, Lou, Louie, Lowes, Ludeg, Ludovicus, Ludvig, Ludwig, Lui, Luigi, Luis.

Lowell From the Old English, *lufu*, 'love, praise'. **Variants:** Loyal, Loyte.

Loyal From the Latin, *legalis*, 'legal, true, faithful', via the Old French, 'loyal'. **Variant:** Loy.

Luce *See* Lucania *under girls;* and also Lucius.

Lucian *See* Lucius.

Lucius *See* Lucia *under girls*; and also Luke. Lucifer is the archangel who was cast out of heaven for leading a revolt of the angels. **Variants:** Lu, Luc, Lucais, Lucas, Luce, Luciano, Lucien, Lucio, Luka, Lukas, Luke, Luscious.

Lucky From the Middle English, *lucke*, 'fortune, fate'. Only recently used as a first name, it means good fortune.

Ludovicus Latin form of Louis, introduced to Scotland in the 17th century, where it is still used. **Variants:** Lodowick, Ludovick, Ludovico.

Ludwig From the Old German name, Hluodowig (see Louis). A popular German name, further encouraged last century by the composer, Ludwig van Beethoven (1770–1827), who straddled the change from the classical to the romantic era and continued to compose long after he became deaf in 1801.

Luke English form of Lucius, or 'man from Luciana', after St Luke. The Greek physician, saint and evangelist (1st century) was a companion of St Paul, whom he seems to have accompanied on his missionary trips. He probably wrote the Third Gospel and The Acts of the Apostles. He is patron saint of doctors and, because he was also an artist, of painters. The name has been used in Britain since the Middle Ages but has become really fashionable only in this century.

Lull The English bishop and saint (died 786) was both a scholar and a zealous missionary in Germany whose reputation spread back to his native England.

Lupo *See* Lupita *under girls.* **Variant:** Lupus.

Luther From the Old German, *hluda*, 'famous, renowned', implying a distinguished fighter. The German leader of the Reformation, Martin Luther (1483–1546), was an Augustinian monk who, shocked by the splendour of the papacy at Rome, nailed to the chapel door of Wittenberg Castle a list of 95 reasons against the sale of papal indulgences, or honours. Three years later, in 1520, he launched the Protestant Reformation. He also translated the New Testament into German, founded the Lutheran churches and defied the rule of celibacy by marrying in 1525. A more recent fighter for reform was the black American clergyman, Martin Luther King (1929–68), who pressed for black rights and preached non-violence, but whose assassination provoked widespread rioting. **Variants:** Lotario, Lothaire, Lothar, Lothario, Lother, Lothur, Lutero.

Lutherum English gypsy name, meaning 'slumber'.

Luzerne From the Latin, *lucerna*, 'lamp', also implying a guiding light, or instructor. **Variants:** Luc, Lucerne, Luz.

Lyde From the Old English, *hlith*, 'hill'. **Variant:** Lydell.

Lyn Male form of Lynn. **Variants:** Lin, Linn, Linnie, Linley, Linly, Linwood, Lynford, Lynley, Lynn, Lynton, Lynwood.

Lyulf From the Old English name, Ligulf, from *lig*, 'flame', and *wulf*, 'wolf'. Still found in parts of Scotland today. **Variants:** Ligulf, Liulf, Lyolf.

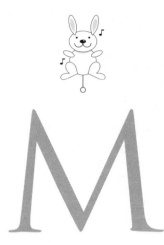

M

Mabry Cornish, male form of Mabel.

Mac From the Gaelic, 'son'. Used as an independent name and also as a prefix, such as in Maclean, 'son of Leander', MacArthur, 'son of Arthur'. The prefix can be applied to any name and is especially common in the ancient families and clans of Ireland and Scotland. Charles Macintosh invented rubberised cloth for waterproof coats. **Variant:** Mack.

Macabee From the Hebrew, *makab*, 'hammer'. A Jewish dynasty of kings, high priests and patriots (2nd – 1st centuries BC). One of the medieval mystery plays was the biblical story of the slaughter of the Macabees, which may have spread the name in Britain. **Variant:** Maccabee.

Macbeth Patronymic of Beth, from Elizabeth. A Scottish name made royal and famous by King Macbeth (died 1057), who killed Duncan to gain the throne of Scotland but was later killed by Duncan's son, Malcolm.

Shakespeare publicised the story in his tragedy, *Macbeth* (1606).

Mace Either from the Old French, *masse*, 'club, mace', symbolic of power and authority, or from the Latin, *macir*, 'mace', the highly valued aromatic spice that grows around a nutmeg seed and is used in perfumes and cooking. **Variants:** Maceo, Macey, Mack, Mackey, Macy.

Macon From the Old English, *macian*, 'to make, create, perform'.

Madison Metronymic of Maude, from Matilda. James Madison (1751 – 1836) helped compose the American constitution and the Bill of Rights and was later President, from 1809 to 1817. His memory is perpetuated in the grand Madison Avenue, Square and Gardens in central New York. **Variants:** Maddie, Maddy, Son, Sonny.

Madoc From the Welsh, *mad*, 'fortunate'. An old Welsh name. **Variants:** Maddoc, Madoch.

 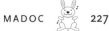

Magen From the Hebrew, 'protector'.

Magnus From the Latin, *magnus*, 'great, considerable, noble, important, mighty'. Used by the Danish royal family; Magnus I (died 1047) was king of both Denmark and Norway when Danish influence was strong in Britain. The Irish form is Manus. **Variant:** Manus.

Magus From the Latin, *magus*, 'learned man, magician, wizard'. Among the Zoroastrians, or fire-worshippers, of Persia, magi were the priests. In the Bible, the three Magi were the three 'wise men from the East' who brought gifts to the child Jesus (Matthew 2). St Augustine later named them (see Balthasar). St Magnus of Orkney (died 1116), a prince of Orkney, was renowned for his virtue and piety.

Mahir From the Arabic, 'industrious'.

Mailen From the Latin, *macula*, 'mesh, chain mail', symbolising protection during the tougher tests of life.

Maimon From the Arabic, 'good luck, good fortune'. The Spanish Jewish doctor and rabbi, Moses ben Maimon Maimonides (1135–1204), known as Rambam, codified Jewish law and philosophy in his writings. **Variant:** Maimum.

Major From the Latin, *major*, 'greater', better than great (*see* Magnus). The name implies importance and status over one's fellow men. **Variant:** Mayor.

Malachai From the Hebrew, 'my angel'. In the Bible, the last of the minor prophets, living during the 5th century BC–Hosea was the first. The Irish St Malachy (c. 1094–1148) was Abbot of Banger, Armagh, Derry, then papal legate for Ireland, and founded the first Cistercian monastery there, at Millifont. In England, an Old Testament name popular after the Reformation. **Variants:** Mal, Malachi, Malachy.

Malcolm From the Gaelic, *mael Colum*, 'servant of St Columba'. The reign of Malcolm III (1031–93), or Malcolm Canmore, 'big-head', King of Scotland for 36 years, marked Scotland's change from Celtic and Culdee to feudal and Roman Catholic. Much of this was due to his wife, Margaret, who was both queen and saint. An extremely popular name in Scotland that spread through Britain much later. The conductor, Sir Malcolm Sargent (1895–1967) was conductor-in-chief for the London Promenade Concerts from 1957 to 1967. **Variants:** Mal, Maolcolm.

Maldon From the Old English, *mael*, 'council, conversation', and *denn*, 'dell', thus 'sheltered meeting place'. **Variants:** Malden, Malton.

Malik From the Arabic, 'master'.

Malise From the Gaelic, 'servant of Jesus'. A name mostly confined to Ireland.

Malory From the Old French, *mallart*, 'male wild duck', the ancestor of the domestic duck of Britain.

Mamo Hawaiian, meaning 'saffron flower'.

Manchu Chinese, meaning 'pure'.

Mandel Male form of Amanda, or from the Old French, *amande*, 'almond'. **Variant:** Mandy.

Mander English gypsy name, meaning 'from myself'.

Manford From the Old English, *ford*, 'shallow river-crossing', thus someone who lives by a ford, perhaps an oblique reference to St Christopher.

Manfred From the German name, Manifred, from the Old High German, *fridu*, 'peace',

 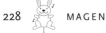

thus 'man of peace'. Carried to Britain by the Normans, but never in great favour. **Variants:** Fred, Freddie, Freddy, Manifred, Mannie, Manny, Mannye.

Manger From the Old French, *mangeoire*, 'manger, eating trough for animals'. In the Bible, this farm word was given religious significance when Joseph and the pregnant Mary had to sleep in the stable of an inn at Bethlehem, where Jesus was born and laid in the manger (Luke 2).

Manheim From the Old High German, *heim*, 'home', thus 'man of the home, servant'.

Manipi North American Indian, meaning 'a walking wonder'.

Manley From the Middle English, *leye*, 'meadow, pastureland', thus 'guardian of the fields'. **Variant:** Manly.

Manning From the Old English, *mann*, 'to station, guard, operate, care for', as in 'manning a ship', implying responsibility and protection. **Variants:** Manny, Manvel, Manville.

Mansur From the Arabic, 'helped by God, divinely assisted'.

Marden From the Old English, *mare*, 'sea', and *denn*, 'sheltered place', thus 'dell near the sea'. **Variant:** Marsden.

Marin From the Latin, *marinus*, 'belonging to the sea, sea-coast, sailor'. **Variants:** Marina, Mariono, Marr, Marriner.

Marion Male form of Mary. Also, a form of Mark. An unusual compound is Marjoe, combining Mary and Joseph, the parents of Jesus. **Variants:** Mari, Marian, Mario.

Mark From the Roman god, Mars, possibly from *mar*, 'to shine'. In Roman mythology, he was the son of Juno's union with a fabulous flower and this cult was even more important than Jupiter's. This was because he was the father of Romulus and Remus, the ancestors of Rome, and god of both agriculture and war, the two major Roman preoccupations. A name borne by numerous great Romans including Mark Antony (see Anthony), Cicero and a prominent Roman family (see Marcella). The month of March and the fourth planet from the sun after the Earth are named after him too. St Mark the Evangelist (1st century) wrote the Second Gospel, probably while he was in Rome with St Paul. He is believed to have been the first Bishop of Alexandria whose relics were brought to Venice in 829 – hence the dedication of the great church there. The memoirs of the Venetian, Marco Polo (c. 1254 – 1324), describe his extensive travels while working as a diplomat for the Mughal emperor, Kublai Khan. In Britain, an early notable Mark was the character in Arthurian legend who was King of Cornwall and uncle of Tristram. The saint and evangelist kept the name popular throughout the Middle Ages, to be revived in the last century. The American novelist, Samuel Langhorne Clemens (1835 – 1910), took the pen name Mark Twain and won fame with *Tom Sawyer* (1876) and *Huckleberry Finn* (1884). *See also* Marion and Martin. **Variants:** Marc, Marceau, Marcel, Marcelino, Marcellino, Marcello, Marcellus, Marcelo, March, Marco, Marcos, Marcus, Marcy, Marek, Mari, Marilo, Mario, Marion, Marius, Markos, Markus, Mars, Marsh, Marshe, Martin.

Marlin From the Old English, *mare*, 'sea'. **Variants:** Mar, Mario, Marle, Marlis, Marlo, Marlow, Marlowe, Marne, Marnin.

Marlon From the old French meaning 'wild falcon'. The name has become well known following American actor Marlon Brando.

Marnin From the Hebrew, 'one who brings joy and songs'.

Marques From the French, *marque*, 'emblem, flag, distinguishing mark'. **Variant:** Marquette.

Marquis From the Old French, *marchis*, 'marches, frontier districts', meaning their ruler. In the British nobility, the rank between Duke and Earl. **Variant:** Marquess.

Marshall From the Old French, *mareschal*, 'groom', but then elevated to mean a high office in the royal household, law courts or the armed services, always demanding great responsibility and organising powers. **Variants:** Marsh, Marshal, Marshe.

Martin French form of the Latin name, Martinus, 'warlike' (*see* Mark). Several early saints popularised the name but, above all, the widespread fame of Martin of Tours (c. 315–97), a mixture of extremely active missionary and recluse. When active, he was Bishop of Tours and founded monasteries at Ligugé and Marmoutier, making him the father of monasticism in France. His preaching drew extra crowds because of his reputation as a miracle-worker. The many British churches dedicated to him include St Martin-in-the-Fields, Trafalgar Square, London. Martin Luther put the name in vogue with the Protestants; and Sir Martin Frobisher (1535–94), who sought a north-west passage in the Canadian Arctic, made it popular with scientists and explorers. The name suffered a decline in the 17th century and then enjoyed a revival in the 19th. **Variants:** Mart, Martainn, Martel, Marten, Martie, Martijn, Martine, Martinet, Martinho, Martino, Martlet, Martoni, Marty, Martyn, Mertil, Mertin.

Marvell From the Latin, *mirabilis*, 'wonderful, extraordinary, marvellous', implying astonished admiration and wonder. **Variants:** Marvel, Marvelle.

Marvin From the Old English name, Maerwine, from *maer*, 'famous', and *wine*, 'friend', thus 'famous friend'. **Variants:** Marve, Marven, Marwin, Mervin, Mervyn, Merwin, Merwyn, Myrwyn. *See also* Titus.

Marx A German form of Mark. The German philosopher and journalist, Karl Marx (1818–83), who wrote the *Communist Manifesto* (1848) with Friedrich Engels, came to live in London where he wrote the influential *Das Kapital* (1867). He believed that violent revolution by the proletariat was necessary to create a classless society. The Marx Brothers were the great American family of comedians whose films included *Duck Soup* (1933) and *A Night at the Opera* (1935). The brothers were Harpo, Chico, Zeppo, Gummo and Groucho, but their real names were Arthur, Leonard, Herbert, Milton, and Julius.

Maskil From the Hebrew, 'educated, learned'.

Mason From the English meaning 'one who works with stone'.

Massing From the Old English, *maes*, 'battle', and *ing*, 'belonging to', meaning a place where soldiers' families live. **Variant:** Massey.

Masud From the Arabic, 'fortunate, lucky'.

Mato North American Indian, meaning 'brave'.

Matthew From the Hebrew name, Matisyahu, 'gift of God', via the Greek name, Mattias, and the Latin name, Matthaeus. A name spread swiftly by the Apostle and evangelist, St Matthew (1st century), whom Christ called from his job as a tax collector for the Romans. He is traditionally the author of the First Gospel. The name was popular in the Middle Ages, when the historian and monk, Matthew Paris (c. 1200–59), wrote his *Chronica Majora*, a history of the world from the Creation. The Puritans favoured the purer form Matthias, because the saint was believed to have been chosen to replace Judas Iscariot as Apostle. **Variants:** Macey, Mack, Mat, Mata, Mateo, Mathern, Mathias, Mati, Matia, Matiah, Matias, Matok, Matomon, Matt, Mattaeus, Mattathias, Matteo, Matteus, Matthaus, Matthias, Matti, Mattie, Mattieu, Matty, Mayo.

Maurice Either from the Greek, *Mauros*, 'Moor', meaning someone from Mauritania, now Morocco, but later used loosely for a dark-skinned person. Or from the Old English, *merisc*, 'marsh, low-lying land'. The Roman soldier and saint was martyred in Switzerland in 286, giving his name to the smart ski resort, St Moritz. A name found in Britain in the 13th century but then mostly confined to Wales where its influence has been maintained by prominent churchmen. **Variants:** Maryse, Maur, Maurey, Mauricio, Maurie, Maurise, Maurits, Maurizio, Maury, Meuriz, Morets, Morey, Morie, Moritz, Moriz, Morrey, Morrie, Morris, Morry, Morus. *See also* Morris.

Maximilian From the Latin, *maximus*, 'greatest, biggest, best', as compared with Magus and Major. Maximilian I (1459–1519), Emperor of the Holy Roman Empire, was named after the Roman military commander, Quintus Fabius Maximus. He attempted to live up to his name by passing his life almost constantly at war to enlarge his territory. He greatly improved the empire's administration, patronised the arts, enjoyed archery and soldiery and was considered the 'first knight of his age'. A name found occasionally in Britain, usually in families of German origin such as that of the caricaturist, wit and writer, Max (Maximilian) Beerbohm (1872–1956). **Variants:** Mac, Mack, Maks, Massimiliano, Massimo, Max, Maxey, Maxie, Maxim, Maxime, Maximilianus, Maximilien, Maximino, Maxwell, Maxy.

Maynard From the Old High German name, Maganhard, from *magan*, 'power', and *hart*, 'strong, hard', implying a powerful strength of physique and character. A name introduced by the Normans. The influential British economist, John Maynard Keynes (1883–1946), believed that government spending could encourage consumer spending and relieve unemployment. **Variants:** May, Mayne, Menard.

Mazal-tov From the Hebrew *mqzal-tov*, 'lucky star'. Stars have always been associated with human fortune, good and bad, and astrologers continue to study the heavens and assess the moments when lucky and unlucky stars are influential.

McKenzie From Scots Gaelic meaning 'son of the handsome one'.

Medric From the Old English, *maed*, 'meadow', and *rice*, 'wealthy, ruler', thus 'flourishing meadow'. **Variants:** Mead, Meade, Medard, Medford.

Meged From the Hebrew, 'sweetness, goodness, near perfection'.

Meinhard From the German, *hart*, 'heart', thus 'my beloved'.

 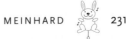

Meir From the Hebrew, *ohr*, 'radiant, shining'. **Variants:** Mayer, Meier, Meir, Meiri, Meyer, Myer.

Melchior From the Hebrew, *melech*, 'king'. In the Bible, one of the three Magi (*see* Balthasar). **Variants:** Melchisadek, Melchizedek.

Melville From the Old English, *mylen*, 'mill', thus 'village with a mill', hence Meldon, 'sheltered mill' and Melford, 'mill by the ford'. **Variants:** Mel, Melbourne, Melburn, Meldon, Melford, Melton, Melville, Melwood. *See also* Milton.

Melvin From the Old English, *mael*, 'council', or *mylen*, 'mill', and *wine*, 'friend', thus either 'friendly meeting' or 'mill-worker'. **Variants:** Malvin, Mel, Mell, Vinny, Vynnie.

Menachem From the Hebrew, 'comforter'. **Variants:** Manasseh, Mann, Mannes, Menasseh, Menahem, Mendel.

Menelaus In Greek mythology, King of Sparta and brother of Agamemnon, the elopement of whose wife, the beautiful Helen, with the Trojan Paris, led to the 10-year Trojan war. **Variant:** Mene.

Mercury In Roman mythology, the messenger of the gods, the counterpart to the Greek god, Hermes. In astronomy, the planet closest to the sun.

Meredith From the Welsh name, Meredydd, 'great chief, defender of the sea'. In use since the 7th century. **Variants:** Merideth, Merri, Merry.

Merle *See under girls.*

Merlin From the Welsh name, Myrddin, probably contracted from Carmarthen, 'sea-hill fort'. In Arthurian legend, the wizard who used his powers of necromancy – prophesying by calling up the dead – to give advice to Arthur. But later Vivien, the Lady of the Lake, seduced him and entangled him in a thorn bush, where he still sleeps. **Variants:** Marlin, Marlon, Merle, Merlo, Merlon.

Merrick From the Old English, *mare*, 'sea', and *rice*, 'ruler, power', thus 'ruler of the sea'. Hence Merton, 'seaside town'. **Variants:** Meril, Merle, Merrill, Merrington, Merton, Meryl, Myril, Myrl.

Merripen English gypsy name, meaning both 'life' and 'death'.

Merrit From the Latin, *meritum*, 'deserving, valued'. **Variant:** Merritt.

Methuselah From the Hebrew, *thuselah*, 'messenger'. In the Bible, the patriarch who lived to the age of 969, having fathered his first child, Lamech, aged 187 (Genesis 5). Thus a name implying longevity and popular from the 16th to 18th centuries. The name is also given to a huge champagne bottle that holds the equivalent of eight standard bottles. *See also* Enoch.

Michael From the Hebrew name, Micah, 'who can be like God?' In the Bible, the archangel is messenger to the Jews in the Old Testament, then appears in the New Testament as leader of the heavenly host in the war against Satan and as the weigher of souls at the Last Judgement. He was a highly revered saint in the Middle Ages, seen as protector of Christians, soldiers and therefore crusaders. After Pope Gregory I saw a vision of him above Castel san'Angelo during the plague in Rome, countless hilltop chapels and churches were dedicated to him. He is patron saint of soldiers. The royal character of the name comes from nine Byzantine emperors, five Rumanian kings and the Tsar of Russia

(1596–1645) who founded the Romanov dynasty. Artistic character comes from Michelangelo Buonarroti (1475–1564), the Florentine painter, sculptor and architect whose works include the painted ceiling of the Sistine Chapel in Rome. Today, the most famous Michael is probably Mickey Mouse, the Walt Disney cartoon character who made his debut in *Plane Crazy* in 1928. A popular name in Britain since the 12th century and especially popular in Ireland today. **Variants:** Maguel, Micah, Micha, Michail, Michal, Micheil, Michel, Michelangelo, Michele, Michiel, Michon, Mick, Mickey, Mickie, Micky, Miguel, Mihal, Mihaly, Mikael, Mikas, Mike, Mikel, Mikey, Mikhail, Mikkel, Misha, Mishca, Miska, Mitch, Mitchel, Mitchele, Mitchell, Mitchiel, Mychal.

Midgard From the Old Norse, 'midway place'. In Norse mythology, the middle of the universe, where mankind lived in a vast fortress built by the gods and encircled by a giant serpent. **Variants:** Midgarth, Midge, Midrag, Mithgarthr.

Miles From the Old German, *mil*, 'beloved, gentle', via the Old English, *milde*, thus a male form of Mildred. Also a form of Michael. In Ireland, the name took a double meaning, 'beloved' and 'servant of Mary'. Carried to Britain by the Normans, it was revived by the Victorians, and more recently made popular following Jazz saxophonist Miles Davis. **Variants:** Milan, Mills, Milo, Myles.

Milileilani Hawaiian, meaning 'to praise, give thanks'. **Variant:** Mili.

Milton From the Old English, *mylen*, 'mill', and *tun*, 'village, town', thus 'the village or town mill'. Hence Miller, the old occupational name. The poet, John Milton (1608–74), won his job as Cromwell's Latin secretary for foreign affairs with his essay in defence of regicides. Among his poems are the epics *Paradise Lost* (1667) and *Paradise Regained* (1671). **Variants:** Millard, Miller, Mills, Milt, Miltie, Milty, Mull, Muller. *See also* Melville.

Minor From the Latin, *minor*, 'less, younger'. A name given to the youngest child. **Variant:** Meena.

Minos In Greek mythology, the king of Crete and son of the supreme god, Zeus, and Europa. He commanded the cunning Daedalus to build the Labyrinth to house the Minotaur, a monster that was half-bull and half-man and lived off human flesh. **Variant:** Minot.

Minster From the Old English, *mynster*, 'monastery church'. **Variant:** Minter.

Mircea From the Latin, *mirari*, 'wonderful, astonishing'; see Marvell. **Variants:** Miro, Miroslav, Mirro.

Misu North American Indian, meaning 'rippling water'.

Mitford From the Middle English, 'small, shallow river-crossing'.

Modred From the Latin, *mordere*, 'to bite, consume'. In Arthurian legend, Modred, or Mordred, was the nephew of King Arthur and knight of the Round Table who led a rebellion against his uncle and mortally wounded him; see Arthur. **Variants:** Modris, Mordred.

Mohammed From the Arabic, *muhammed*, 'praised, glorified'. The prophet (570–632) who founded Islam was a rich merchant of the ruling tribe of Mecca. After a vision in the cave of Mount Hera telling him to teach the true religion, he began his work in

Yathrib, renamed Medina, 'city of the prophet', and in 630 conquered Mecca. **Variants:** Mahomet, Mohammad, Muhammad, Muhammed.

Mohan From the Hindu, 'delightful'.

Monford From the Old English, *munt*, 'mount, hill', and *ford*, 'shallow river-crossing', thus 'mountain ford'. **Variants:** Montford, Mountford.

Monita Italian, from the Greek, *monis*, 'alone'. A name suitable for an only child.

Monroe Scottish, from *mon*, 'man', and the French, *roue*, 'wheel', thus 'turner'. Like Barber, an old occupational name. **Variants:** Monro, Munro, Munroe. *See also* Marilyn.

Montague French form of the Latin, *mons*, 'mountain, big hill' and the French, *aigu*, 'pointed'. Like Howard, an aristocratic name taken up by the rest of society in the last century. **Variants:** Mante, Monte, Montgomery, Monty.

Moon Male form of Mona, or a direct use of the word 'moon'. For other moon names, see Phoebe under girls.

Mordecai From the Babylonian name, Marduk. In Assyro-Babylonian mythology, Marduk was god of water and thus of crops; was responsible for the organisation of the universe; was god of life; created man; healed the sick, and determined men's fates and fortunes. **Variants:** Marduk, Mord, Mordechai, Mordkhe, Mordy, Mort, Mortie, Morty.

Morgan From the Welsh name, Morcant, from *mawr*, 'great', and *can*, 'bright', thus 'brilliance'. Also akin to another Welsh name, Morien, 'sea-born'. A name still mainly restricted to Wales where it has enjoyed consistent popularity.

Morris From the Old English, *mor*, 'uncultivated open land, marshland', or from the Latin, *Maurus*, 'Moor' (see Maurice). Morris dancing, traditional English country dancing, comes from the second meaning. One of the main forces behind the medieval revival and then the Arts and Crafts Movement in the last century was William Morris (1834–96), who wrote *In Defence of Guenevere* (1858), founded a firm of craftsmen dedicated to handmade rather than mass-produced goods (1861), and was a founding spirit of the Socialist League (1884). **Variants:** Mo, Moor, Moreton, Morey, Morgan, Morrey, Morrie, Morrison, Morry, Morse, Mort, Mortimer, Morton, Morty, Myrton. *See also* Morgan.

Moses From the Hebrew, *mosheh*, possibly meaning 'saved from the water'. In the Bible, the baby Moses was found abandoned in a cradle floating among bullrushes. He later led the Israelites out of Egypt and received the Ten Commandments from God on Mount Sinai, the basis of Mosaic Law (Exodus 20). A popular Puritan name. **Variants:** Moe, Moise, Moises, Moke, Mose, Moshe, Mosheh, Moss, Moy, Moyes, Moys, Moyse, Moyses, Mozes. *See also* Maimon.

Mozart From the Italian, *mozzare*, 'to cut off, to take one's breath away'. Possibly an old Italian occupational name for a cheese seller. Undoubtedly, the most famous bearer of the name is Wolfgang Amadeus Mozart; *see* Amadeus.

Muraco North American Indian, meaning 'white moon'. For other moon names *see* Phoebe *under girls*.

Murdoch From the Gaelic name, Muireadhach, 'leader of the sea, sailor'.

 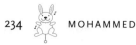

Variants: Muireadhach, Murdock, Murtagh, Murtaug, Murtaugh.

Murphy From the Celtic, *muir*, 'from the sea'. A name so popular in Ireland that it became the slang word for the Irish staple food, the potato. Another discouraging association for the name is the phrase 'Murphy's Law',

meaning 'if anything can go wrong, it will'. **Variants:** Meriadoc, Morty.

Murray Scottish, from the Celtic, *mor*, 'sea'. The name of an ancient noble Scottish clan.

Myron See Myrna under girls. **Variants:** My, Ron, Ronnie, Ronny.

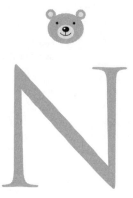

Naaman *See* Naama *under girls.*

Nabil From the Arabic, 'prince, noble'. **Variants:** Nadiv, Nagid.

Naboth From the Hebrew, 'prophecy'.

Nadar *See* Nadia *under girls.* **Variant:** Nader.

Nahum From the Hebrew, 'consoling'. In the Bible, the 7th-century BC prophet who predicted the fall of Nineveh. A name used since the Reformation. **Variants:** Nehemiah, Nemiah, Nemo.

Namid North American Indian, meaning 'star dancer', referring to the legend of the coyote who wanted to dance with the stars.

Namir From the Arabic, 'leopard'.

Naphtali From the Hebrew, 'wrestler'. In the Bible, one of the 12 sons of Jacob, born to Bilhah, the handmaid of Jacob's wife, Rachel (Genesis 30). **Variants:** Naftali, Naftalie, Naphthali.

Napoleon From the Greek name, Neapolis, 'new town'. The Italian town, Naples, is a contracted form. It was the Emperor of France and King of Italy, Napoleon Bonaparte (1769–1821), who made the name a legend and had cakes, coins, cities and children named after him. A brilliant general and skilled politician, he proclaimed himself Consul (1799), then Emperor (1804) and continued to pursue his military ambitions until he was finally defeated at Waterloo and exiled to St Helena. His *Code Napoléon* is the basis of modern French law. His wife and adviser was Josephine. **Variants:** Leon, Nap, Napoleon, Nappie, Nappy.

Narain From the Hindu name, Narayana, one of the names of Siva, the god of creative energy.

Narcissus *See* Narcissa *under girls.*

Nasser From the Arabic, 'victorious'. In the Qur'an, one of the 99 names for God.

Nathaniel From the Hebrew name, Nathan, 'he gave', thus 'gift of God'. In the Bible, Nathan was the prophet who carried God's message to King David reprimanding him after he had arranged Uriah's death so that he could marry his widow, Bathsheba. After he repented, she gave birth to Solomon (2 Samuel 12). In the New Testament, Nathaniel is one of the 12 Apostles, also called Bartholomew. Its Old Testament associations made the name popular after the Reformation. **Variants:** Nat, Natal, Natale, Nataniel, Nate, Nathan, Nathanael, Neal, Niel, Noel, Nowell.

Nav English gypsy name, meaning 'name'. **Variant:** Nev.

Nayati North American Indian, meaning 'wrestler'.

Negev From the Hebrew, 'south, southwards'.

Neil From the Gaelic names Niul and Niall, from *niadh*, 'champion', or from the Old Norse name, Niel, a form of Nicholas. Neil has been popular since the Middle Ages. Despite losing an eye and an arm, Horatio Nelson (1758–1805) was the most distinguished admiral of his age, whose greatest triumph was to destroy French naval power at the Battle of Trafalgar (1805), preventing an invasion. Thus his name, 'Neil's son', also became a first name. **Variants:** Neal, Neale, Neall, Nealson, Neaton, Neely, Neill, Neils, Neilson, Neilus, Nels, Nelsi, Nelson, Nial, Niall, Niel, Niels, Nil, Niles, Nils, Nilson, Niul, Nyles.

Neot Almost nothing is known of the saint who gave his name to towns in Cornwall and Cambridgeshire, but he later became associated with Arthurian legend; *see* Arthur.

Nestor In Greek mythology, the king of Pylos and the oldest and most experienced of the rulers at the seige of Troy, thus a name implying both longevity and wisdom.

Nevada From the Spanish for 'snow' or 'white as snow'. Nevada is also the name of an American state.

Neville From the French, *neuville*, 'new town'. A name carried to Britain by the Norman family of de Nevil who settled here and held a succession of high public posts for generations. The British politician, Neville Chamberlain (1869–1940), was Conservative Prime Minister from 1937 to 1940. Having advocated appeasement of Hitler to prevent war, he finally declared war on Germany and later resigned. A Christian name first found in the 17th century, but only recently widespread. **Variants:** Nev, Nevil, Nevile, Nevill.

Nevin From the Old English, *navu*, 'middle', used to describe the hub of a wheel, thus a name implying someone who is the centre and strong supporter of events. **Variants:** Nefen, Nev, Neven, Nevins, Niven.

Newell From the Latin name, Novellus, 'young, new'. **Variant:** Nowell.

Newton From the Middle English, *newe*, 'new', and *toun*, 'town', thus 'new town'. A name made lastingly famous by Isaac Newton who is supposed to have developed his theories on gravity after an apple fell on his head. **Variants:** Newgate, Newland, Newman, Niland.

Nicholas From the Greek, *nike*, 'victory', and *laos*, 'people', thus 'people's victory'. In Greek mythology, Nike was the winged goddess of victory. The name was popularised in Christian times by various saints of whom the 4th-century Nicholas has been one of the most consistently popular in Europe. As patron saint of sailors, children, merchants and pawnbrokers, his name has been constantly in use for kings, subjects, places, popes and churches. The only known fact is that he was Bishop of Myra in Lycia. A healthy legend was developed, including extensive biographies that recount miracles of saving girls from prostitution, boys from death, just men from the gallows and sailors from rocks. As Santa Claus, patron saint of children, his festival on December 6 was the occasion for the exchange of presents, which in many countries now takes place on Christmas Day – Santa Claus is also known as Father Christmas. **Variants:** Claus, Cola, Colas, Cole, Colet, Colin, Collet, Collett, Colley, Collis, Colly, Klaas, Klaus, Nic, Niccolo, Nick, Nickie, Nicky, Nico, Nicol, Nicolai, Nicolas, Nicolaus, Nicole, Nicolo, Nicy, Niel, Nike, Niki, Nikita, Nikki, Nikola, Nikolai, Nikolaos, Nikolas, Nikolaus, Nikolos, Nilo. *See also* Colin.

Nicodemus From the Greek, 'the people's conqueror', the hero who led the people to their victory. The Greek monk, St Nicodemus of the Holy Mountain (c. 1748 – 1809), was a considerable scholar, mystic, hagiographer, canonist and ascetic. His *Philokalia*, a collection of Greek spiritual writing, has been lastingly influential, especially in the Eastern Orthodox Church. A highly fashionable name in the Middle Ages, only falling entirely out of favour in the last century. *See also* Nicholas.

Nigel Either from the Icelandic name, Njal, or a short form of Daniel. When the Normans introduced it to Britain, the Saxons understood it to come from the Latin, *nigellus*, 'black, dark', and therefore added the 'g'. The name is also similar to the Middle English

word, *night*, 'night, dark'. A popular medieval name. **Variants:** Nidge, Nig, Nye.

Niles A variation of Nicholas from the English meaning 'champion of the people'. Also seen as Nyles.

Ninian The missionary and saint (died 432) seems to have trained in Rome and then returned to convert many Picts, working from his base at Candida Casa, in Galloway. The name is now mostly confined to Scotland. **Variants:** Nennius, Ninian, Ninidh.

Nir From the Hebrew, *nir*, 'ploughed field', implying industry and fruitfulness, hence Niral, 'cultivated field of the Lord'. **Variants:** Niral, Niria, Nirel.

Nissan From the Hebrew, *nais*, 'banner, flag, emblem'. **Variants:** Nisi, Nissi, Nissim.

Nitis North American Indian, meaning 'good friend'. **Variant:** Netis.

Niv From the Arabic, 'speech'.

Noah From the Hebrew, *noah*, 'long-lived'. In the Bible, Noah is the man chosen by God to build the ark and thus save himself, his family and a pair of all living creatures from the destructive Flood (Genesis 5 – 9). When the rains stopped, a dove returned to Noah bearing an olive leaf, showing that the waters were subsiding and God had forgiven mankind. Like other Old Testament names, popular in the 17th century, but falling out of favour by the 19th. **Variants:** Ark, Noach, Noak, Noe.

Noam *See* Naomi *under girls*.

Noble From the Latin, *nobilis*, 'celebrated, renowned, famous' and 'born into nobility'. **Variant:** Noda.

THE BIRTH CERTIFICATE

A child's birth is recorded in a register. The registers are kept locally but there is also a full set of copies of registrations for England and Wales in London. In the early 1970s, the copies of births, marriages and deaths entries were moved out of Somerset House, a fine Thameside building, to St Catherine's House – but the phrase 'at Somerset House' is still often used to refer to the records. People often lose their birth certificates, but it is easy to obtain copies from St Catherine's House. There are two ways to do this, both requiring a form to be completed. In person, the Public Search Room is open Monday to Friday, 8.30 am to 4.30 pm. A full copy of the certificate currently costs £5.00; a shortened one, giving just the name, place and date of birth, costs £3.00. By post, a completed form needs to be returned with £13.00 for a full certificate or £11.00 for a shortened one. Further information is available from: Office of Population Censuses and Surveys, St Catherine's House, 10 Kingsway, London WC2B 6JP (01-242 0262).

Noel *See* Natalie *under girls.* **Variant:** Nowell.

Noga From the Hebrew, 'celebrated, a star'.

Nolan From the Celtic, 'famous, noble', or a form of Northland, from North. **Variant:** Noland.

Norbert *See* Norberta *under girls.* The reformer and preacher, St Norbert (c. 1080–1134), founded the Premonstratensian Order of Canons near Laon, France, which swiftly spread through northern Europe, spreading his name with it. **Variants:** Bert, Bertie, Berty, Norb, Norbie, Norby.

Norman From the Old English, *north*, 'north', thus someone from the north, hence the Normans who lived in northern France. In Britain, the name was originally confined to Scotland. The fashion designer Norman Hartnell (1901–79), after designing utility clothes during World War II, became official dressmaker to the Queen who in gratitude knighted him in 1971. **Variants:** Norm, Normand, Normann, Normie, Norrie, Norris, Norry.

North From the Old English, 'north', hence Northrope, 'north farm'; Norval, 'north valley', and Norwood, 'north wood'. The newspaper baron, Alfred Charles William Harmsworth, 1st Viscount Northcliffe (1865–1922), was a pioneer of popular journalism in Britain. He founded the *Daily Mirror* (1903) and, with his brother, drove the circulation of the *Daily Mail* up to a million, the first daily newspaper to hit that mark. **Variants:** Nolan, Noland, Northcliffe, Northcote, Northrop, Norton, Norval, Norwood.

Noy *See* Noya *under girls.*

Nuncio From the Latin, *nuntius*, 'announcer, bearer of news'.

Nur *See under girls.* **Variants:** Nahir, Nuri, Nuria.

Nye From the Middle English, 'islander, island'. **Variant:** Nyle.

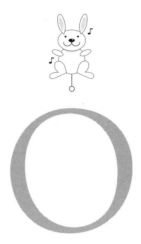

O

Obediah From the Hebrew, *eved*, 'servant', thus 'servant of God'. In the Bible, one of the 12 minor prophets. Obadiah Slope is the ambitious chaplain in Anthony Trollope's novel, *Barchester Towers* (1857). Popular from the 17th to 19th centuries. **Variants:** Abdias, Obadiah, Obadias, Oban, Obe, Obed, Obie, Oby.

Ocean A popular modern name that refers to the sea.

Octavius *See* Octavia *under girls*. **Variants:** Octave, Octavio, Otavio.

Odam From the Middle English, 'son-in-law'.

Odell *See* Odelia *under girls*; also Odo. Also from the Danish, *od*, 'otter', an animal valued for its rich dark brown fur. **Variants:** Dale, Dell, Obert, Od, Odbert, Odd, Ode, Odey, Odie, Odo, Ody, Otho.

Odilo The French saint (c. 962–1048) was Abbot of Cluny for 54 years and united and centralised the Cluniac houses, instigating an annual day of prayer for the dead, All Souls' Day (November 2), the day after All Saints' Day.

Odin In Norse mythology, Odhinn is the supreme god who presides over the creation of the universe and of mankind, the northern counterpart of Woden. He is also the specific god of wisdom, law, art, war and the dead. He is handsome, charming, eloquent, a great poet and, although married to Frigg, enjoys countless amorous adventures – as does she. **Variants:** Ode, Odie.

Odo From the Old English, *ead*, 'rich'. St Odo of Cluny (879–942) was the second Abbot of Cluny, who reformed, enlarged and increased the power of the order, aided by his own sympathetic yet strict character. The name was carried to Britain by the Normans and swiftly became popular. *See also* Otto. **Variants:** Aodh, Audo, Oddie, Oddo, Oddy, Odey, Odinal, Ody, Otes, Othes, Otho, Otis, Ottes, Otto.

Odysseus *See* Odessa *under girls.*

Oedipus In Greek mythology, the abandoned son of Laius and Jocasta who murdered his father and married his mother without knowing they were his parents. Thus, in Freudian psychology, an Oedipus complex is a young son's hatred of his father and sexual desire for his mother.

Ofer From the Hebrew, 'young deer', implying gentleness and agility. **Variant:** Opher.

Offa The King of Mercia (died 796) issued the first Anglo-Saxon coinage, established diplomatic relations with Charlemagne, ruled most of England south of the Humber, and defended his western border from the Welsh by building Offa's Dyke.

Og In the Bible, the giant King of Basham who was saved from the Flood by climbing onto the roof of Noah's ark. He was later killed by Moses, just as he was hurling a mountain at the Israelites (Deuteronomy 3). In John Dryden's political satire, *Absalom and Achitophel* (1681), Og is the name given to the writer Thomas Shadwell, a contemporary whom Dryden intensely disliked.

Ogden From the Old English, *ac*, 'oak', and *denn*, 'sheltered place', thus 'oak tree valley'; hence Oakley, 'field of oaks'. The humorist Ogden Nash (1902–71) is best known for his epigrammatic verse, such as, 'The cow is of the bovine ilk; one end is moo, the other, milk'. **Variants:** Oak, Oakes, Oakie, Oakleigh, Oakley, Oaks.

Ogier From the Old German name, Audagar, from *auda*, 'rich', and *gar*, 'spear', implying a famous warrior. Introduced by the Normans and popularised in the Middle Ages by romantic tales of Ogier, one of Charlemagne's knights. **Variants:** Oger, Ogier.

Olaf From the Old Norse name, Anleifr, 'ancester, remains'. The king and saint, Olaf I of Norway (995–1030), was a zealous Christian who was driven out and killed by King Knute, making him a national hero-saint and symbol of independence. The name was brought to Britain by the Danes and became immediately popular – hence the churches in London, York and elsewhere dedicated to St Olave. **Variants:** Olav, Olave, Ole, Olen, Olif.

Oleg *See* Olga *under girls.* **Variant:** Ole.

Olin *See* Holly *under girls.* **Variant:** Olney.

Oliver See Olive under girls; or from the Old Norse name, Anleifr (*see* Olaf). Introduced to Britain by the Normans and popularised in the Middle Ages by the romance, *Song of Roland*, in which Roland and Oliver are the two most chivalrous royal officers of Charlemagne. Totally out of fashion after Oliver Cromwell, it was brought back in by Dickens' novel *Oliver Twist* (1838) and by the 19th-century medieval revival. **Variants:** Alvar, Noll, Nollie, Nolly, Olivero, Olivier, Ollie, Olvan.

Omar From the Arabic, 'long life' or 'most high'. The Persian poet and mathematician, Omar Khayyam (c. 1050–1123), reformed the Islamic calendar and wrote the *Ruba'iyat*, made famous in the West through Edward Fitzgerald's 1859 translation. The name was thus introduced to Britain in the last century. **Variant:** Omri.

Ona From the Greek, *onos*, 'ass, donkey', implying a beast of burden but also a clumsy and ignorant person. **Variants:** Onny, Oona.

Onan From the Turkish, 'prosperous'.

 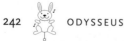

Opal *See under girls.*

Oral From the Latin, *os*, 'mouth', meaning speech. A name implying someone who is articulate and intelligent.

Orban From the Latin, *orbis*, 'circle, globe', meaning a planet or satellite and carrying the association of influence and power, hence the orb and sceptre symbolising sovereign power.

Orde From the Latin, *ordo*, 'regular, proper, ordered, logical, peaceful', the opposite of chaos. The word also implies 'beginning', as at the start of life. **Variant:** Ordell.

Oren From the Gaelic, 'pale', meaning a pale complexion; or from the Hebrew, 'tree', hence *orental*, 'tall tree'. **Variants:** Oran, Orenthal, Orin, Orren.

Orestes From the Greek, *oros*, 'mountain'. In Greek mythology, an oriad was a mountain nymph; Orestes was the character who showed extreme, if violent, loyalty towards his father's honour; *see* Electra. **Variants:** Orest, Oreste.

Orien *See* Oriana *under girls*. **Variants:** Orie, Orin, Orion, Oris, Oron, Orono, Orrin.

Original From the Latin, *origo*, 'beginning, source, birth, lineage'. A name given to the first-born son from the 16th to 18th centuries.

Orlando *See* Oriel *under girls*; also a form of Roland. Orlando is the hero of Shakespeare's comedy, *As You Like It* (1599), brother of Oliver and in love with Rosaline. The novel *Orlando* (1928), based on the character and family history of Victoria Sackville-West, was Virginia Woolf's greatest commercial success. **Variants:** Arland, Arlando, Land, Lannie, Lanny, Orlan, Orland, Orleans, Orley, Orlin, Orlo, Orval, Orville.

Orlov Russian form of Orlando. A name whose romantic and political associations stem from Grigory Grigoryevich, Count Orlov (1734–83). As the lover of the Tsarina, Catherine the Great, he engineered the coup that brought her to power and was then her trusted adviser, although his aim to free the serfs was never realised.

Ormond From the Old Norse, *orme*, 'serpent'. In Norse mythology, a vast serpent encircled the fortress-like Earth. Or from the French, *orme*, 'elm tree'. **Variants:** Orma, Orman, Ormand.

Orpheus From the Greek, *ous*, 'ear'. In Greek mythology, the poet and musician whose works could move even inanimate objects. When his wife Eurydice died, he went down to the underworld, where his musical lyrics charmed Pluto, god of Hades, to release her back into life again on condition that he did not look back until he touched earth. As he was about to place his foot on earth, he turned back to check that she was behind him – and she vanished instantly. The name implies entrancingly beautiful sounds. *See also* Otis.

Orson From the Latin, *ursus*, 'bear', the male form of Ursula. **Variants:** Sonnie, Sonny, Urson.

Osbert An Old English name derived from the Old Norse, *aesir*, 'the gods', anglicised to *os*, 'god'; and from *beorht*, 'bright', thus 'illustrious god'. Hence Osgood, 'benevolent god'; Osbourne, 'divine strength', and Osric, 'divine ruler'. 'Os' was the prefix for the names of the Northumbrian royal family and Osbert was first popular in the north before becoming widespread during the Middle Ages, revived along with other old names in the last century. **Variants:** Obgood, Osborne, Osric, Ossie, Ossy.

 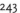

Oscar From the Old English, *os*, 'god', and *gar*, 'spear', thus 'divine spear', implying incredible strength. An Old English name, like Osbert. When James Macpherson (1736–96) published with great success what he claimed were poems by the legendary Gaelic bard, Ossian, he revived that form of the name. More recently, the Irish-born writer, Oscar Wilde (1854–1900), whose real name was Fingal O'Flahertie Wills, achieved his reputation with essays, poems and witty plays, such as *The Importance of Being Earnest* (1895). The American team of Oscar Hammerstein (1895–1960) and Richard Rodgers wrote a string of hit musicals such as *Oklahoma!* (1943) and *The Sound of Music* (1959). Oscar as the nickname for the prestigious American Academy Award is said to have arisen from someone's observation that the trophy looked like his Uncle Oscar. **Variants:** Oke, Oskar, Ossie, Ossy, Ozzie, Ozzy.

Osiris In Egyptian mythology, god of the underworld who was therefore responsible for rebirth, resurrection, after-life and fertility, including the all-important annual flooding of the Nile to make the crops grow.

Osmand From the Old English, *os*, 'god', and *mund*, 'protection', thus 'protected by God'. Hence Osman, 'servant of God', and Oswin, 'friend of God'. The Norman St Osmund (died 1099) was a strict disciplinarian. As William the Conqueror's chancellor, he was involved in the Domesday Book survey and, as Bishop of Salisbury, he completed building the cathedral. Like Osbert, an Old English name that survived the Norman arrival. **Variants:** Esmand, Esme, Osman, Osmond, Osmund, Oswin, Oz. *See also* Otto.

Oswald From the Old English, *os*, 'god', and *weald*, 'wood, forest', thus 'god of the forest'. Oswald of Northumbria (c. 605–42), king and saint, won back Northumbria from the Welsh and was a close friend of St Aidan who came as a missionary to his people, a combination that made him a popular hero-saint. A second British saint, Oswald of Winchester (c. 925–92), was Bishop of Worcester, founded the great monastery at Ramsey and stimulated English monasticism. The politician Oswald Ernald Mosley (1896–1980) founded the British Union of Fascists in 1933. **Variants:** Ossie, Osvald, Oswal, Oswaldo, Oswall, Oswold, Oz, Ozzie, Ozzy, Waldo, Waldy.

Otis From the Greek, *ous*, 'ear', implying someone who not only has a good ear for music and literature but who takes and gives advice. **Variant:** Otes. *See also* Orpheus.

Otto German form of Odo, from the Old High German, *otho*, 'prosperous'. Otto I (912–73), known as Otto the Great, was both King of Germany and Emperor of the Holy Roman Empire, a strong Christian and patron of the arts. The name also comes from the Turkish, *Osman*, the tribe that rose in power to produce Othman I (1259–1326), also called Osman. He founded the Ottoman dynasty and the powerful empire that lasted for almost 700 years, ending in 1923. Despite its royal character, the name has never been very popular in Britain, and the murderously jealous hero of Shakespeare's tragedy *Othello* (1604) did not help either. **Variants:** Odo, Osman, Othello, Othman, Othmar, Otho, Ottmar.

Overton From the Middle English, *over*, 'higher, above', and *toun*, 'town, village', thus the higher of two towns, or a hillside town.

Ovid From the Latin, *ovul*, 'egg', an ancient symbol of life. The Roman poet, Publius Ovidius Naso (43 BC–18 AD), known as Ovid, wrote romantic poetry and also the *Metamorphoses*, a collection of legends in which gods and humans change their forms.

Owen Welsh form of Eugene. **Variants:** Bowen, Bowie, Ewan, Ewen, Owain, Owayne, Ovin, Uwen, Ywain.

Oz From the Hebrew, 'strength'. The American journalist Lyman Frank Baum (1856–1919) wrote the highly successful children's fairytale, *The Wizard of Oz* (1900), whose musical version (1901) was followed by the award-winning film starring the five-year-old Judy Garland (1939). **Variants:** Ozzie, Ozzy. *See also* Osmand.

Ozni From the Hebrew, *ozen*, 'ear'. *See also* Otis.

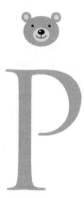

Paco North American Indian, meaning 'eagle'.

Padget *See* Page *under girls*. **Variants:** Padgett, Page, Paige.

Painton From the Latin, *pagus*, 'country, country people', thus 'country town'. A name introduced by the Normans. **Variants:** Pagan, Paganel, Pain, Paine, Pannet, Pyne.

Pal English gypsy name, meaning 'brother'.

Palmer *See* Palma *under girls*.

Pan From the Greek, *pan*, 'all'. In Greek mythology, the satyr with a human torso and goat's legs, horns and beard. His specific duties as a rural god were to preside over the fertility of goats and ewes. He teased the forest nymphs and permitted hunters to kill wild beasts. The Roman counterpart is Faunus. *See also* Peter.

Pancho Spanish, from the Latin, *penna*, 'feather, plume', a symbol of gaiety and celebration. **Variant:** Panchito.

Paris In Greek legend, the son of Priam, King of Troy, who was the mortal selected to settle the gods' dispute over who was the fairest among Athena, Hera and Aphrodite. The first bribed him with promises of power, the second with military victory and the third with her own beauty and the promise of the fairest mortal woman for his enjoyment. He gave Aphrodite the prize, the golden apple. Paris' abduction of Helen caused the Trojan war.

Parish From the Greek, *paroikos*, 'neighbour', thus 'district, parish'. **Variants:** Parrie, Parrish, Parry.

Parke From the Middle English, *parc*, 'enclosure', often meaning a well-tended public garden with trees and flowers. Paradise, the best park of all, is an ancient Persian word, meaning 'walled-in park'. **Variants:** Park, Parker, Parkman.

Parley From the Latin, *parabola*, 'discourse', implying debate and discussion to create peace.

Parry From *ap-Harry*, 'son of Harry', the Welsh patronymic of Harry (*see* Harold).

Parson From the medieval Latin, *persona ecclesiae*, 'person of the church', that is, the clergyman who takes care of a parish.

Partha From the Greek, *parthenos*, 'virgin', meaning someone who is new to the world. In Athens, the Parthenon temple on the Acropolis is dedicated to Athena, the virgin goddess of wisdom.

Pascoe Male form of Pascal. A popular medieval name, revived in the last century. **Variants:** Pascal, Pasco, Pasqual, Pesach.

Patrick From the Latin, *patricius*, 'patrician, member of the Roman nobility'. The patron saint of Ireland (c. 385–461), son of a deacon and grandson of a priest, who changed his name from Sucat when he was ordained. After pirates captured him and took him to Ireland, he worked as a slave herdsman but studied religion all the while. He then escaped to the continent where he trained to be a bishop, only to return to Ireland as a missionary. Although other missions had gone before, it was Patrick who spread and consolidated the Gospel in Ireland, establishing the first episcopal see at Armagh in 444. Although now extremely fashionable, his name was so revered in Ireland until the 17th century that it was hardly used. But it was common in Scotland from early times, where it was interchangeable with Peter. It was probably from Scotland that the name reached England. **Variants:** Pad, Paddie, Paddy, Padraig, Padriac, Padrig, Pat, Paton, Patrice, Patricio, Patrizio, Patrizius, Patsy, Patten, Patti, Pattie, Pattison, Patty, Paxton, Payton, Peter, Peyton.

Patrin English gypsy name, referring to a trail of leaves or grass that is left for others to follow and thus implying a leader. The name **Pattin** means 'leaf'.

Paul From the Greek, *paulos*, 'small'. Of several saints, it is the Apostle (died c. 67) who encouraged the name's use. A firm Pharisee and persecutor of Christians, Saul had a vision on the road to Damascus of Christ rebuking him and telling him to preach. He was converted, baptised, changed his name to Paul and went on three principal missionary journeys, described in the Bible in his Acts of the Apostles and several epistles. His tireless work and religious thought had a powerful and formative influence on nascent Christianity. Six popes have taken the name Paul. St Paul's Cathedral, London, is dedicated to him, as well as over 300 English churches. The British St Paulinus of York (died 644) was with the second band of missionaries sent from Rome. He converted King Edwin of Northumbria and large numbers of his subjects. More recently, the Spanish painter, Pablo Picasso (1881–1973) was the dominant figure in 20th-century art, whose protests against war and fascism produced the painting *Guernica* (1937) and twice earned him the Lenin Peace Prize. Despite its strong Christian links, the name became really popular only in the 17th century. **Variants:** Pablo, Pail, Paley, Pall, Paolo, Paulie, Paulinus, Paullus, Paulos, Paulot, Paulus, Pauly, Pavel, Pawley, Pol, Poul, Powel, Powle.

Paxton From the Latin, *pax*, 'peace', thus 'town of peace'. **Variants:** Payton, Paz.

Pelagius *See* Pelagia *under girls.*

Pelham From the Latin, *pellis*, 'skin, hide, pelt', thus 'town with a tannery'.

Penini *See* Penina *under girls.*

Penn Either from the Latin, *penna*, 'quill, pen', implying a writer or clerk, or from the Old German, 'commander'. **Variants:** Pennie, Penny, Penrod.

Pentecost *See under girls.*

Pepin From the Old German, 'petitioner'. Pepin III (c. 715–68), known as Pepin the Short, was King of the Franks and father of Charles the Great, known as Charlemagne. **Variants:** Peppi, Peppie, Peppy, Pipi.

Pepper From the Sanskrit, *pippali*, 'berry'. The highly prized dried berries of the *Piper nigrum* vine are a fundamental spice in most cuisines. To find this and other spices was the stimulus for the early explorers and their royal patrons. The name implies a spicy and high-spirited character.

Percival A name invented by the 12th-century French writer, Chrétien de Troyes, for the hero of his romance based on the Welsh hero, Peredur, 'warrior of the cauldron'. The French warrior later became the naive and good knight of the Round Table in Arthurian legend, who finally glimpsed, but did not reach, the Holy Grail. The name was revived in both Malory's and Tennyson's epics and then in Richard Wagner's opera, *Parsifal* (1882). Percy Bysshe Shelley (1792–1822) was a leading English Romantic poet. **Variants:** Parsifal, Perceval, Percy. *See also* Arthur.

Peregrine From the Latin, *peregrinus*, 'foreigner', meaning someone who travels in other lands. A name found in Britain since the 13th century.

Peretz From the Hebrew, 'blossom, burst forth'. **Variant:** Perez.

Peter From the Greek, *petra*, 'rock'. Of the many saints Peter, the leader of the Apostles (died c. 64) spread the name most of all. When the fishermen brothers, Peter and Andrew, were called to be Christ's disciples, Jesus changed Peter's original name from Simon bar Jonah to Kapha, Aramaic for 'rock', to indicate that Peter was to be the rock on which Christ would build Christianity. He finally went to Rome where traditionally he was the first bishop – and therefore pope – before being martyred. The mother church in Rome is dedicated to him and countless kings, churches, cities and citizens are named after him – but no pope since has ever presumed to take his name. Peter I (1672–1725), Tsar of Russia and known as Peter the Great, transformed his country into a major European power; fought the Turks, Persians and Swedes and founded the Russian navy. In Britain, the name was first Piers, as in the poet Piers Plowman, before Peter was adopted in the 14th century. Since it was associated with Rome, the name was ousted when England became Protestant. It was revived to high fashion only this century, probably helped by the perpetually youthful fairytale character, Peter Pan, created by James Barrie (*see also* Wendy). The compounds include **Peter Paul**. **Variants:** Farris, Ferris, Parlett, Parnell, Parren, Parry, Peader, Pearce, Peder, Pedro, Peirce, Per, Perkin, Pernell, Perren, Perry, Pete, Peterus, Petey, Petko, Petr, Petros, Petrus, Petur, Pier, Pierce, Pierre, Piers, Pieter, Pietr, Pietrek, Pietro, Piotr, Petits, Pettis, Pettus, Rock, Rockey, Rockie, Rocky. *See also* James.

Petit From the French, *petit*, 'small, delicate'.

Phelim From the Irish, *feiolin*, 'constantly good'. *See also* Felix.

Philander *See* Philana *under girls*.

Philbert *See* Philberta under girls. **Variant:** Philibert.

Philemon From the Greek, *philema*, 'kiss'. In Ovid's collection of legends, *Metamorphoses*, Philemon and Baucis are poor cottagers who entertain the disguised gods, Jupiter and Mercury, so beautifully that the gods transform their cottage into a grand temple with the couple as priest and priestess. They further grant the devoted couple's wish to die together. When that happens, they turn into an oak and a linden tree whose branches are forever intertwined. A name popular with the Puritans. **Variant:** Philo.

Philip See Philippa under girls. As with Peter and Paul, the Apostle (1st century) spread the name more than the other saints Philip. It was Philip who asked Christ at the Last Supper, 'Lord, show us the Father', to which Christ replied: 'He that hath seen me hath seen the Father' (John XIV). He is thought to have preached the Gospel in Asia Minor. The name's strong royal associations include six French and five Spanish rulers. Philip II (382–336 BC), King of Macedonia, defeated the Greeks with his powerful army and was father of Alexander the Great. The powerful and devout Philip II (1527–98), King of Spain and the extensive Spanish Empire, married Mary I of England. The name was introduced to Britain by the Normans and spread swiftly, but fell into Protestant disfavour after Mary I's reign. It enjoyed a revival in the last century. Today, Prince Philip (born 1921), Duke of Edinburgh, is the husband of Queen Elizabeth II. **Variants:** Felip, Felipe, Felippe, Filippo, Hippolytos, Lipp, Lippo, Pepe, Phelps, Phil, Philipot, Philipp, Philippe, Philippus, Phillip, Phillipp, Phip, Pip, Pippo.

Philmore From the Greek, *philos*, 'loving', and the Welsh, *mor*, 'sea', thus 'lover of the sea'.

Phineas From the Egyptian, 'dark-skinned, negro'. Found in Britain in the 16th and 17th centuries. **Variants:** Phinhas, Pinchas, Pinchos, Pincus, Pini, Pink, Pinkus, Pinky.

Phoebus *See* Phoebe *under girls*. **Variants:** Feibush, Feivel, Feiwel.

Phoenix From the Greek, *phoinix*, 'purple'. In Egyptian mythology, the fabulous bird who lives for 500 years and then makes a pyre of spices, sings a sorrowful song and sets light to the pyre to burn itself up. As the bird is reduced to ashes, it is re-born into new life.

Pias English gypsy name, meaning 'fun'.

Piers *See* Peter.

Pirro Spanish, from the Greek, 'with flaming hair'.

Pius From the Latin, *pius*, 'dutiful, devout, loyal, kind, conscientious, respectful', thus an appropriate name to have been chosen by 12 popes. St Pius V (1504–72) was noted for his rigorous character and his somewhat ruthless reforms, which included approving the Inquisition and excommunicating Queen Elizabeth I. St Pius X (1835–1914) rose to the post from poverty and was noted for his single-minded goodness and simplicity. **Variant:** Pitkin.

Placid *See* Placida *under girls*. **Variant:** Placido.

Plato From the Greek, *platus*, 'broad, flat'. The Greek philosopher, Plato (428–347 BC) was an Athenian aristocrat and devotee of Socrates who founded and taught at the Academy. His *Dialogues* and *Republic* have been a major influence on Western thought. **Variant:** Platon.

Poco From the Italian, *poco*, 'little'.

Pomeroy From the French, *pomme*, 'apple', thus a gardener who tends the orchards; *see also* Gardiner. **Variants:** Pom, Pommie, Pommy, Roy.

Pompey From the Latin, *pampinus*, 'young vine shoot, vine leaf'. Gnaeus Pompeius Magnus (106–48 BC), known as Pompey the Great, was a great Roman general and statesman. More recently, Georges Jean Pompidou (1911–74), the French statesman who succeeded de Gaulle as President in 1969, now has a massive arts complex named after him in Paris. **Variant:** Pompeyo.

Pope From the Greek, *papas*, 'father, bishop'. In the Christian church, the pope is Bishop of Rome and head of the Roman Catholic Church, seen by many as Christ's vicar on earth in the tradition of St Peter.

Porter From the Latin, *portare*, 'to carry', thus the keeper of the gate, one who guards, helps and looks after people. Like Barber, an old occupational name.

Pov English gypsy name, meaning 'earth'.

Powell From *ap-Howell*, 'son of Howell', the Welsh patronymic of Howell.

Prentice Archaic form of 'apprentice', from the latin, *apprendere*, 'to understand'. Someone who serves an apprenticeship is learning and training for his future career.

Presley A popular modern name reflecting the immense popularity of the singer Elvis Presley.

Preston From the Old English, *preost*, 'priest', and *tun*, 'town, village', thus 'priests's town' and hence Prescott, 'priest's cottage'. At Preston in Lancashire Cromwell defeated the Royalists in 1648; and at Prestonpans in Scotland Charles Edward Stuart, known as Bonnie Prince Charlie, defeated the English in 1745. **Variants:** Prescott, Scott, Scottie, Scotty.

Priam In Greek mythology, the King of Troy. His 50 children included Paris whose abduction of the beautiful Helen precipitated the 10-year seige of Troy. When the Greeks cunningly stole inside the gates of Troy in a wooden horse, they slew the old king.

Price A patronymic, meaning 'son of Rice'; *see* Richard.

Priestley From the Latin, *presbyter*, 'elder', via the Old English, *preost*, 'priest, elder of the church'.

Primo *See* Prima *under girls*. **Variant:** Prime.

Prince From the Latin, *princeps*, 'the most distinguished, the first, the chief, the principal'. Either a member of a royal family or someone who is outstanding, the prince of his class.

Prior From the Latin, 'first, superior, better, more excellent', implying precedence. In the church, an abbey prior ranks directly under the abbot. In Renaissance Florence, a prior was a ruling magistrate.

Proctor From the Latin, *procreator*, 'producer, creator, author'.

Prospero From the Latin, *prosperare*, 'to make things succeed, to make someone happy, fortunate and prosperous'. In Shakespeare's comedy, *The Tempest* (1611), Prospero is the rightful Duke of Milan who regains his kingdom by exercising his magic arts from his mysterious island, confounding his enemies. **Variant:** Prosper.

Puck In British folklore, another name for Robin Goodfellow (see Robert). In Shakespeare's play, *A Midsummer Night's Dream* (1596), Puck is the mischievous sprite serving Oberon who gives Bottom his ass's head.

Purnal From the Latin, *pirum*, 'pear'. In botany, the many fruit trees belonging to the rose family, with glossy leaves, white blossoms and luscious fruits. Because the tree is long-lasting, it is a symbol of longevity in China.

Purvis From the Latin, *providere*, 'to foresee, look after, provide'. A purveyor may supply information he has gleaned or, more usually, he stocks and supplies food.

Putnam From the Latin, *putator*, 'pruner', someone who prunes trees, implying attentive upkeep of the symbolic garden of life; *see also* Gardiner.

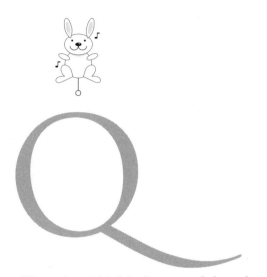

Quentin From the Latin, *quintus*, 'fifth', and thus the male form of Quinta. Revived in the last century with the success of Sir Walter Scott's novel, *Quentin Durward* (1823). **Variants:** Quenton, Quincy, Quinn, Quint, Quintin, Quintus. *See also* Fabius.

Quirinal In Roman mythology, the son of Mars. After his human life as Romulus, founder of Rome, Mars deified him and called him Quirinus. **Variant:** Quirinus.

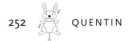

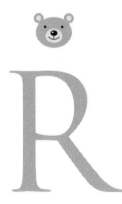

R

Rabi *See* Rabia *under girls.*

Rachamin From the Hebrew, 'compassion, understanding, kindness'.

Radburn From the Old English, *read*, 'red', and *burne*, 'stream, fountain', thus 'stream with red-coloured stones'. Hence Radcliffe, 'red cliffe' and Radley, 'red meadow'. **Variants:** Rad, Radborne, Radbourne, Radcliffe, Radclyffe, Raddie, Raddy, Radley.

Radomil Czech, meaning 'love of peace'.

Rafferty Irish, from the Gaelic, *rabhartach*, 'rich and prosperous'. **Variants:** Rafe, Raff.

Rainer *See* Raine *under girls*. **Variants:** Rain, Raine, Raines, Rains.

Raja From the Sanskrit, *rajan*, 'king'. **Variants:** Raj, Raja.

Raleigh From the Old English, *ra*, 'roe deer', and *leah*, 'grassland, meadow'. The dashing Sir Walter Raleigh (c. 1554–1618) encouraged the name. **Variants:** Rawley, Rawly.

Ralph From the Old English, *raed*, 'counsel, advice', and *wulf*, 'wolf', thus 'fearless adviser'. An old English name that survived the Conquest. Nicholas Udall (1505–56) wrote the earliest known English comedy, *Ralph Roister Doister*, for his pupils when he was headmaster at Eton. Raoul is the French form, found in Britain since the Middle Ages. *See also* Randolph. **Variants:** Raaf, Rafe, Raff, Ralf, Ralston, Randolph, Raoul, Raoulin, Rauf, Rauffe, Raul, Rawley, Relman.

Ramsey From the Old English, *hraefn*, 'raven', or *ram*, 'male sheep', and *eq*, 'island'. The Scot, James Ramsay Macdonald (1866–1937), became Britain's first Labour Prime Minister in 1924. **Variants:** Ram, Ramsay.

Ran *See under girls.* **Variant:** Ren.

Ranan From the Hebrew, 'fresh, luxuriant'. **Variant:** Raanan.

 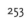

Randolph From the Old English name, Randwulf, from *rand*, 'shield', and *wulf*, 'wolf', implying courageous protection. The statesman, Randolph Churchill (1849–95), father of Winston Churchill, was leader of the 'Fourth Party' of Conservative members of parliament who sought social and constitutional reform. An old English name that not only survived the Normans but grew in popularity, overtaking the formerly popular Randal. **Variants:** Dolph, Rand, Randal, Randall, Randell, Randi, Randl, Randle, Randolf, Randy, Rankin, Raoul.

Ranen From the Hebrew, 'singing with joy'. **Variant:** Ranon.

Ranger From the Middle English, *range*, 'wanderer', meaning a man who roves the forests, such as a game-keeper or forest warden. **Variants:** Rainger, Range.

Ransom From the Latin, *redemptio*, 'release, rescue, redemption'.

Raphael From the Hebrew, *raphael*, 'God has healed'. In the Apocrypha, St Raphael is one of the seven archangels; he is patron saint of travellers and doctors. But the name was lifted to fame by the Renaissance painter, Raffaelo Santi (1483–1520), known as Raphael, who produced his serene masterpieces in Florence and then Rome, where he decorated several rooms in the Vatican. Thus a name found during the English Renaissance until the 17th century. **Variants:** Rafael, Rafaelle, Rafaello, Rafe, Raffaello, Rafi.

Rastus *See* Erasmus.

Raven From the Old English, *hraefn*, 'raven'. The raven on the flag of the Danish Vikings symbolised war-like power. The jet black plumage of the bird makes the name suitable for a dark-complexioned boy; someone of 'raven beauty' has dark eyes and hair.

Ravi Indian name, meaning 'sun'.

Ravid From the Hebrew, 'jewellery, adornment'.

Ravinder From the Old French, *rapine*, 'mountain torrent, rush of water'. As water is a symbol of life, the name implies an almost violent energy and enthusiasm for life.

Raviv *See* Ravital *under girls*.

Ray From the Old English, *ree*, 'stream, river'. **Variants:** Reigh, Reo, Rey, Rio, Riordon. *See also* Raymond.

Rayburn From the Old English, *ra*, 'roe deer', and *burn*, 'stream, fountain', thus 'a stream where deer go'. **Variants:** Burn, Burnie, Burny, Ray, Rayford.

Raymond From the Old English name, Raginmund, from *ragen*, 'wisdom, advice', and *mund*, 'guardian'. A name introduced by the Normans and raised to great popularity with crusading families because of two 13th-century saints, Raymond of Toulouse and Raymond Nonnatus. It then fell out of fashion, to be revived in this century. **Variants:** Raimondo, Raimund, Raimundo, Ramon, Ray, Raymund, Raynard, Rayner, Reamonn.

Raynor From the Old German name, Raganher, from *ragan*, 'wisdom, advice', and *harja*, 'army, people'. Introduced by the Normans, the name remained in favour until the 15th century. **Variants:** Ragnar, Rainer, Ray, Rayner.

Razi *See* Raz *under girls*. **Variants:** Raz, Raziel.

Read Male form of Reade. The German form is Rhoten. **Variants:** Reade, Red, Redd, Redding, Redmond, Redmund, Reed, Reid, Reidar, Rhoten, Rodman.

Redford From the Old English, *read*, 'red', and *ford*, 'shallow river crossing', meaning a crossing where the stones are a red colour. **Variants:** Ford, Red, Redd.

Reeves From the Old English, *gerefa*, 'assembly'. A reeve was a high-ranking Anglo-Saxon officer and, later, a steward of a manor. Thus, like Barber, an old occupational name.

Regan From the Old High German, *ragin*, 'wise', or from the Latin, *rex*, 'king', via the Gaelic, 'little king'. **Variants:** Reagan, Reagen.

Reginald From the Old High German name, Ragenweald, from *regen* and *weald*, both meaning 'power, strength, mightiness', and thus 'great warrior'. The Normans reinforced the name's popularity, as did one of the heroes of the Charlemagne romance, Reynold or Rinaldo, a cousin to Roland. The 'g' somehow fell out of the name in the 15th century, to be put back in by the Victorians. Ronals was the usual form in Scotland. **Variants:** Ranald, Reg, Reggie, Reginauld, Regnault, Reinald, Reinaldo, Reinaldos, Reinhold, Reinold, Reinwald, Renaldo, Renaud, Renault, Rene, Rex, Reynaldos, Reynold, Reynolds, Rinaldo, Rinold, Ronald.

Remus From the Latin, *oar*, implying 'as swift as possible'. In Roman mythology, the twin brother of Romulus. In Christianity, St Rémi (c. 438–533), or Remigius, was Bishop of Rheims aged 22 and later baptised Clovis I, King of the Franks. **Variants:** Remer, Remy.

Renaldo From the Spanish meaning 'wise and powerful ruler'. Alternatives include Rinaldo (Italian), Ronaldo (Portuguese) and Roald (Norwegian).

Renatus From the Latin, *renascor*, 'to be born again, to rise up, to spring up again', meaning the new life of another generation. A name first popular in France, where St Reni, or Renatus, was Bishop of Anger in the 5th century; then carried to Britain and used by the Puritans. **Variant:** Rene.

Renfred From the Old High German name, Raganfrid, from *ragin*, 'wisdom, advice', and *fridu*, 'peace', thus 'wise and peaceful counsel'. Introduced by the Normans, the name fell out of use in the 17th century.

Reuben From the Hebrew, *rue-ben*, 'behold, a son'. In the Bible, Jacob's eldest son by his wife Leah, and thus ancestor of one of the 12 tribes of Israel. When Leah found that Jacob loved her younger sister Rachel much more than herself, she prayed to God and was rewarded with a son, while Rachel was barren (Genesis 29). A name found in Britain since the 17th century. **Variants:** Reuven, Revie, Ribbans, Rouvin, Rube, Ruben, Rubens, Rubin, Ruvane. *See also* Peter.

Reuel From the Hebrew, 'friend of God'. **Variant:** Ruel.

Rex From the Latin, *rex*, 'king, ruler, leader'. Only recently used as a first name. **Variants:** Regino, Regis, Rexer, Rexford, Reynaud, Reyner.

Reynard From the Old High German name, Reginhart, from *ragin*, 'wise', and *hart*, 'strong, bold, brave'. A name combining two favourite medieval qualities in a man and suitably given to the cunning hero of the medieval beast-epic, *Reynard the Fox*, a satire of contemporary life; *see also* Chanticleer. **Variants:** Rainardo, Ray, Raynard, Regnard, Reinhard, Reinhart, Renard, Renart, Renaud, Renke, Rey, Reynaud, Reynauld, Reyner.

Rhodric From the Greek, *rhodon*, 'rose', and the Old English, *rici*, 'wealth, power'. As a rose symbolises love and beauty, the name means 'fine and caring ruler'. **Variant:** Rohn.

Rhys From the Welsh, 'rashness'. In Arthurian romance, King Rhyence of North Wales trimmed his coat with the beards of his dead rivals, but was slain before he could add King Arthur's. However, the name's popularity in Wales is due to the royal Rhys family who stopped the Normans at the borders. The wild success of Margaret Mitchell's novel, *Gone with the Wind*, which was filmed in 1939 starring Clark Gable as the hero Rhett Butler, brought that form into vogue. **Variants:** Race, Rase, Ray, Reece, Reese, Rey, Rhett, Rhyence, Rice, Royce.

Richard French form of the Old High German name, Richart, from *richi*, 'powerful, wealthy, ruling', and *hard*, 'strong'. Another manly combination of qualities, carrying royal associations through three kings of England. A name introduced by the Normans and swiftly popular. Richard I (1157–99), known as Coeur de Lion, 'Lionheart', led the Third Crusade (see Leonard); Richard II (1367–1400) bravely faced the Peasants' Revolt when aged only 14; and Richard III (1452–85) seized the throne from the rightful heir, Edward V, and imprisoned him and his brother in the Tower of London. In Christianity, St Richard of Chichester (1197–1253) was the reforming, charitable and yet strict Bishop of Chichester. In the arts, the German composer, Richard Wagner (1813–83) took opera to a new level with his four-part epic that revived interest in German mythology, *The Ring of the Nibelung*, first performed in its entirety at Bayreuth in 1876 – someone who is 'Wagnerian' is grand and dramatic in behaviour. In politics, Richard A. Butler (1902–82), known from his initials as Rab, was Minister for Education when the 1944 Education Act was passed providing free education for all. Richard has been one of the top ten favourites since medieval times, apart from a dull patch in the 18th century. Quantities of nicknames grew up for it, including the first rhyming nickname, Hick for Dick. **Variants:** Aric, Arick, Dic, Diccon, Dick, Dickie, Dicky, Dix, Dixey, Dixie, Dixy, Dizzy, Hicks, Hickson, Hudd, Hudde, Hudi, Hudson, Rab, Ric, Ricardo, Riccardo, Ricoo, Rice, Rich, Richardo, Richardon, Richart, Richie, Richy, Rici, Ricci, Rick, Rickey, Ricki, Rickie, Ricky, Rico, Riik, Riocard, Ritchie, Rocco. *See also* Thomas.

Rida From the Arabic, 'favoured'. **Variant:** Raza.

Rider From the Middle English, *ridde*, 'to clear, make space, rescue', thus someone who clears land. Like Barber, an old occupational name. Sir Henry Rider Haggard (1856–1925) was the British novelist who wrote *King Solomon's Mines* (1885) and *She* (1887). **Variants:** Rid, Riddle, Ridgeley, Ridley, Ryder, Ryerson. *See also* Eric.

Riley *See* Rilla *under girls*. **Variants:** Reilly, Ryley.

Rimon *See* Rimona *under girls*. **Variant:** Rimmon.

Ring From the Old English, *hring*, 'ring', meaning a ring of precious metal. Although a ring symbolises the circle of eternity, there are countless other meanings too. Worn on the forefinger, it means boldness; on the middle finger, dignity; on the wedding finger, love; on the little finger, strong spirit. The Romans exchanged betrothal rings, the origin of engagement and wedding rings. In the Church, priests wear a ring on the forefinger which represents the Holy Ghost. Episcopal rings have stones according to rank: sapphire for a cardinal, amethyst for a bishop or abbot. In mythology, rings are constantly popping up: the enchanted ring of Agramant; Luned's ring that made the wearer invisible and Ogier's ring which brought back youth. *See also* Richard.

Rio From the Spanish meaning 'river'.

Riordan From the Gaelic, 'bard, royal poet'.

Ripley *See* Ripa *under girls.* **Variants:** Lee, Leigh, Rip.

Ritter From the German, *reiter,* 'mounted warrior, knight'. **Variant:** Rit.

Rivers *See* River *under girls.* **Variants:** Riverton, Rivington.

Roarke From the Gaelic, 'famous ruler'.

Robert From the Old German name, Hrodebert, and the Old English name, Hreodbeorht, both from *hrothi,* 'fame', and *berhta,* 'bright'. Robert has been highly popular since the Norman Conquest. Two legends made the form Robin popular in Britain: Robin Hood, the hero-outlaw who has been protecting pretty ladies and robbing the rich to give to the poor since at least the 14th century; and Robin Goodfellow, also known as Hobgoblin or Puck, a capricious elf who roamed England in the 16th and 17th centuries. And, in Scotland, Robert Macgregor (1671–1734), known as Rob Roy, became a bandit when he was outlawed for not paying his debts: he was immortalised in Sir Walter Scott's novel (1818). Robert Peel (1788–1850) was twice Conservative Prime Minister and established the Metropolitan Police Force in 1829. The form Rupert was anglicised from the German name, Rupprecht, introduced in the 16th century.

Variants: Bob, Bobbie, Bobby, Dob, Dobb, Dobbs, Dobs, Dobson, Hab, Hob, Hobs, Hobson, Hodge, Hodges, Hopkins, Hopson, Hutchins, Rab, Riobard, Rip, Rob, Roban, Robard, Robart, Robb, Robben, Robbie, Robby, Robers, Roberto, Roberts, Robertson, Robin, Robinson, Robson, Robyn, Rori, Roric, Rory, Roy, Ruberto, Rupert, Ruperto, Ruprecht, Nob, Nobbie, Nobby.

Rochester From the Old English, *roche,* 'stone', and the Latin, *castrum,* 'fortress'. The Kent seaport was a Roman stronghold. In Charlotte Brontë's novel, *Jane Eyre* (1847), Edward Rochester is the hero who engages Jane as governess and then falls in love with her. **Variants:** Chester, Rock, Rocky.

Rockwell From the Old English, *roche,* 'rock', and *wella,* 'well', thus 'a well in the rocks'; or from the Old English, *roccain,* 'to cradle, rock', thus 'to rock gently'. The French saint, Roche (14th century), healed victims of the plague while on his pilgrimage to Rome and is therefore still invoked against disease. **Variants:** Roarke, Rocco, Rock, Rocker, Rochie, Rockne, Rocky.

Roderick From the Old German name, Hrodric, from *hrothi,* 'fame', and *richi,* 'wealthy, powerful, ruling', thus 'famous ruler'. **Variants:** Rod, Rodd, Roddie, Roddy, Roderic, Roderich, Roderigo, Rodrigo, Rodrique, Rori, Roric, Rory, Rurik, Ruy. *See also* Rory.

Rodney From the Old English, *hreod,* 'reed', thus 'island of reeds'. Admiral George Brydes, Lord Rodney (1719–92) took his title from the Somerset village of Rodney Stoke. His success at the battle of Dominica (1782) led to Rodney being taken up as a first name. **Variants:** Rod, Rodd, Roddy.

Roger From the Older English name, Hrothgar, from *hruos*, 'fame' and *ger*, 'spear', thus 'renowned warrior'. The Normans brought two Old German versions of the name with them, Ruodiger and Hrodger, making the name a favourite during the Middle Ages, so common that the diminutive Hodge became a type-name for an agricultural labourer. A period of disfavour was followed by a revival of the name in the last century. **Variants:** Dodge, Hodge, Rodge, Rodger, Rodgers, Rog, Rogelio, Rogerio, Rogers, Roj, Rozer, Rudiger, Rugero, Ruggerio, Rutger, Ruttger.

Roland From the Old High German, *hrothi*, 'fame', and *landa*, 'land', thus 'renowned throughout the land'. Roland (Orlando in Italian) was the most famous of all Charlemagne's knight-officers and his nephew. Reputed to be eight feet tall and the epitome of chivalry, he was tragically slain at Roncesvalles (778). His legend was popularised and exaggerated in the 12th-century *Song of Roland*, making the name extremely fashionable. **Variants:** Orlando, Rolando, Rolla, Rollan, Rolland, Rollen, Rollin, Rollo, Rowland.

Rolf From the Old German name, Hrodulf, from *hrothi*, 'fame', and *wulf*, 'wolf', thus 'renowned for bravery and courage'. Introduced by the Normans but quickly superseded by Ralph, to be revived only recently. **Variants:** Rolf, Rollo, Rolph, Rolphe, Roulf.

Rollo *See* Earl, Errol, Roland and Rolf.

Romain French form of Roman, from the Latin, *Romanus*, 'citizen of Rome'. The French writer and pacifist, Romain Rolland (1866–1944), wrote the 10-volume novel, *Jean Christophe* (1904–10), was influenced by Tolstoy and Gandhi, and was awarded the Nobel Prize for literature in 1915.

Romeo From the Italian name, Romolo, from the Latin, *Romanus*, 'citizen of Rome'. A name made lastingly famous and romantic by Shakespeare in his tragedy, *Romeo and Juliet* (1595), the plot of which was set in Verona and based on a story by the Italian, Matteo Bandello. **Variants:** Romallus, Roman, Romanus, Romeo, Rommie, Romney, Romolo.

Romi *See* Romia *under girls*.

Romulus In Roman mythology, Romulus and Remus were the twin founders of Rome, sons of Mars and the vestal virgin, Rhea Silvia, who was killed for having conceived, leaving the boys to be suckled by a she-wolf. When the twins got down to founding Rome they quarrelled over the plans; Romulus slew his brother and became first king of Rome. At his death, Mars carried him up to heaven in a flaming chariot where he was worshipped by Romans as Quirinus.

Ronald *See* Reginald. **Variants:** Ranald, Roald, Ron, Ronel, Ronello, Roni, Ronnie, Ronny, Roone.

Ronan An Irish name meaning 'little seal'. Famous Ronans include the singer Ronan Keating.

Roone From the Old English, *run*, 'mystery, secret consultation, magic sign, rune'.

Rory The Irish version of the Gaelic name, Ruadidhri, from *ruadh*, 'red'; the Scottish version is Roderick. Roger is another translation.

Ross Male form of Rose, or from the Scottish Gaelic, 'peninsular'. The Dutch form, Roosevelt, 'field of roses', is found in the USA, used in honour of Franklin Delano

Roosevelt (1882–1945) who as Democratic President from 1933 to 1945 fulfilled his promise of the New Deal, while his wife Eleanor laboured for human rights. **Variants:** Roosevelt, Roscoe, Rosey, Rosie, Rossano, Rossie, Rossy, Roswald, Royce.

Roswell From the Old German name, Roswald, from *hros*, 'horse', thus 'mighty horseman', meaning a skilled equestrian warrior.

Rowan *See* Rowena *under girls.* **Variants:** Rooney, Rowen, Rowney.

Rowland From the Old English, *rhu*, 'rugged land'; also another form of Roland. **Variants:** Ragnar, Rowby, Rowe.

Roy Usually from the Gaelic, *ruadh*, 'red', rather than from the French, *roi*, 'king' (*see* Leroy). **Variants:** Royal, Roye, Royle, Royston. *See also* Robert.

Ruby *See under girls.*

Rudolph From the Old High German name, Hrodulf, from *hruod*, 'fame', and *wulf*, 'wolf', meaning 'famous for boldness and courage'. Rudolf I (1218–91), King of Habsburg, became Holy Roman Emperor in 1273 and enlarged his territories to form a power base for his Habsburg descendants which lasted for over six centuries, ending only in 1918. More recently, the Italian actor, Rudolf Valentino (1895–1926), born Rodolpho

Guglielmi di Valentina d'Antonguolla, was the top idol of the silent screen in the 1920s, whose string of romantic films included *The Sheik* (1921) and *Blood and Sand* (1922). **Variants:** Raoul, Raul, Rodolfo, Rodolph, Rodolphe, Rodolpho, Rodulfo, Rolf, Rolfe, Rollo, Rolph, Roul, Rudi, Rudie, Rudolf, Rudolfo, Rudy. *See also* Rolf.

Rudyard From the Old Saxon, *rod*, 'red', and *gyrd*, 'pole'. The British writer, Joseph Rudyard Kipling (1865–1936) was brought up in India where he acquired his rich source material for his novels (*see* Kim). **Variants:** Rudd, Ruddie, Ruddy, Rudel, Rudy, Rutledge, Rutter.

Rufus Male form of Rufina. A name often given to red-heads, with royal approval. Otto II of Germany (955–83) and William II of England (c. 1056–1100) were both nicknamed Rufus. **Variants:** Rush, Ruskin, Russ, Rusty.

Rupert *See* Robert.

Russell French form of Rufus, from *roux*, 'red'. The politician, John, 1st Earl Russell (1792–1878), fought for Parliamentary reform and was twice Prime Minister. Like Spencer, an old aristocratic name taken up as a smart first name in the last century. **Variants:** Russ, Russel. *See also* Bertram.

Ryan From the Gaelic, 'little king'. **Variant:** Ryen.

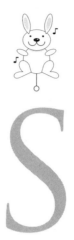

S

Saadia *See* Saada *under girls.* **Variants:** Saadiah, Saadya.

Sabas The Cappadocian St Sabas (439–532) was an outstanding monk of his time whose example and teaching was practised in the monastery he founded, Mar Saba, now one of the oldest occupied monasteries in the world.

Sabath From the Hebrew, *shabbat*, 'rest'. In the Bible, God created the world in six days and then rested on the seventh, which he blessed and sanctified (Genesis 2). **Variant:** Shabbetai.

Sabin *See* Sabina *under girls.* **Variant:** Savin.

Sacheverell Possibly from the French, *sans cheveral*, 'without leather'. Popular in 18th-century Britain because of the Tory preacher, Dr Sacheverall (1674–1724), who toured rural districts. William Sacheverall (1638–91) was a founder of the Whig party, and the Sitwell family use the name to this day in his honour. **Variant:** Sacheverall.

Sagi From the Aramaic, 'mighty, strong'.

Sakima North American Indian, meaning 'king'.

Salathiel An ancient Babylonian name, whose later Hebrew version, Shaltiel, means 'requested of God'. Found in Britain from the 16th to 18th centuries. **Variant:** Sealtiele.

Sale *See* Salena *under girls.* **Variants:** Sal, Zales.

Salem *See* Salome *under girls.* **Variants:** Shalom, Shelomi, Shlomi, Sholom.

Salim From the Arabic, 'flawless, perfect'. **Variant:** Selim.

Salvador From the Latin, *salvus*, 'preserved, saved, unharmed, well'. **Variants:** Sal, Sallie, Sally, Salvador, Salvator, Sauveur.

Sami From the Arabic, 'exalted, high up'.

Samir *See* Samira *under girls.*

Samson From the Hebrew, *shemesh*, 'sun', thus 'child of the sun'. In the Bible, an Israelite judge of extraordinary strength whose lover, Delilah, betrayed him to the Philistines. The name thus suggests considerable physical strength. The Welsh bishop, St Samson (c. 490 – c. 565), founded an abbey at Dol in Brittany and had a strong cult following there and in Cornwall. After the Reformation vogue for Old Testament names, it fell out of use. **Variants:** Sam, Sammie, Sammy, Sampson, Sams, Sansom, Sanson, Sansone, Shem.

Samuel From the Hebrew, *schama*, 'hear', thus 'heard by God', meaning the answer to prayers for a child. In the Bible, the powerful Hebrew judge and prophet living in the 11th century BC who anointed Saul the first king of Israel (I Samuel 10). The poet and critic, Samuel Taylor Coleridge (1772 – 1834) was a leading poet of the English Romantic movement, best known for his poem, *The Rime of the Ancient Mariner* (1798). A favourite Reformation name whose popularity has survived until today. **Variants:** Sahm, Sam, Sami, Samm, Sammie, Sammy, Samy, Uel.

Sancho From the Spanish meaning truthful and sincere. In Miguel de Cervantes' story, *Don Quixote* (1605 – 15), Sancho Panza is the cunning and practical servant of the hero, a middle-aged landowner who dons knight's armour and sets out to right the world's wrongs. **Variants:** Sanchez, Sancho.

Sanford From the Old English, *sand* and *ford*, 'sandy river crossing'. **Variant:** Sandy.

Santiago Spanish, from *San Diego*, 'St James', a revered saint in Spain. *See* James.

Saphir Male form of Sapphire. **Variant:** Sapir.

Sardis From the Latin, *sardius*, 'carnelian'. A red, translucent, semi-precious stone. Carnelian is a name given to girls.

Sarto Italian, from the Latin, *sartor*, 'mender'. Like Barber, an old occupational name. The Renaissance painter, Andrea del Sarto (1486 – 1530), was a Florentine who studied under Raphael and painted mostly serene religious and classical subjects.

Saturnino Male form of Saturnia.

Saul From the Hebrew, *shaul*, 'asked for, borrowed'. In the Bible, a tall and good man of the Benjamite tribe whom Samuel anointed first King of the Israelites, to be succeeded later by his son, David (I Samuel 9). In the New Testament, Saul changed his name to Paul when he was baptised. A name used since the 17th century, but never touching the popularity of Paul. **Variants:** Paul, Saulo, Shaul, Sol, Sollie, Solly, Zollie, Zolly.

Saville Male form of Sybil.

Sawyer From the Middle English, *sawer* and *sawyer*, 'someone who saws'. Like Barber, an old occupational name. The publication of Mark Twain's novel, *Tom Sawyer* (1876), revived Sawyer as a first name. **Variants:** Saw, Sawyere.

Saxon From the Old High German, *sahso*, 'knife'. The Saxons, a West Germanic people, invaded England with the Angles and Jutes in the 5th and 6th centuries. As Anglo-Saxons, they were the dominant power until the Normans arrived in 1066. **Variants:** Sax, Saxe.

Sayer A contraction of the Old German word, *sigiheri*, from *sigu*, 'victory', and *harja*, 'army', people', thus 'victorious people'. Popular in medieval Britain, falling out of favour with the Tudors. **Variants:** Saer, Say, Sayers, Sayre, Sayres.

Scipio From the Latin, *scipio*, 'staff, walking stick'. Two great Roman generals were called Scipio. The first, whose full name was the mouthful Publius Cornelius Scipio Africanus Major (234–183 BC), defeated Hannibal and his elephants in 202 BC. The second, who had much the same string of names but switched Major for Minor (c. 185–129 BC) was responsible for the final destruction of Carthage in 146 BC.

Scott From the Old English, *Scot*. The ancient Gaelic-speaking people lived in Ireland before moving across to Scotland, to which they gave their name, in the 6th century. **Variants:** Scot, Scoti, Scottie, Scotty.

Seabrook From the Old English, *sae*, 'sea', thus a place where a brook flows into the sea. **Variants:** Seabern, Seaman.

Sean Irish form of John. **Variants:** Eoin, Shane, Shanen, Shannon, Shanon, Shaughn, Shaun, Shawn, Shoon.

Sear From the Old English, *sear*, 'battle'. **Variants:** Searle, Sears, Serle, Serlo.

Sebastian From the Greek, *sebastos*, 'venerable'. Almost nothing is known about the Roman martyr and saint but his popularity generated the romantic legend of a boy from Gaul rising to be an officer of the imperial guard in Rome under Diocletian, only to be martyred with arrows when his faith was discovered. A favourite French and Spanish name, and found in Britain since at least the 16th century. **Variants:** Basti, Bastian, Bastiano, Bastien, Seb, Sebastien, Steb.

Sebert From the Old High German, *sigu*, 'victory', and *beraht*, 'bright, illustrious', thus 'notable victory'. **Variant:** Sebold.

Segel From the Hebrew, *segula*, 'treasure'. A popular name for Jews because the Israelites are called 'the treasured people' in the Bible.

Segev From the Hebrew, 'majestic'.

Selden From the Old English, *seldlic*, 'wonderful, strange, rare'. **Variants:** Seldon, Don, Donnie.

Selig From the Old English, *saelig*, 'blessed, holy'. A popular 18th and 19th century Jewish name. **Variant:** Zelig.

Selwyn From the Old English name, Selewine, from *sele*, 'house', and *wine*, 'friend', thus 'friend of the family', or from *saelig*, 'blessed', thus 'blessed, valuable friend'. A name found mostly in Wales, possibly helped by George Augustus Selwyn (1809–78), Bishop of New Zealand and Lichfield and founder of Selwyn College, Cambridge. **Variants:** Selwin, Win, Winnie, Winny, Wyn, Wynn.

Senior From the Latin, *senior*, 'older', from *senex*, 'old'. Thus suitable for the first son of a family.

Septimus See Septima *under girls*. For Romans, a seventh son was regarded as especially lucky. The Roman general, Lucius Septimus Severus (146–211), consolidated the eastern frontiers of the empire and then came to Britain where he extended Hadrian's Wall, then died while planning a campaign against the Scots. **Variant:** Sep.

Seraf See Seraphina *under girls*. **Variants:** Serafino, Seraph.

Sereno See Serena *under girls*.

Serge From the Greek, *serikos*, 'silk'. Despite its meaning, the serge made in Britain is a worsted wool. **Variants:** Sergei, Sergi, Sergio, Sergiu.

Serle From the Old German name, Sarilo, from *sarva*, 'armour'. Found in pre-Norman Britain, then in high vogue with the Normans. **Variants:** Sarilo, Serill.

Sergent From the Old French, 'one who serves', usually meaning a non-commissioned officer in the forces. **Variants:** Sargent, Seargent.

Seth From the Hebrew, 'appointed'. In the Bible, Adam and Eve's third son, conceived after their eldest son Cain slew his brother, Abel (Genesis 4).

Seton From the Old English, *sae*, 'sea', and *tun*, 'town, village', thus 'seaside town'. Hence Seward, 'defender of the sea'. **Variant:** Seward.

Sevilen From the Turkish, 'beloved'.

Sewal From the Old English name, Sigeweald, from *sigu*, 'victory', and *weald*, 'strength'. Widespread in Britain until the 16th century. **Variants:** Sewall, Sewell.

Sexton From the Middle English, *segerstane*, 'sexton', the church officer who looks after the fabric of the church, its contents, the bells and the graveyard.

Sextus From the Latin, *sextus*, 'sixth'. Like Septimus, a number name, suitable for a child born on the sixth day, week, month or year – or for the sixth child.

Seymour From the Old English, *sae*, 'sea', and *mor*, 'marshland, moor', thus 'wild coastal land'. **Variant:** Seymore.

Shaanan From the Hebrew, 'peaceful'. **Variants:** Shanen, Shannon, Shanon.

Shafer See Shifra under girls. **Variants:** Shapir, Shefer.

Shamir From the Hebrew, 'diamond'. In Jewish legend, the shamir was the tiny creature who could even cut through diamonds, the hardest stones of all, and who was used to cut the stones for Solomon's Temple.

Shamus Irish form of James. **Variants:** Seamus, Seumas, Seumus, Seusmas.

Sharif From the Arabic, 'honest'.

Sharon *See under girls.*

Shaw From the Old English, *scaega*, 'the far edge', that is, the woods beyond some cultivated land.

Shearman From the Old English, *sceran*, 'to cut', thus 'cloth cutter'. Like Barber, an old occupational name. **Variant:** Sherman.

Shelley From the Old English, *scylf*, 'rugged rock, pinnacle', and *leah*, 'meadow', thus 'rocky hilltop field'. A name promoted by the British Romantic poet, Percy Bysshe Shelley (*see* Percival). **Variants:** Shell, Shelly.

Shem From the Hebrew, 'name'. In the Bible, the older brother of Ham and Japheth, who were born when Noah was some 500 years old (Genesis 5). **Variant:** Shammai.

Shep From the Old English, *scep*, 'sheep'. **Variants:** Shap, Ship, Skip.

Shepherd From the Old English, *scep*, 'sheep', and *hirde*, 'heard', thus 'shepherd'. An old occupational name that implies tending and caring. It also carries the Christian symbolism of Christ as the Good Shepherd who gave his life for his sheep (John 10).

The cartoonist and illustrator, Ernest Howard Shepard (1879–1976) contributed to *Punch* and illustrated A. A. Milne's children's books about Christopher Robin. **Variants:** Shep, Shepard, Sheppard, Shepperd.

Shepley From the Old English, *scep*, 'sheep', and *leah*, 'meadow, grassland', thus 'sheep pastureland'. **Variants:** Shapley, Ship, Shipley.

Sheraga From the Aramaic, 'light'. **Variants:** Sheragal, Shraga, Shragal.

Sherill From the Old English, *scir*, 'area of land, countryside', and *hyll*, 'hill'. *See also* Shirley *under girls*. **Variant:** Sherrill.

Sherira From the Aramaic, 'strong'.

Sherwood From the Old English, *scir*, 'area of land, countryside', and *wudu*, 'forest, wood'. Hence Sherlock, 'enclosed area of land'; Sheriff, 'district officer'; Sherman, 'resident of the area', and Sherwin, 'friend of the district'. Sherwood Forest was one of the haunts of Robin Hood. Sir Arthur Conan Doyle gave the name Sherlock Holmes to his fictional detective, whose character he based partly on Dr Joseph Bell who worked in Edinburgh Infirmary. **Variants:** Sheriff, Sherlock, Sherman, Shermie, Shermy, Sherry, Sherwin, Sherwynd, Win, Winnie, Winny, Wood, Woodie, Woody.

Shing Chinese, meaning 'victory'.

Sholto From the Gaelic name, Sioltaich, 'shower'. A name used by the Douglas family in Scotland who are thought to descend from a man named Sioltaich Dhu Glas.

Shushan Male form of Susan.

Sidney An anglicised version of the French, *Saint Denis*, which in turn comes from Dionysius. The family arrived from Anjou during the reign of Henry II and the name established itself in Britain speedily. Sir Philip Sydney (1554–85), whose name was also written Sidney, was a true man of the English Renaissance: poet, critic, soldier and courtier. The name was especially popular at the turn of this century. **Variants:** Sid, Syd, Sydney. *See also* Spencer.

Siegfried From the Old High German, *sigu*, 'victory', and *frithu*, 'peace'. In Norse legend, Sigurd, later called Siegfried, is the hero who loves Brunhild but instead marries Gudrun while under the influence of a love potion. A popular medieval legend, revived by Wagner, which encouraged a revival of the name. *See also* Brunhild. **Variants:** Siffre, Sig, Sigfrid, Sigurd, Sigvard.

Siegmund From the Old High German, *sigu*, 'victory', and *mund*, 'guardian, protector'. **Variants:** Siegmond, Sig, Sigismondo, Sigismund, Sigismundo, Sigmund, Sigsmond.

Signe *See* Signa *under girls*.

Silas From the Aramaic, *sh-ol*, 'to borrow'; or from the Latin, *silus*, 'snub-nosed, with a turned-up nose', or from Silvanus. In the Bible, St Silus is one of St Paul's companions. In one of her best novels, *Silas Marner* (1861), George Eliot's hero is a village weaver who selflessly brings up the abandoned baby daughter of the local squire's son. First used during the Reformation, the name did not fall out of favour until the twentieth century. **Variants:** Silo, Silus.

Silver *See under girls*.

Silvester Male form of Sylvia. The name of three popes. St Silvester I (died 335) has acquired two good legends: that he baptised Emperor Constantine; and that the emperor in return made the see of Rome supreme over all others in Italy. The name was popular during the Middle Ages and is still used today. **Variants:** Silvan, Silvano, Silvanus, Silvio, Sly, Sy, Sylvan, Sylvanus, Sylveanus, Sylvester, Vesta, Vester.

Simcha From the Hebrew, 'joy'. **Variants:** Simha, Sisi, Sissi.

Simen English gypsy name, meaning 'alike', to comment on the similarity of a parent and child.

Simon Greek form of the Hebrew name, Shimeon, from *shama*, 'he heard', although the Greek word, *simos*, means 'snub-nosed'. In the Old Testament, Simeon is the second son of Jacob and Leah and thus ancestor of one of the 12 tribes of Israel (Genesis 29). In the New Testament, the six Simons include the devout old man, Simeon, who speaks the Nunc Dimittis when he sees the child Jesus (Luke 2); and Simon Peter, the chief Apostle, known as Peter. Of the several saints Simon, the strangest life was led by Simeon the Stylite (c. 390–459), who punished himself with various austeries and fastings and then spent 36 years living on a platform at the top of a pillar, making him the first and most famous of the pillar ascetics. A popular name until the Reformation, then revived in this century to become very fashionable. **Variants:** Imon, Cimon, Shimone, Si, Silas, Sim, Simeon, Simi, Simie, Simmie, Simone, Simp, Simpson, Sims, Sy, Ximenes, Ximenez.

Sinclair Contraction of 'Saint Clair'. Sinclair Lewis (1855–1951) satirised middle-class America in his many novels, such as *Main Street* (1920), and in 1930 was the first American to win the Nobel Prize for literature. *See* Clarence.

Sinbad Sinbad the Sailor is a hero of the Persian tales, *A Thousand and One Nights*, who discovered the Valley of Diamonds during his seven great voyages. *See also* Aladdin.

Siva From the Sanskrit, meaning 'auspicious'. For Hindus, the third member of the Trinity who symbolises both creative and destructive energy. He appears in many forms, such as Nataraj, 'Lord of the Dance'. **Variants:** Shiva, Siv. *See also* Narain.

Sivan See Sylvia under girls.

Siward From the Old English name, Sigeweard, from *sigu*, 'victory', and *weard*, 'protector', thus 'guardian of victory'; or from *sae*, 'sea', and *weard*, 'guardian'. A common pre-Conquest name that survived until the 14th century.

Skelly From the Gaelic, 'storyteller'.

Skipper From the Middle Dutch, *schipper*, 'ship's captain'. Thus, like Barber, an old occupational name. In poetry, Skipper's daughters are white-crested waves. **Variants:** Skip, Skipp, Skippie, Skippy.

Smith From the Old English, 'smith, blacksmith, someone who works at a forge'. Thus, like Barber, an old occupational name. **Variant:** Smithy.

Snowden From the Old English, *snaw*, 'snow', and *denn*, 'sheltered place'.

Socrates The Greek philosopher (c. 469–399 BC) believed that goodness is knowledge, evil is ignorance and, therefore, no one ever knowingly does wrong. For this he was accused of atheism and the corruption of young people, and condemned to death. His pupils, Plato and Xenophon, passed on his theories.

 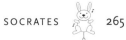

Sol From the Latin, *sol*, 'the sun, sunshine'. In the solar system, the sun is the source of all energy and the centre of the nine planets: Mercury, Venus, Earth, Mars, Jupiter, Saturn, Uranus, Neptune and Plato. Sol is the common personification of the sun who, like the Greek god Helios, is shown in paintings riding his chariot across the sky. The Athenian lawyer Solon (c. 638–558 BC) was one of the Seven Sages of Greece, whose reforms became the basis of Greek law and included the abolition of serfdom and of privilege by birth. *See also* Heli.

Solomon From the Hebrew, *shalom*, 'peace', thus 'man of peace'. In the Bible, the King of Israel (died c. 930 BC) who succeeded his father David; he built the Temple at Jerusalem and was credited with great wisdom. Thus the name implies wisdom and was a nickname for James I of England and Charles v of France. Solomon's Seal, like the Star of David, is a six-pointed star or amulet in the shape of a hexagram believed to possess magical and mystical powers. **Variants:** Salamon, Salman, Salmen, Salmon, Salo, Saloman, Salome, Salomon, Salomone, Selman, Shelomo, Shlomo, Sol, Sollie, Solly, Solmon, Suleiman, Zalman, Zalmon, Zelmen, Zelmo, Zollie, Zolly. *See also* Jedaiah and Lemuel.

Somerby From the Middle English, *sombre*, 'over', and *by*, 'village, town', thus 'town across the fields, nearby town'.

Songan North American Indian, meaning 'strong'.

Sorrell From the Old French, *sorel*, 'light chestnut-brown colour'.

Spalding From the Old English, *spald*, 'split', and *ing*, 'meadow', thus a meadow divided by a river or path.

Spark Male form of Sparkle. **Variants:** Sparke, Sparkie, Sparky.

Speed From the Old High German, *spuot*, 'prosperity, wealth, success'.

Speer From the Old High German, *sper*, 'spear'. The long-handled weapon was originally used for hunting animals and for defence, so implying both keeper and protector.

Spencer From the Middle English, 'steward, butler', meaning dispenser of food and supplies in a household. Like Barber, an old occupational name. Edmund Spenser (c. 1552–99) began his epic poem, *The Faerie Queene*, when he was aged 28. It combines medieval allegory, romance and Arthurian legend, and makes constant reference to Elizabeth I who is given a series of names: Gloriana, Mercilla, Astraea and Belphoebe. The Spencer family rose under Robert Spencer (died 1627), reputedly the richest man in England, and later acquired the title of Dukes of Marlborough. In 1812, one of their relations, Spencer Perceval, became the only Prime Minister of Britain to be assassinated. Like Russell, Sidney and others, this noble and famous family surname was taken up as a first name in the last century. The American actor, Spencer Tracy (1900–67), began his impressive film career with *Up the River* (1930), continued with such glories as *Father of the Bride* (1950) and ended in the year of his death with *Guess Who's Coming to Dinner*, the last of many films in which he co-starred with Katherine Hepburn. **Variants:** Spence, Spens, Spense, Spenser.

Spike From the Latin, *spica*, 'point, spike' and also 'ear of corn'. Spica is the brightest star in the constellation Virgo.

Spiro From the Latin, *spiro*, 'I breathe', implying the breath of life.

Sproule From the Middle English, *sproul*, 'energetic, active'. **Variant:** Sprowl.

Squire From the Old French, *esquier*, 'esquire'. In the Middle Ages, a high-born young man serving under a knight; later, any man's attendant.

Stacey Male Irish form of Anastasia. **Variant:** Stacy. *See also* Eustace.

Stafford From the Old English, *staef*, 'walking stick', and *ford*, 'shallow river crossing', thus a stick to help cross a ford. The British lawyer and Labour politician, Stafford Cripps (1889–1952), was ambassador to Moscow (1940–42), minister for aircraft production (1942–5) and Chancellor of the Exchequer (1947–50).

Stanhope From the Old English, *stan*, 'stone', and *hopen*, 'hope', or *hoppen*, 'hop'. A stanhope is a high stone from which to get a distant view. The stanhope – a light, open, horse-drawn carriage – was invented by an English clergyman, Reverend Fitzroy Stanhope (1787–1864). Stancliff means 'rocky cliff' and Stanford, 'stony river crossing'. **Variants:** Ford, Hope, Stan, Stancliff, Stanford.

Stanislav From the Slavic, 'glory of the camp'. St Stanislaus of Cracow (1030–c. 1079) was a greatly revered saint who made the name very popular in Poland. Konstantin Stanislavsky (1863–1938) was the controversial Russian actor-producer who began to encourage actors to develop their own idea of the characters they were playing. **Variants:** Estanislau, Stan, Stanislao, Stanislas, Stanislaus, Stanislaw, Stanislus.

Stanley From the Old English, *stan*, 'stone', and *leah*, 'meadow, grassland', thus 'stony meadow'. Hence Stanfield, 'stony field', and Stanton, 'stony town'. Stanley Baldwin (1867–1947), Conservative Prime Minister 1923–9 and again 1935–7, presided over the passing of the Trades Dispute Act (1927) after the General Strike, and the political events leading up to Edward VIII's abdication. **Variants:** Stan, Stanfield, Stanleigh, Stanly, Stanton.

Stedman From the Old English, *stede*, 'place, farmstead', thus 'owner of a farmstead'.

Stephen From the Greek, *stephanos*, 'crown'. In the Bible, St Stephen (died c. 35) was one of the seven men chosen to help the Apostles spread the Gospel. Renowned for his preaching and miracles, he was brought before the Jewish council as a blasphemer and stoned to death. St Stephen Harding (died 1134) came from Dorset and became a monk at Cîteaux in France. With the saints Alberic and Robert he founded the Cistercian reform, became abbot of Cîteaux and founded a dozen more houses. He drew up the Charter of Charity defining Cistercian aims, which embodies his own austerity, simplicity and high ideals. **Variants:** Esteban, Estes, Estien, Estienne, Estiennes, Estvan, Etiennes, Stefan, Stefano, Stepan, Stephan, Stephanus, Stepka, Stevan, Steve, Steven, Stevie, Stevy.

Sterling From the Old English, *steorra*, 'star'. In early British coinage, some of the early Norman pennies bore a small star. **Variant:** Stirling.

Stiggur English gypsy name, meaning 'gate'.

Stockton From the Old English, *stoc*, 'tree trunk', and *tun*, 'town', thus 'town near the felled trees'. Hence Stockwell, 'well by

 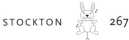

the tree stump' and Stockley, 'meadow with tree stumps'.

Stoke From the Middle English, *stoke*, 'village'.

Storm *See under girls.*

Storr From the Old Norse, *storr*, 'great one'.

Strahan From the Gaelic, *strathan*, 'poet, wise man'.

Stratford From the Old English, *straet*, 'street', and *ford*, 'shallow river-crossing'. The name of Shakespeare's birthplace, Stratford-upon-Avon, Warwickshire.

Stringfellow An old occupational name for a man who used to string bows. Later used for a man who strings musical instruments.

Strom From the Greek, *stroma*, 'mattress, bed'.

Struther From the Gaelic name, Strathair, 'stream'.

Stuart Scottish, from the Old English word, 'steward, keeper'. A name brimful with royal character. Both Stuart and Stewart were the family name of the royal house of Scotland (1371–1707), of England (1603–1707) and then of Britain for seven years (1707–14). Like other Scottish clan names, it was taken up as a first name in the last century. **Variants:** Steward, Stewart, Stu.

Styles From the Latin name, Stilus, from *stilus*, 'writing, composing, style, pen'. A name that implies eloquence in speech and fluency in language.

Sudi From the Swahili, 'luck'.

Sucat From the Gaelic, 'warrior'. St Patrick was baptised Sucat, but changed his name when he was ordained.

Sullivan From the Old English, *syl*, 'plough', and *ban*, 'high place', thus 'hilltop field'. **Variants:** Sullie, Sully.

Sully From the Old French, 'stain'. Réné François Armand Sully-Prudhomme (1839–1907) was the French poet who won the first Nobel Prize for literature in 1901.

Sultan From the Arabic, *sultan*, 'prince, ruler'. **Variant:** Zoltan.

Sunny *See Sol, and Sunny under girls.*

Sutcliff From the Old English, *suth*, 'south', thus 'south cliff'. Hence Suffield, 'south field' and Sutton, 'southern town'.

Sutherland From the Old Norse, Suthrland, the Viking's name for the Shetland Islands and northern Scotland.

Sven From the ancient Swedish tribe, the Sviars, who gave their name to Svealand, their home, later called Sweden; or from the Old Norse, *sveinn*, 'boy' (*see* Swain). **Variants:** Svarne, Svend, Swen.

Swain From the Old Norse, *sveinn*, 'boy, attendant'. In medieval Britain, a young boy attending a knight, a farmworker such as a shepherd or, in pastoral poetry, a young country lover or sweetheart.

Sweeney From the Gaelic name, Suidhne, 'little hero'.

Swithin From the Old English, *swith*, 'strong', thus 'strong man'. Little is known about the popular St Swithin (died 862), except that he was Bishop of Winchester and a trusted adviser for the Wessex kings, Egbert and Ethelwulf. **Variant:** Swithun.

Syshe From the German, *suss*, 'sweet'.

 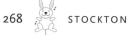

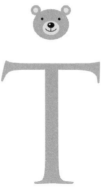

Tabbai From the Aramaic, 'good'.

Tabib From the Turkish, 'doctor, physician'.

Tabor From the Persian, *tabirah*, 'drum'. **Variants:** Tab, Tabb, Tabbie, Tabby.

Taffy Welsh form of David.

Taft From the Old English, *taf*, 'river'. **Variants:** Taffie, Taffy.

Tahir From the Arabic, 'pure'. **Variant:** Taher.

Tal *See* Tali *under girls*.

Talbot Possibly a contraction of the Old English, 'Botolph's River', or of the Old French name, Taillebotte, 'cutter of faggots'. The ancient English family, Talbot, gave their name to the large, intelligent hound with an exceptional sense of smell. **Variants:** Talbert, Tallie, Tally.

Talcott From the Old English, *tal*, 'lake', thus 'lakeside cottage'. Hence Taldon, 'hilltop lake, lakeside hill'. **Variants:** Taldon, Talmadge.

Talia *See under girls.*

Talmai *See under girls.* **Variants:** Talmie, Telem.

Talman From the Aramaic, 'deprive, oppress, injure'. **Variant:** Talmon.

Talor *See under girls.*

Tamir Male form of Tamar. **Variant:** Timur.

Tancred From the Old German name, Thancharat, from *thane*, 'think', and *radi*, 'counsel, advice'.

Tanner From the Old English, *tannere*, 'a tanner', a man who treats skins and hides to make leather. Like Barber, an old occupational name. **Variants:** Tan, Tann, Tannie, Tanny.

Tannhauser The 13th-century German lyrical poet who was so popular that a romantic legend grew up around him in the 16th century. Having spent a voluptuous year with the goddess Venus in the land of Venusberg, he returned to Earth to ask the pope's forgiveness. When pardon was refused, he went back in despair to pass the rest of his life with his beloved goddess. Wagner's opera (1845) revived the legend in the last century.

Taro Japanese, meaning 'big boy'. A name given to the first-born male in a family.

Tarver From the Old English, *tawien*, 'to soften and whiten hides'. Thus a process of leather-making; like Barber, an old occupational name.

Tas English gypsy name, meaning 'bird's nest'.

Tate From the Middle English, *tayt*, 'cheerful, spirited'. **Variant:** Tait.

Tavi From the Aramaic, 'good'. **Variants:** Tov, Tovi, Tuvia.

Tavish From the Irish Gaelic, 'twin'. **Variants:** Tav, Tavis, Tevis.

Tawno English gypsy name, meaning 'small, tiny'.

Taylor From the Middle English, *taillour* and *taylour*, 'tailor, maker of clothes'. Like Barber, another old occupational name. Also given to girls. **Variant:** Tailor.

Taz From the Persian, *tast*, 'basin, goblet, draught of liquor'; or from the Middle English, *tas*, 'pile, heap'. **Variant:** Tazwell.

Teague From the Gaelic, *tadhg*, 'poet', the anglicised nickname for an Irishman. A name mostly confined to Ireland. **Variants:** Tadhgh, Taig, Teige, Thady.

Telford From the Latin, *tellus*, 'earth, globe, territory', and *ford*, 'shallow river-crossing'.

Tem English gypsy name, meaning 'country'.

Teman From the Hebrew, *yamin*, 'right side'. Since the south is to the right of a person facing east where Jerusalem lies, the name also means south. **Variant:** Temani.

Temple *See* Templa *under girls*. **Variants:** Temp, Templeton.

Tennyson A patronymic, 'son of Tenny', from Denis. The English poet, Alfred, Lord Tennyson (1809–92), was one of three tall, handsome poet brothers and one of 12 children, who became Poet Laureate in 1850. He published *The Lady of Shalott* aged 23 and his later works included *Ulysses, Maud* and *The Idylls of the King* (1859). This last was an epic based on the Arthurian legend and was an instant and widespread success, selling 10,000 copies in the first week of publication. It doubtless revived and popularised the names of the numerous Arthurian heroes and heroines: Arthur, Bedivere, Galahad, Gareth, Gawain, Geraint, Lancelot, Merlin, Pelleas and Percival for boys; Elaine, Enid, Ettare, Guinevere, Lynette and Vivien for girls. Queen Victoria, an ardent fan of his work, knighted him in 1883. **Variants:** Tennis, Tenny, Sonny.

Tenzin From the Tibetan meaning 'the protector of Dharma'. Alternatives include Tenzing.

Terence From the noble Roman family, Terentius. The great and influential Roman playwright, Terence (c. 190–159 BC), started as a North African slave in the house of a Roman senator and took his name when he became a free man. However, the name is mostly found in Ireland where it is a translation of the Gaelic names Turlough and Toirdhealbhach. **Variants:** Tel, Telly, Terencio, Terrance, Terrel, Terrence, Terris, Terry, Terryal, Torn, Torrance, Torrence, Torrey, Tory.

Thadford From the Old English, Thad, a form of Theodore, and *ford*, 'shallow river crossing', thus 'Thad's ford'.

Thalmus From the Greek, *thallein*, 'to blossom, bloom'. The new growth of green shoots and flowers is an ancient symbol for rebirth and springtime of life.

Thanatos *See* Thana *under girls*. **Variants:** Than, Thann.

Thane From the Old English, *thegan*, 'man'. An Anglo-Saxon thane held land from the king: a Scottish thane ranked with an Earl or was the chief of his clan and a king's baron. **Variants:** Thaine, Thayne.

Thatcher From the Old English, *thaec*, 'thatch'. Thus, like Barber, an old occupational name. **Variants:** Thacher, Thatch, Thaxter.

Thelmus *See* Thelma *under girls*. **Variant:** Thel.

Theobald From the Old German name, Theudobald, from *theuda*, 'people', and *bald*, 'bold'. The Old English name Theodbeald was reinforced by the Normans who brought the German version and it has never entirely died out. The name Tybalt was given to the cunning cat in the medieval epic, *Reynard the Fox* (*see* Reynard) – hence the name Tibby or Tabby for a cat – and later given to the aggressive character who is killed by Romeo in Shakespeare's *Romeo and Juliet* (1595). **Variants:** Tebald, Ted, Tedd, Teddie, Teddy, Thebault, Theo, Thibaud, Thibault, Thibaut, Tibald, Tibbald, Tibold, Tiebout, Toiboid, Tybalt.

Theodore *See* Theodora *under girls*. Of the quantity of saints, Theodore of Canterbury (c. 602–90) is of great importance for Britain and therefore for the name's use. He was a 60-year-old Greek monk when the pope appointed him Archbishop of Canterbury. He presided over the first council of the whole English church, held at Hertford in 672; greatly improved church organisation and administration; and his African abbot, St Adrian, gave the Canterbury school a lasting reputation. The name was taken up by the Puritans, becoming a favourite with the 19th-century Tractarians. **Variants:** Fedor, Feodor, Feodore, Fyoder, Tad, Tadd, Taddeo, Taddeus, Taddeusz, Tadeo, Ted, Tedd, Teddie, Teddy, Telly, Teodor, Teodoro, Thad, Thaddaus, Thadeus, Thaddeus, Thaddy, Thady, Theo, Theodor, Theodoric, Theodoro, Theodosius, Tod, Todd, Tudor.

Theodoric From the Old German name, Thiudoricus, from *theuda*, 'people', and *richi*, 'wealth, power, ruler', thus 'people's ruler'. Theodoric the Great (c. 454–526), King of the Ostrogoths, established the Italian kingdom whose power lasted until the 6th century. A name found in the Middle Ages in Britain, then revived in the 18th century with the nickname Terry. **Variants:** Derek, Dieter, Dietrich, Dirk, Ted, Tedd, Teddy, Teodorico, Terry, Theo, Theodore, Thierr.

Theophilus *See* Theophila *under girls*. A name taken up and popularised in post-Reformation Britain. **Variant:** Theophillus.

Theron From the Greek, *ther*, 'wild beast', thus 'hunter'. **Variant:** Tharon.

Theros From the Greek, *theros*, 'summer'.

Thomas From the Aramaic, *t'ome*, 'twin'. Several notable saints have borne the name. In the Bible, the Greek apostle, Didymus, 'twin', is known as St Thomas (1st century). It was to him that Christ said at the Last Supper, 'I am the way, the truth, the life' (John 14). Some believe that he was later a

 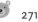

missionary to South India and was martyred there. The bishop, saint and martyr, Thomas of Canterbury (1118–70), born Thomas Becket, was soldier, diplomat, statesman and close friend to Henry II who appointed him Archbishop of Canterbury. Quarrels between church and state grew, and one day Henry's soldiers murdered Thomas, making his shrine at Canterbury one of the top pilgrimage centres in Europe from that moment for 400 years. Then there were also St Thomas of Hereford (c. 1218–82); the theologian St Thomas Aquinas (c. 1225–74); and the humanist, St Thomas More (1478–1535), who wrote *Utopia* (1516) and was beheaded for refusing to take the oath repudiating papal authority. The name moved out of monasteries when the Normans arrived and St Thomas of Canterbury ensured it rose to be one of the most common names in Britain from the 13th century onwards. The phrase of nicknames, 'Tom, Dick and Harry', meaning 'all sorts of people', testifies to the long-lasting popularity of all three names: Thomas, Richard and Henry. **Variants:** Forma, Maso, Tam, Tamas, Tamlane, Tamsen, Tamson, Thom, Thoma, Thompson, Tip, Tom, Tomas, Tomaso, Tome, Tomie, Tommie, Tommy. *See also* Sawyer.

Thor *See* Thora *under girls*. **Variants:** Terrell, Thork, Thorn, Thorold, Tirrell, Tore, Torin, Torre, Turrell, Tyrell, Tyrus.

Thornton From the Old English, *thorn*, 'thorn, thornbush', and *tun*, 'town, village', thus 'town near the thornbushes or hawthorn trees'. Hence Thorndike, 'thorny embankment'. **Variants:** Thorn, Thorndike, Thornie, Thorny.

Thorpe From the Old English, *thorp*, 'village, farmstead, hamlet'.

Thoth In Egyptian mythology, the god of the moon, wisdom and learning, represented as a man with the head of an ibis or baboon. He invented both numbers and time, giving him a magician's powers.

Thron From the Greek, *thronos*, 'raised seat', that is, one indicating importance. Gods, rulers, popes and bishops all sit on thrones, symbolising their position of authority and power.

Thurman An Old English compound, meaning 'servant of Thor', god of thunder. Hence Thorold, 'Thor's strength'; Thorwald, 'Thor's forest'; Thunderbird, 'Thor's bird'; Thurgood, 'Thor is good'; and Thurlow, 'Thor's hill'. These early names survived the Conquest and only fell out of favour in the 15th century. *See also* Thor. **Variants:** Thorold, Thorwald, Thunderbird, Thurgood, Thurlow, Thurmon.

Thurstan From the Danish name, Thorstein, meaning 'Thor's stone, Thor's jewel'. A pre-Norman name that has survived in the north of England until today. *See also* Thor. **Variants:** Thorstein, Thorston, Thruston, Thurstain, Thurston.

Tiberius *See* Tiberia *under girls*.

Tibon *See* Tivona *under girls*.

Tibor *See* Tybal *under girls*.

Tiger From the Greek, *tigris*, 'tiger'. One of the largest cats, the tiger is known for its beauty, cunning and, when provoked, ferocity. **Variant:** Tige.

Tilden From the Old English, *tilian*, 'to cultivate, plough', and *denn*, 'sheltered place', thus 'fertile and well-protected field'. **Variant:** Tilly.

THE LONG AND THE SHORT OF IT

───────────   🐨   ───────────

Eb, Ib, Jo, Job, Jon, Mac, Pip, Tim and Tom may be short names. But the 33rd President of the USA did better than all of them: the middle name of Harry Truman was 'S' from birth. At the other end of the scale, the longest-known first name has 598 letters. It was given to an American baby girl in 1979 expressly to muddle the computers of the federal bureaucracy. But she is known by her nicknames – Snow Owl and Oli.

───────────────────────────────

Timon The benevolent hero of Shakespeare's play, *Timon of Athens* (c. 1607), is based on a story in Plutarch's life of Mark Antony. Through his unthinking generosity, the rich and noble Athenian becomes penniless. When his former friends spurn him, he entertains them at a banquet of bowls of water before going to live in a cave. There he finds a hoard of gold, news spreads, flatterers arrive again, but the old man dies before he returns to Athens.

Timothy From the Greek name, Thaddeus, from *time*, 'honour, respect', and *theos*, 'god'. In the Bible, St Timothy (died c. 97) was converted by St Paul and became his companion and helper. He was also the first Bishop of Ephesus. However, the name was taken up in Britain only after the Reformation. **Variants:** Tim, Timmie, Timmy, Timofei, Timoteo, Timothee, Timotheus, Tymon.

Tinsley From the Old English, *din*, 'defence', and *leah*, 'meadow', thus 'fortified field, fort near the field'.

Titus Possibly from the Greek, *tito*, 'day, sun'. In early Greek mythology, the 12 strong giant-like rebellious Titans symbolised power by force and were the children of the supreme god Uranus and Gaea. At their mother's instigation, they overthrew Uranus and made Cronus king. When Zeus overthrew Cronus, he waged a long war with the Titans. The Roman emperor, Titus Flavius Vespasianus (9–79), known as Vespasian, rectified the empire's finances, reformed the army, patronised the arts, began building the Coliseum and, with his son and successor, Titus, captured Jerusalem in 70. The allegations of the English clergyman and agitator, Titus Oates (1649–1705), that there was a Roman Catholic plot (the 'Popish Plot') to murder Charles II led to the execution of many Catholics and the Test Act of 1678 excluding Catholics from Parliament. The writer and artist, Mervyn Peake (1911–68), made Titus the hero of his fantasy Gothic Trilogy, *Titus Groan* (1946), *Gormenghast* (1950) and *Titus Alone* (1959). **Variants:** Titan, Toto, Totos.

Tobbar English gypsy name, meaning 'road', referring to the path or road of life.

Tobias From the Hebrew, 'God is good'. The hero of the Old Testament apocryphal book, Tobit, was a captive Hebrew in Nineveh. The book was a medieval favourite, keeping the name popular until after the 17th century, and it has recently undergone a revival. **Variants:** Tavi, Tivon, Tobe, Tobey, Tobiah, Tobie, Tobin, Tobit, Toby, Tobye, Tobyn.

Todd From the Middle English northern word, *tod*, 'fox'. The bushy-tailed animal is known for his cunning, craftiness and mischievousness. **Variants:** Tad, Tod, Toddie, Toddy.

Toller From the Greek, *telos*, 'toll, tax'. Originally, a payment to a ruler or lord who in return provided protection. Later, tolls were levied on roads, fords, the miller's mill and market stalls.

Topaz *See* Topaza *under girls*.

Torbert From the Old English, *torr*, 'rocky peak, hilltop', and *beorht*, 'bright, shining', thus 'sunny peak'. **Variant:** Topper.

Torrance *See* Terence. **Variants:** Tore, Torey, Torr, Torrence, Torry.

Toussaint From the French, 'all saints'. Pierre Dominique Toussaint l'Ouverture (c. 1743–1803) was the Haitian revolutionary who expelled the British and Spanish from his island in 1798.

Townsend From the Old English, 'edge or end of the town'. **Variants:** Town, Townie.

Toy *See* Toyah *under girls*.

Tracey From the Latin, *tractare*, 'to manage, handle, lead, investigate, follow'. Also given to girls. **Variant:** Tracy.

Trahern From the Old Welsh, 'strong as iron'.

Travis From the Old French, *travers*, 'crossroads'. **Variants:** Traver, Travers.

Tray *See* Trahern

Trevor From the Welsh name, Trefor, 'great homestead'. The name is now popular in both Wales and England. **Variants:** Trefor, Trev, Treva.

Trini From the Latin, *trinitas*, 'three, triad, Trinity'. In Christian theology, the Trinity is the union of the three divine elements, God, Christ and the Holy Ghost. It is celebrated especially on Trinity Sunday, the first Sunday after Pentecost. Thus a suitable name for a child born on this day. **Variant:** Trinity.

Tristam From the Latin, *tristis*, 'sorrowful, mournful'; or from the Celtic name, Drystan, 'tumult, noise'. In medieval legend, the romance of Tristam and Isolde had two versions, one with a happy ending, the other sad (see Isolde). A name found in Britain by the 12th century. **Variants:** Drest, Driscoll, Drust, Drystan, Tristan, Tristram.

Troth From the Middle English, *trouthe*, 'faithfulness, honesty, loyalty'. To plight one's troth was to make a solemn declaration of love and betrothal for marriage.

Troy According to Greek legend, the great city of the Trojans, ruled over by King Priam whose son, Paris, abducted the beautiful Helen, thus precipitating the 10-year long war with the Greeks that ended in the city's destruction. A favourite Greek and Roman story, given full treatment by Homer (8th century BC) in his epic *The Iliad* – Ilium was another name for Troy. According to archaeological fact, the very ancient city of Troy has had ten major periods of occupation, beginning with the Early Bronze Age. **Variant:** Troilus. *See also* Cressida.

Truman From the Old English, *getriewe* and *treowe*, 'steadfast, loyal, trustworthy, constant', thus a 'totally loyal and reliable man'. **Variant:** Truett.

Tucker From the Middle English, *tukee*, 'clothfinisher, fuller'. Like Barber, an old occupational name. In 17th-and 18th-century fashion, a tucker was a piece of lace put on the neck-line of a lady's dress. Friar Tuck is the jolly chaplain and steward in the Robin Hood legend. **Variants:** Tuck, Tuckie, Tucky.

Tullis From the Latin, *titulus*, 'title of honour or of a book, reputation, fame'. Marcus Tullius Cicero (106 – 43 BC) was a leading Roman orator, scholar and statesman (*see* Cicero). **Variants:** Tule, Tull, Tulley, Tullos, Tully.

Turlough From the Irish name, Toirdhealbhach, usually translated as Terence or Charles.

Turner From the Latin, *tornare*, 'to turn on a lathe', thus 'turner'. Like Barber, an old occupational name. *See also* Joseph.

Tycoon Japanese, from *taikun*, 'prince, great lord'. The Shogun kings were described to foreigners as 'taikuns'. Today, a tycoon is an industrial, not a royal, prince.

Tydeus In Greek mythology, one of seven chieftains who went on an expedition to Thebes and killed 50 Thebans single-handed before being slain himself.

Tynan From the Gaelic meaning 'the dark one'.

Tyrone Either from the Greek, *turannos*, 'absolute ruler, illegal sovereign', later meaning just an oppressive ruler or prince, or from the Gaelic, 'Owen's land' (*see* Eugene). **Variant:** Tyron.

Tyson From the Old French, 'firebird'.

Tzevi From the Hebrew, *tz'vee*, 'deer'. **Variants:** Tzvi, Zevi, Zeviel, Zvi.

U

Udell From the Old English, *iw* and *eow*, 'yew', thus 'yew-tree valley'. **Variants:** Del, Dell, Udale, Udall.

Ulem *See under girls.*

Ull In Norse mythology, Thor's stepson, whose name means 'magnificent'. The handsome, skilled hunter was so popular with the other gods that he replaced the supreme Odin for a while, before retiring to Sweden with his magic bone which enabled him to cross seas and oceans.

Ulric From the Old English name, Wulfric, from *wolf*, 'wolf', and *rice*, 'wealthy, powerful, ruler', thus 'strong and powerful ruler'. St Ulric of Augsburg (890–973) was a good man who was an exemplary Bishop of Augsburg for 50 years. The name survived the Conquest and is still found today. **Variants:** Ric, Rick, Ricki, Ricky, Ulf, Ulfa, Ull, Ulrich, Ulrick, Ulu.

Ultimus *See* Ultima *under girls.*

Ulysses The Latin form of Odysseus. Hiram Ulysses Grant (1822–85), known as General Grant, was commander of the victorious Vicksburg campaign (1862–3) in the American Civil War and was then elected Republican President in 1868 and 1872. **Variants:** Uileos, Ulick, Ulises, Uluxe.

Umberto From the Italian, *terra d'ombra*, 'umber', an earthy colour.

Upton From the Old English, *tun*, 'town, village', thus 'upper town'.

Uranus From the Greek, *ouranos*, 'heaven'. In early Greek mythology, the supreme god. He personified the sky and was both husband and son of Gaea, and father of the Cyclops and the Titans. His name is given to the seventh planet from the sun. *See also* Brian and Titus.

Urban From the Latin, *urbanus*, 'citizen of a town'. Eight popes took the name.

Uriah *See* Urit *under girls*. In the Bible, Uriah is the husband of the beautiful Bathsheba, with whom King David is deeply in love. He is finally ordered to lead the battle in which he dies, thus clearing the way for David. The name was taken up during the Reformation but only gained fame when Dickens created the cunning villain, Uriah Heep, for his novel, *David Copperfield* (1849–50). **Variants:** Uri, Urie, Uriel, Yuri.

Urian Welsh, possibly from *urbigenos*, 'town'. A name found in both Wales and England during the Middle Ages. **Variant:** Urien.

Ursel Male form of Ursula. **Variant:** Urshell.

Utgard In Norse mythology, Utgard-Loki is an invisible giant who lives with other giant gods in his castle at Utgard.

Uzi From the Hebrew, 'my strength'.

 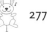

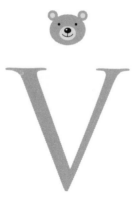

V

Vada From the Latin, *vadum*, 'ford, shallow water'.

Vail From the Latin, *valles*, 'valley, vale'. **Variants:** Val, Vale.

Valentine *See under girls.* **Variants:** Val, Valentijn, Valentin, Valentinian, Valentino, Vallie.

Valerius *See* Valerie *under girls.* **Variants:** Valerian, Valerio, Vallery, Vallie.

Vali In Norse mythology, one of the sons of the supreme god, Odin. The day he was born he avenged the death of his brother, Balder, who had been the gods' favourite. **Variants:** Valle, Vallie, Walerian.

Vander From the Dutch, *van der*, 'from the, belonging to'. Hence Van Dyck, 'from the dike'. The Flemish painter, Anthony Van Dyck (1599–1641), was a pupil of Rubens, then worked extensively for Charles I painting numerous portraits of the royal family and courtiers.

Vane From the Dutch and German, *von*, 'from, belonging to'. **Variants:** Van, Vanne, Von.

Vaughan From the Celtic, 'small'. **Variant:** Vaughn.

Vedie From the Latin, *vidi*, 'I saw', implying understanding and appraisal. It was Julius Caesar who wrote, *Veni, vidi, vici*: 'I came, I saw, I conquered'.

Venice Male form of Venetia. **Variants:** Vean, Ventan, Vinicio.

Venn From the Gaelic, *gwen*, 'fair'.

Verdo *See* Verdi *under girls.* **Variants:** Verda, Verdi, Verle, Verlin, Verlon, Vernal, Virl, Virle, Viron.

Vere *See* Verena *under girls.* The Vere family arrived with the Normans. Like many surnames, it was used as a first name by members of the family, then by outsiders.

Vered From the Hebrew, 'rose'.

Vernon From the Latin, *vernalis*, 'vernal, belonging to spring', implying a blossoming youth. With Russell and Cecil, another 19th-century surname converted to a first name. **Variants:** Lavern, Laverne, Laverno, Varney, Vern, Verne, Vernice, Verrier.

Veston From the Latin, *vestis*, 'clothing', referring to clergymen's garments, and the Old English, *tun*, 'town, village', thus 'town of churches'.

Vibert From the French, *vie*, 'life', and the Old English, *beorht*, 'shining, bright, illustrious'.

Victor See Victoria under girls. A name found in 13th-century Britain but only widespread and fashionable since the French Revolution and then the reign of Queen Victoria. **Variants:** Vic, Vickie, Viktor, Vito, Vittorio.

Vidar In Norse mythology, one of the sons of Odin, the supreme god. Although very taciturn and almost slow-witted, he was the hero whose great feat was to surpass Odin's courage and kill the wolf Fenrir.

Vincent From the Latin, *vincere*, 'to conquer, be victorious'. Several saints bear the name including the martyr, Vincent of Saragossa (died 304). He is the most revered Spanish martyr, with little fact but much legend attached to him. Despite the saints, the name gained popularity only in the last century. **Variants:** Vin, Vince, Vincente, Vine, Vinicent, Vinnie, Vinny, Vinson. *See also* Louise and Vedie.

Virgil From the Latin, *virginalis*, 'maidenly, like a virgin'. The Roman poet, Publius Vergilius Maro (70–19 BC), known as Virgil or Vergil, wrote the *Aeneid*, which recounts Aeneus' wanderings after the fall of Troy, the founding of Rome and the Julian dynasty. **Variants:** Verge, Vergit, Virge, Virgie, Virgilio.

Virginius See Virginia *under girls*.

Virtue From the Latin, *virtus*, 'manliness', the sum of all the excellences: strength, bravery, aptness, worthiness, moral perfection. As expected, a favourite with the Puritans.

Vitas See Vita *under girls*. A name brought to Britain by the Normans as Vitalis or by the French as Viel. **Variants:** Vida, Vidal, Viel, Vitalis.

Vivian See Vivien *under girls*. **Variants:** Bibiana, Fithian, Phythian, Vivien, Vyvyan.

Vladimir From the Slavonic, 'world prince'. The saint and sovereign, Vladimir I (c. 965–1015), grandson of St Olga, was the first Christian ruler of Russia. From his capital at Kiev, he extended his territory to stretch from the Ukraine to the Baltic Sea. After his conversion, he turned from bloodthirsty and dissolute prince to zealous but generous Christian. **Variants:** Ladimir, Ladislas, Ladislaw, Laidslaw, Vladmir.

Volley From the Latin, *volare*, 'to fly'. **Variants:** Vollon, Volney.

 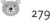

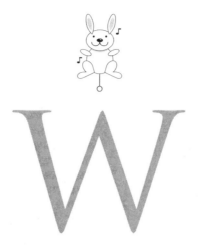

W

Wadell From the Old English, *wadan*, 'to wade'. Hence Wadsworth, 'manor with a shallow lake', the name of the American poet, Henry Wadsworth Longfellow (1807–82). **Variants:** Wade, Wadsworth.

Wagner From the Old Dutch, *wagenaar*, 'waggoner, waggon driver, charioteer'. Thus, like Barber, an old occupational name implying leadership. Phoebe, goddess of the moon, is often called the charioteer. (*See also* Richard).

Waights From the Old English, *waad*, 'road'.

Wainwright From the Old English, *waegen*, 'waggon, open vehicle', and *wryhta*, 'carpenter, joiner', thus 'waggon-maker'. Like Barber, an old occupational name. **Variants:** Wain, Wayne, Wright.

Walbert From the Old English, *wall*, 'wall, rampart, defence', and *beorht*, 'bright, illustrious', thus 'strong, good wall'. **Variants:** Walber, Wilber, Wilbert.

Walker From the Old English, *wealcere*, 'fuller of cloth'. *See* Fuller.

Wallace From the Middle English names, Walisc and Waleis, from the Old English, *wealas*, 'foreigner, stranger'. The name Welsh was first given to the native British people as distinct from the Anglo-Saxons (*see* Saxon) and only later applied to the people living in Wales. Wallace is the Scottish form, raised to popularity in the last century in honour of the patriot, William Wallace (c. 1272–1304). As Wallis, given to girls. **Variants:** Wal, Wall, Wallache, Wallas, Wallie, Wallis, Wally, Walsh, Welch, Welsh.

Walter From the Old German name, Waldhar, from *vald*, 'rule', and *harja*, 'folk, people'. A favourite Norman name which has maintained its popularity. A Walter Mitty is someone who fantasises about his triumphs while in reality achieving very little, from the hero of *The Secret Life of Walter Mitty* by James Thurber (1894–1961). **Variants:** Gauthier,

Gualterio, Gualtiero, Valdemar, Wald, Waldemar, Walden, Waldo, Waldron, Wallie, Wally, Walt, Walther, Wat, Watkins, Watley, Watly, Watson, Waud, Wilt, Wolli, Wollie, Wolly. *See also* Scott.

Waltheof From the Old English name, Wealdtheof, from *weald*, 'power, rule', and *theof*, 'thief'. A name that survived the Conquest and was still used in the 17th century in northern England.

Walton From the Old English, *wall*, 'wall, defence, rampart', and *tun*, 'town, village', thus 'fortified town'. The work of the British composer, William Turner Walton (1902–83) includes the extravaganza, *Façade* (1923) and the oratorio *Belshazzar's Feast* (1931). **Variants:** Wallie, Wally, Walt. *See also* Isaac.

Wapi North American Indian, meaning 'lucky'.

Ward From the Old English, *weardian*, 'to guard, defend, protect'. **Variants:** Warde, Warden, Worden.

Warner From the Old German name, Warinhari, from the name Varin and *harja*, 'folk'. As Garnier, the name was introduced by the Normans and flourished until the 14th century, to be revived this century. **Variants:** Garnier, Wernher.

Warren From the Old German folk name, Varin. Introduced by the Normans as Guarin or Warin but out of favour by the 14th century, to be revived recently. **Variants:** Varner, Vaney, Walena, Ware, Waring.

Warwick From the Old English, *gwawr*, 'hero', and *wic*, 'village', thus 'village hero'. Richard Neville, Earl of Warwick (1428–71), was called the Kingmaker because during the Wars of the Roses he first secured the throne for Edward IV of the York house, then switched sides and put Henry VI of Lancaster back in charge. When he was killed in battle, his death generated another switch and Edward regained power.

Washington From the Old English village name, meaning 'home of the Wassa people'. The American general and statesman, George Washington (1732–99), commanded the forces during the War of Independence (1775–83) and became the first President of the United States in 1789. The capital of the United States, founded in 1800, was named after him, as was the American writer and diplomat, Washington Irving (1783–1859). **Variants:** Wash, Washburn.

Watly From the Old English, *watul*, 'wattle', a fence or wall of interlaced twigs and branches.

Wayland From the Old English, *weg*, 'way, path, journey', thus 'land beside the road'. Common metaphors for a man's life are a long and varied journey or a winding path. In mythology, Wayland Smith was the English name for the Norse figure, Wolund, the supernatural smith and lord of the elves who finally escaped his master by flying away in a feather robe. The location of his legendary forge was in Berkshire. **Variants:** Land, Way, Walen, Weyland.

Wayne From the Old English, *waun*, 'meadow'; from Wainwright, or from Wayland. **Variants:** Dwaine, Wene.

Weaver From the Old English, *waeg-faru*, 'waterside path'. A name with the double symbolism of life as a river and a winding path. **Variant:** Wharton.

Webster From the Old English, *webba*, 'weaver'. **Variants:** Web, Webb, Weeb.

 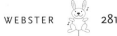

Welcome *See under girls.*

Wellington From the Old English, *welig*, 'willow', or *wella*, 'well', and the Gaelic, *dun*, 'hill, hill-fort'. The British soldier and statesman, Arthur Wellesley, 1st Duke of Wellington (1769–1852), known as the Iron Duke, defeated Napoleon at the Battle of Waterloo (1815) and was Prime Minister from 1828 to 1830. He had the redwood tree, a waterproof boot and the capital of New Zealand named after him. **Variants:** Welby, Weldon, Wells, Wellwood, Welthy, Welton.

Wen English gypsy name, meaning 'winter'.

Wendell *See* Wenda *under girls.* **Variants:** Wendayne, Wendel, Wendelin, Wentford, Wynn.

Wesh English gypsy name, meaning 'woods, forest'.

Wesley From the Old English, *west*, 'west', and *leah*, 'meadow, grassland'. The English preacher and evangelist, John Wesley (1703–91), founded Methodism, wrote many hymns and had a large following among the working class. **Variants:** Lee, Leigh, Wellesley, Wes, West, Westbrook, Westcott, Westleigh, Westley, Weston.

Whitfield From the Early modern English, *whyt*, 'very small, particle', thus 'tiny field'. **Variants:** Whitcomb, Whitelaw, Whitley, Whitney, Whittaker.

Wilber German form of Gilbert, or from the Old English, *wileg*, 'willow', or *wella*, 'well', and *beorht*, 'bright'. A name popular in the USA. **Variants:** Wilbert, Wilbur, Wilburh, Wilburn, Wilburt, Wiley, Wilford, Wilgburh, Willard, Willmer, Wilmar, Wilmer, Wilt, Wilton, Wilver, Wylie.

Wilder From the Old English, *wildeornes*, 'wilderness', implying that someone is lost, perplexed, bewildered.

Wilfred From the Old English name, Wilfrith, from *willa*, 'wish', and *frith*, 'peace', thus 'desire for peace'. The popular and influential St Wilfrith (c. 634–709), Bishop of York, was the first Englishman to take a lawsuit to the courts in Rome and had around 50 churches dedicated to him. He made the name very fashionable until the Conquest, and it was revived in the last century by the Tractarians. **Variants:** Wilfred, Wilfrid, Wilfried, Wilfredo.

William From the Old French name, Willaume, and the Old High German name, Willahelm, from *wilja*, 'desire, hope', and *helm*, 'helmet, guardian', thus 'resolute protector'. A name with strong English royal and cultural connections: William I (c. 1027–87), known as William the Conqueror, conquered England in 1066, defeating Harold at Hastings and establishing the Norman line. His second son succeeded him as William II (c. 1056–1100), known as William Rufus. Then came William III or William of Orange (1650–1702) and, finally, William IV (1765–1837). Not surprisingly, William vies with John as the top favourite name from the 11th to the 19th centuries. In the Tudor period, a big boost came from William Shakespeare (1564–1616), known as 'The Bard'. Born the son of a leather craftsman in Stratford-upon-Avon, he married Anne Hathaway at the age of 18. A decade later he was an established actor and playwright in London, working at the popular Globe theatre. His extraordinary output ranges from the comedy *As You Like It* (1598) to the tragedies *Hamlet* (1600) and *Macbeth* (1605). In Switzerland, the popular legend of William

Tell recounts how the hero was sentenced to shoot an apple off his son's head. Having done so, he shot the bailiff who had given him the punishment. William Ewart Gladstone (1809–98) was Liberal Prime Minister four times, during which he introduced national education in England, the secret ballot for parliamentary elections, and fought for Home Rule for Ireland. **Variants:** Bill, Billie, Billy, Guglielmo, Guillaume, Guillemot, Guillermo, Guillim, Guillot, Gwylim, Liam, Wil, Wile, Wilem, Wilhelm, Will, Willard, Wille, Willem, Willi, Williamson, Willie, Willis, Willmer, Willy, Wilmar, Wilmer, Wilmot, Wilson.

Willoughby From the Old English, *welig*, 'willow', and *by*, 'dwelling, village', thus 'house beside willow trees'.

Winfred Male form of Winifred. **Variants:** Winford, Winfrid.

Winston From the Old English, *winnan*, 'to win, gain by working, defeat, conquer', and *tun*, 'town, village', thus 'victorious town'. Sir Winston Leonard Spencer Churchill (1874–1965) became a Conservative member of parliament at the age of 26, was Chancellor of the Exchequer (1924–9) and Prime Minister from 1939 to 1945 and again from 1951 to 1955. He was also a painter and writer, winning the Nobel Prize for literature in 1953. Winston became a first name when a previous Sir Winston Churchill (born 1620), ancestor of the politician, was given his mother's maiden name, and it has been in the family ever since. The form Winnie was popularised by A. A. Milne as Winnie-the-Pooh, Christopher Robin's honey-loving bear. **Variants:** Win, Winfield, Wingate, Winnie, Winny, Winslow, Winthrop, Winton, Wystan.

Witt From the Old English, *hwit*, 'fair, white'. Thus a name suitable for a fair son. **Variant:** Witter.

Woden The Anglo-Saxon name for Odin, supreme god of Norse mythology. Like Thor, a god so popular that his name is a day of the week, Wednesday, 'Woden's day'. Also, another name for Harlequin.

Wolcott From the Old English, *wald*, 'field', thus 'cottage in a field'.

Wolf From the Old English, *wulf*, 'wolf', implying great strength. Hence Wolfgang, 'wolf path' and Wolfhart, 'strong as a wolf'. **Variants:** Wilf, Wolfe, Wolfgang, Wolfhart, Wolfie, Wolfy, Wulf.

Woodrow From the Old English, 'woody hedge'. **Variants:** Wood, Woodie, Woodruff, Woodson.

Woody *See* Woodrow. Woody is a popular nick name.

Worthy From the Old English, *worth*, meaning either 'homestead, enclosed area' or 'price, value' and thus 'valuable'.

Wulfstan From the Old English, *wulf*, 'wolf'. The Bishop of Worcestor, St Wulfstan (1009–95), supported William the Conqueror and fought the slave-trade in Bristol. He was also a good preacher and is considered one of the greatest early English bishops.

Wyatt From the Old English, *gwy*, 'water'. The poet and courtier, Sir Thomas Wyatt (c. 1503–42) was twice imprisoned for allegedly being the lover of Anne Boleyn, wife of Henry VIII. Wyatt Berry Stapp Earp (1848–1929) was an American hunter and gambler who fought Ike Clanton and his

 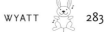

gang at the OK Corral in 1881. **Variants:** Wayman, Wyatte, Wyeth, Wyman.

Wycliffe From the Old Norse, *wyc*, 'village', thus 'village near the cliff'. The religious reformer, John Wycliffe (1329–84), produced the first English translation of the Bible, attacked papal practices and denied transubstantiation. His followers, the Lollards, preached his philosophy. **Variants:** Wyche, Wyck, Wycke.

Wyndham From the Old English, *gewind*, 'spiral', meaning a winding lane, thus 'village with a twisting lane'. The English painter and writer, Wyndham Lewis (1884–1957), was a leading figure in the Vorticist movement and editor, with Ezra Pound, of its magazine, *Blast*.

Wystan From the Old English name, Wigstan, from *wig*, 'battle', and *stan*, 'stone'. St Wigstan (died 849) was the much-loved King of Mercia and so the name is mostly confined to the Midlands. Wystan Hugh Auden (1907–73) was a well-known 20th-century poet, who was Professor of Poetry at Oxford University from 1956 to 1961.

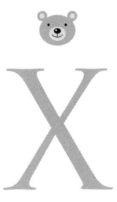

X

Xanthus Male form of Xanthe. In Greek mythology, one of Apollo's many names.

Xavier From the Arabic, 'bright'. St Francis Xavier popularised the name for boys and girls; *see* Francis. **Variants:** Javier, Zever.

Xenophon From the Greek, *xenos*, 'stranger', and *phone*, 'voice', thus 'stranger's voice'. The Greek soldier and historian (c. 430–354 BC) was a pupil of the philosopher, Socrates, and a successful commander who led 10,000 Greeks out of central Persia, a journey recounted in his *Anabasis*. **Variants:** Zeno, Zennie.

Xerxes From the Persian, 'king'. Xerxes I (c. 519–465 BC), succeeded his father, Darius, as King of Persia. He triumphantly defeated the Greeks at Thermopylae, ravaged Athens (480 BC), then was in turn defeated at Salamis and Plataea and finally assassinated.

Xylon From the Greek, *xulon*, 'wood, forest'.

 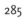

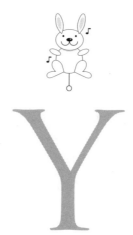

Y

Yadid *See* Yadida *under girls*. **Variants:** Yedid, Yedidia, Yedidiah.

Yagil From the Hebrew, 'rejoice'. **Variant:** Yagel.

Yakir From the Hebrew, 'beloved, honoured'.

Yale From the Old English, *eald*, 'old'.

Yank Possibly from the Dutch, *Janke*, 'John', the derisive name for a Dutchman in the 17th century and then transferred to Dutch arrivals in New England the following century. Later applied to a Unionist soldier during the American Civil War and today a nickname for an American. *See also* John. **Variants:** Yance, Yancy, Yankee.

Yarb English gypsy name, meaning 'fragrant herb'.

Yardley From the Old English, *geard*, 'enclosure, residence'. **Variants:** Lee, Leigh, Yard.

Yarkon *See* Yarkona *under girls*.

Yashar From the Hebrew, 'honest, with high morals'. **Variants:** Yesher, Yeshurun.

Yavin From the Hebrew, 'God will sympathise, understand, judge kindly'. Hence Javniel, 'God will build'; Yedial, 'knowledge of God'; Yehoram, 'God will uplift'; Yehoshafat, 'God will judge'; Yekutiel, 'God will nourish', and Yoram, 'God is uplifted, praised'. **Variants:** Jabin, Jehoram, Joram, Juti, Yadin, Yadon, Yavniel, Yediel, Yehoram, Yehoshafat, Yekutiel, Yoram.

Yehudi From the Hebrew, 'praise'. When King Solomon's kingdom was split, the people living in the southern part, Yehuda (Judah), were called Yehudis, the old word for Jew. **Variants:** Yehuda, Yehudah.

Yigal From the Hebrew, 'God will redeem'. Hence Yivchar, 'God will choose'. **Variants:** Yagel, Yigael, Yigdal.

Yora From the Hebrew, *yore*, 'to teach'. **Variant:** Jorah.

 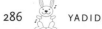

ROYALS SET THE TONE

Royalty has been directly responsible for the popularity of many names. Anne reached its height during the 17th century, when Queen Anne was on the throne. Before then, the Conqueror and his family brought William to instant and long-lasting fame while the several Queen Margarets did the same in Scotland. Henrys, Edwards, Catherines, Georges, Elizabeths and Victorias (and all her children's names) followed. Foreign royals played their part too. Alexandra was introduced into Britain by Edward II's Danish wife, to be royally reinforced much later by another Danish beauty, Edward VII's popular wife. Caroline was introduced by George II's wife. And waves of influence from continental royals have carried Alexandra, Augustus, Charles and Philip to Britain. Princess Anne has probably caused many Zaras in families who had never previously heard the name.

Yorick Danish form of George. A character in Shakespeare's tragedy, *Hamlet* (1602). **Variants:** York, Yorke.

Yucel From the Turkish, meaning 'sublime'.

Yudan From the Hebrew, *din*, 'law, judgement'.

Yukio Japanese, meaning 'snow boy'. In Japan, this implies an independent spirit.

Yule *See* Yullis *under girls.*

Yuma North American Indian, meaning 'son of the chief'.

Yves French form of the Welsh name, Evan, from John. The priest and lawyer, St Yves (1303–47), was a diocesan judge from Brittany, distinguished for his modesty, fairness, incorruptibility and concern for the poor. A name especially popular in Brittany, north-west France.

Note: many names beginning with Y can also begin with I or J.

Z

Zabdi From the Hebrew, *zeved*, 'gift', thus 'my gift'. **Variants:** Zavdi, Zavdiel, Zebdiel.

Zachariah From the Hebrew, 'remembrance of God'. In the Bible, an Old Testament prophet who lived when the Jewish captives returned from Babylonia to Israel in the 6th century BC. And in the New Testament, the elderly husband of Elizabeth and father of John the Baptist (Luke 1). The Greek saint and pope, Zachary (died 752), was noted for his wisdom and understanding and for his fight against trading in Christian slaves. A name found in Britain in the Middle Ages, rising to Puritan popularity in the 17th century. **Variants:** Benzecry, Zacaria, Zaccaria, Zacchaeus, Zach, Zacharias, Zacharie, Zachary, Zack, Zak, Zakarias, Zecharia, Zechariah, Zecharias, Zeke.

Zahid From the Arabic, 'self-denying, ascetic'.

Zahur From the Swahili, meaning 'flower'.

Zakkai From the Hebrew, 'pure, innocent'.

Zamir From the Hebrew, 'song', especially the nightingale's song.

Zebulun From the Hebrew, 'to honour, praise'. In the Bible the sixth son of Jacob and Leah and thus the ancestor of one of the 12 tribes of Israel. **Variants:** Zeb, Zev, Zevulum, Zubin.

Zedekiah From the Hebrew, 'God is goodness'. In the Bible, King of Judah (597–586 BC). Like other Old Testament names with virtuous meaning, popular with the Puritans. **Variant:** Zed.

Zehavi *See* Zehava *under girls.*

Zeira From the Aramaic, 'small'.

Zeke From the Arabic, *zaki*, 'intelligent'.

Zemer *See* Zimra *under girls.* **Variants:** Zemaria, Zemariah, Zemira, Zemirah, Zimran, Zimri.

 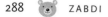

Zeno From the Greek, *sema*, 'sign'. The Greek philosopher, Zeno of Citium (c. 334–262 BC), founded the Stoic school of thought which promoted true goodness and questioned the morality of any material desire, family ties or public honours. **Variants:** Zenas, Zenon, Zenus.

Zephaniah From the Hebrew, 'protected and highly valued by God'. Like Zedekiah, fashionable in the 17th century. **Variant:** Zevadia.

Zephyr *See under girls.*

Zera From the Hebrew, 'seed'. **Variant:** Zerach.

Zerah From the Hebrew, 'morning brightness'.

Zetan Male form of Zeta.

Zeus From the Greek, 'brightness, sky'. In Greek mythology, the supreme god who ruled the heavens. As father, ruler and protector of all, his counterparts are the Roman god, Jupiter, and the German Tiw–hence the day of the week, Tuesday. Like other supreme gods, he is god of the weather, especially thunder. He also maintains law, morals and order, presides over households, protects mortal kings and ensures political freedom. **Variant:** Zenon.

Zev From the Hebrew, *z'ayu*, 'wolf'. Both Zev and Wolf are popular Jewish names because Jacob compared his son, Benjamin, to a wolf when he blessed him. **Variants:** Seef, Seff, Sif, Zeeb, Zeev.

Zia *See under girls.*

Zinn *See* Zinnia *under girls.*

Zion From the Hebrew, *siyon*. The hill in Jerusalem on which David's city, Jerusalem, was built. It became the centre of Jewish life and worship, and then the word for Israel, Judaism, the Christian church, heaven, utopia and, for Rastafarians, the promised land.

Ziv *See* Ziva *under girls.* **Variant:** Zivi.

Zohar From the Hebrew, *ohr*, 'radiant light'.

Zoie Male form of Zoe, from Eve.

Zola From the German, *zoll*, 'toll, tax, price'. The French novelist, Emile Zola (1840–1902), whose real first names were Edouard Charles Antoine, led the realist movement; his works include *Thérèse Raquin* (1867), *Germinal* (1885), and *J'accuse* (1898). **Variants:** Zoilo, Zollie.